Pelvic Organ

Prolapse

THE SILENT EPIDEMIC

Sherrie Palm

Third Edition

POP Publishing and Distribution

PELVIC ORGAN PROLAPSE
THE SILENT EPIDEMIC

MEDICAL DISCLAIMER

The material provided in this book is meant for informational and educational use only. It is not intended to replace guidance or care from health care clinicians. If you believe you have symptoms of pelvic organ prolapse (POP) or any other illness, consult with the appropriate health care professional for diagnosis and treatment. If the insights you receive from your health care clinician do not satisfy your needs, seek advice from additional health care professionals. Neither the author nor publisher is liable for the misuse or misinterpretation of the information provided in this book.

Published by POP Publishing and Distribution
Milwaukee, WI
262-642-4338
info.apops@gmail.com
http://www.pelvicorganprolapsesupport.org/contact/

Softcover 978-0-9855356-3-6
Hardcover 978-0-9855356-4-3

POP Illustrations by Design By Day
Edited by Andrew Siegel, MD
Cover by Hammad Khalid

Manufactured in the United States of America
Third Edition May 2017

ENDORSEMENTS

CLINICIAN:

As a physician, I feel it is truly important for my patients to understand the important issues related to prolapse and urinary incontinence, as well as the options for treating these distressing conditions. With a good understanding of the problem and their options, women can make good informed choices regarding their care. As a surgeon, I spend a lot of time explaining pelvic organ prolapse to my patients.

I am very pleased to see Sherrie Palm doing the same thing from a woman's perspective. As a woman who had to deal with prolapse herself, she shares the inside information on how to recognize prolapse and how to get qualified help for it. This book is a must read for every woman who is concerned about pelvic organ prolapse!

Lennox Hoyte MD, MSEECS
Managing Member
The Pelvic Floor Institute
Tampa, FL/USA
Author: A Patient Guide to Prolapse Repair

At last, pelvic organ prolapse is emerging from the shadows and into the spotlight, as women and their physicians begin to appreciate that prolapse is remarkably common, and perhaps even more importantly that prolapse can be effectively treated, and quality of life restored. Sherrie Palm's tireless work as a patient advocate, and as an author of "Pelvic Organ Prolapse: The Silent Epidemic", continues to play a key role in this transformation of women's healthcare. I recommend Sherrie's book as an essential reference for women impacted by these conditions, or for any individual seeking a better understanding of this remarkably common women's health condition.

Roger P. Goldberg, MD MPH
Director, Division of Urogynecology, Northshore University
HealthSystem
Clinical Associate Professor, Obstetrics and Gynecology
University of Chicago Pritzker School of Medicine
Author: Ever Since I Had My Baby

Sherrie Palm's book, 'Pelvic Organ Prolapse: The Silent Epidemic,' is my single most trusted resource for my patients to gain insight and education for optimal decision making in their care. I keep several copies available in my office at all times and encourage my patients to get a copy of their own.

Vincent Lucente, MD, MBA
The Institute for Female Pelvic Medicine & Reconstructive
Surgery
Allentown, PA/USA

The global prevalence of pelvic organ prolapse (POP) is increasing and has more recently reached community pandemic proportions in women's health. POP is indeed a silent affliction mainly because of inadequate public knowledge, so a much greater epidemic is anticipated if patient information is improved. This, I believe, is the key contribution of Sherrie Palm's book: it serves as a sharp reminder to health policy makers of an impending "prolapse-quake" when more women become aware of the causes, manifestations, consequences and therapeutic options after reading this comprehensive educational package. Whilst not life-threatening, POP has the potential for a significant adverse impact on quality of life, as reported eloquently in the book, and thus the patient perspective has become increasingly important when evaluating the symptoms and treatment outcomes.

As clinicians, our management strategy for POP is often based on the best available scientific evidence and physician-directed guidelines. Sherrie Palm, however, provides us again with a finger-on-the-pulse resource to ensure that the diagnostic and management principles of POP are also women-centered. The growing complexity of biomedical research and clinical practice dictates newer methods of service delivery. As a direct result, health care providers are required to consider person-orientated medical approaches and explore novel models of individualized science-a woman with POP is a case in point. Urogynaecologists who are the perfect and natural advocates for women with POP will thus find the third edition of the seminal monograph 'Pelvic Organ Prolapse: The Silent Epidemic', by Sherrie Palm, extremely enlightening.

Diaa E. E. Rizk, MSc, FRCS, FRCOG, MD, Dip BA,
Professor and Chairman,
Department of Obstetrics and Gynaecology
College of Medicine and Medical Sciences
Arabian Gulf University
Manama, Kingdom of Bahrain

Kudos to Sherrie Palm for her updated 'Pelvic Organ Prolapse: The Silent Epidemic,' which de-stigmatizes and takes out of the closet this important, highly prevalent, but largely hushed issue. Chock full of information, it is uniquely written from the perspective of the patient who by sharing her personal experience will enlighten and benefit women worldwide. A staunch champion of women's pelvic health, Sherrie continues her advocacy with great strides forward with respect to awareness, guidance and support, accelerating the pelvic organ prolapse movement.

Andrew Siegel, MD
Urology Attending, Hackensack University Medical Center
Assistant Clinical Professor Surgery, Division of Urology
Rutgers-NJ Medical School
Hackensack, NJ/USA
Author: The Kegel Fix: Recharging Female Pelvic, Sexual and Urinary Health

Sherrie Palm has a dream: she wants to inform women with POP

*that they are not alone and that many women share the same
condition. Patient information is really important because it helps
people to look for answers. We, as physicians involved in POP
treatment, should help people like Sherrie in their activities
because they help us in our mission: improve the health of our
patients.*

Enrico Finazzi Agrò, MD
Associate Professor of Urology
President of the Italian Society of Urodynamics (SIUD)
Dept. of Experimental Medicine and Surgery
Tor Vergata University
Unit of Functional Urology
Policlinico Tor Vergata University Hospital
Rome, Italy

*Brilliant clinical and personal experience by Sherrie Palm has
given the reader an unbiased, thoughtful, and useful insight into
the issues surrounding pelvic organ prolapse. By being a well-
versed patient advocate she is able to bridge the gaps of
knowledge and experience that the lay person can relate with and
the doctor relate to.*

Red M. Alinsod, MD, FACOG, FACS, ACGE
Urogynecology & Pelvic Reconstructive Surgery
Laguna Beach, CA/USA

*I often get the question about a woman's prolapse: "Why didn't
my doctor find this (prolapse) when he/she did my exam?" And my
answer usually is "If you don't look for it, you won't find it!"
Pelvic organ prolapse is definitely a silent epidemic as Sherrie
points out that lacks awareness among the public - so women with
vague symptoms "down there" don't even know what to ask for
and are ecstatic when someone, usually after multiple doctors'
visits, finally recognizes the problem and can address it. Lack of
awareness has led to the stigma which has plagued this
embarrassing condition. Through the tireless efforts of groups*

such as the Association for Pelvic Organ Prolapse Support, the breakthrough is slowly coming. Urinary incontinence, a similarly embarrassing problem, has largely broken away from this stigma in the last 20 years - it's time pelvic organ prolapse did too!"

Sumana Koduri, MD
Associate Professor of Obstetrics/Gynecology and Urology
Medical College of Wisconsin
Milwaukee, WI/USA

Sherrie Palm is an amazing woman with a lot of energy. She is leading a great movement to break the stigma surrounding pelvic organ prolapse. The 3rd edition of 'Pelvic Organ Prolapse: The Silent Epidemic' is evidence of this. It is filled with great information to help women navigate the healthcare system and to help them make informed decisions, leading to the improvement of the quality of their health and their lives. This is a must read for every woman experiencing pelvic organ prolapse. It is also a great resource for healthcare providers.

Debbie Callif, OT, BCB-PMD
Co-owner Continence & Pelvic Wellness Clinic
Board of Directors Biofeedback Certification International
Alliance, Chair of Pelvic Muscle Dysfunction
Board of Directors International Pelvic Pain Society
Mequon, WI/USA

In a time when data analytics and Triple Aim discussions are shaping priorities and budgets with respect to optimizing health care delivery, this book provides tremendous and timely insights for not only improving the POP patient experience of care, but also is a call for action for clinicians to be able to apply integrated, evidence-based research and approaches for prevention, assessment and treatment that improve patient outcomes and costs across the continuum of care. "Hear Us" has been Sherrie Palm's mission for a number of years. Her tenacious efforts to raise awareness, educate and challenge the health care environment to embrace a multidisciplinary, patient centered delivery of care is resonating. It is my belief that her efforts, over a number of years, are about to fuel dramatic changes in the way we talk about and cultivate an outlook that appreciates the essential need for progress to move from a linear dimension, to one that suddenly explodes with dramatic advancements in the field of POP care. Thank you Sherrie, for awakening us all!

Ms. Karen L. Campbell, RN, BScN
Corporate and Community Health Consultant
Retired Director of Wellness Northern Kentucky University
Cincinnati, Ohio/USA

'Pelvic Organ Prolapse: The Silent Epidemic' is one of the most in depth resources on prolapse I have read. Sherrie covers every possible question for women concerning prolapse with great detail on treatments, surgery, possible complications, and essential questions to ask the surgeon. If you want to learn more about prolapse and treatment options, put this book on your reading list.

Mary O'Dwyer
Women's Health Physiotherapist
Brisbane, Australia
Author: Hold It Sister & Hold It Mama

Sherrie is an accomplished author and a dear friend who has dedicated her career and life to helping women navigate the world of pelvic organ prolapse. I am honored to endorse her latest book, 'Pelvic Organ Prolapse: The Silent Epidemic'. Sherrie has touched so many women around the world suffering from POP issues and has been able to change their lives in so many ways. It is about time that women start talking about intimate issues! Because of the work Sherrie has done, this quite private subject is being brought to the forefront. We now have pharmaceutical companies looking at new devices and therapies that can help women. This book provides a resource for every woman to find minimally invasive solutions through surgical options for managing the condition.

Debra Muth BSN, MSNH, WHNP, BAAHP
Serenity Health Care Center
Waukesha, WI/USA

Sherrie's passion for smashing the stigma and breaking the silence surrounding prolapse is evidenced, not only in her book 'Pelvic Organ Prolapse: The Silent Epidemic', but also from her amazing APOPS Facebook Group (POPS), which she has established. The book has increased credibility for women because of Sherrie's own personal journey with prolapse and the APOPS Facebook group has become a safe haven for women to share their journey with other kindred sisters, as well as an invaluable resource for information as to how to manage prolapse. Well done Sherrie, and thank you for your efforts to bring prolapse out of the closet.

Sue Croft, Physiotherapist,
Brisbane, Australia.
Author: Pelvic Floor Essentials and Pelvic Floor Recovery:
Physiotherapy for Gynaecological Repair Surgery

'Pelvic Organ Prolapse: The Silent Epidemic' is a wonderful collection of information for women looking for support and treatment for pelvic organ prolapse. I recommend it to my patients as an adjunct to physical therapy treatment. Patient education is very important in healing and this is a great resource.

Beth Shelly, PT, DPT, WCS, BCB PMD
Beth Shelly Physical Therapy
Moline, IL/US/USA

Sher provides an excellent resource for women and health professionals. Within that resource is an abundance of support and knowledge provided through her wisdom, experience and loving heart.

Patricia Koehler Lawn, CSW, CHt
Certified Practitioner of

Holographic Memory Resolution
Pewaukee, WI/USA

PATIENT:

Sherrie Palm is an extraordinary advocate for women who are navigating POP. Her initiative to found the APOPS advocacy agency and to write this book has changed lives, and continues to change lives every day. Like most women, I had not heard of POP until I was diagnosed. Because of the stigma attached to the symptoms, I remained silent, isolated and lost. As soon as I began reading this book, I immediately felt understood. Sherrie's knowledge, energy and passion to help women navigate this tough condition is palpable throughout the book. It is frequently said that knowledge is power, I think that is a great way to describe this book. With each chapter the reader will gain knowledge and become empowered. This book also addresses the impact POP has on our quality of life, which is so validating, and that is priceless!

Sherrie is such an inspiration as she continues her crusade to educate women, healthcare providers, and academics about the impact that POP has on lives. She understands that impact and she has dedicated her life to educating others and to obliterating the stigma attached to POP. I am so grateful for this book, for APOPS, and for Sherrie. This book is a must read for all women, as we are all vulnerable to issues affecting the pelvic floor.

Thank you, Sherrie Palm, for modeling passion, compassion, tenacity, and persistence, and for encouraging and empowering women to use their voice…because it is true - every voice matters.

Mary Pippen
Kentucky/USA

Living with a POP diagnosis can be a frightening and lonely time. With no education of its existence, POP is truly a 'silent epidemic,' Organizations like APOPS are giving voice to the concerns and needs of an up-until-now voiceless population. Becoming a member of Sherrie's APOPS support group has empowered me to advocate for myself as I make my way through this POP journey."

Cathy Carlin
Minnesota/USA

Sherrie Palm is a warrior out to vanquish the ignorance and shame surrounding pelvic organ prolapse. She has designed the quintessential weapon in her organization, Association for Pelvic Organ Prolapse Support, and women of the world are fortunate to have her as an ally. I was one of those women; confused and disheartened by the alarming changes in my nether regions. Fortunately, I was somehow guided to Sherrie and the extensive information available on the APOPS site. Her tireless guidance was integral in helping me through this very challenging time in my life. APOPS is the preeminent source promoting education of women dealing with pelvic organ prolapse and the medical professionals responsible for preventing, diagnosing and treating POP. Sherrie and APOPS are indispensable in the effort to initiate and support research on the condition, and are vital liaisons between the medical community and the government agencies that regulate the related industries. We are all lucky to have Sherrie as our advocate!"

Jacqueline Munera
Florida/USA

Sherrie Palm is a fearless, superbly informed, and tireless advocate for women who suffer from pelvic organ prolapse (POP). She is willing to speak out for all of us who are affected by this humiliating and debilitating condition, which, as she emphasizes, can be easily screened for, and managed. As Sherrie notes, this is a "silent epidemic" affecting millions of women globally. It impacts our sexuality, our continence, our ability to lift, carry, laugh, eliminate, and move. For many women, POP decides for us how many children we can bear.

Women whose jobs depend on heavy lifting – women who serve in the military, who wait tables, who stock shelves, cater food and do any sort of heavy labor find themselves forced to choose between long-term health, career and income. In this way, POP is also an "invisible" disability with economic consequences for these women and their families. We deal with our humiliating symptoms in silence – either not knowing why we have them, or being fully aware but feeling equally powerless in the face of non-invasive medical devices that have scarcely changed since antiquity, or highly complex surgical procedures that can carry considerable risk. The other solution we have is neatly packaged diapers in pastel boxes at the local drugstore. We are half the world, birth the world and deserve better information, options and treatment.

So many women – whether new mothers or squarely on the other side of menopause – say "If I only knew" when they learn that POP is the root of their physical pain, sexual dysfunction, and fecal and urinary incontinence. Sherrie's life work is to make sure more and more women know how to prevent and manage POP. And thanks to the information in this book, the medical community is becoming more sensitized.

Since POP results from tears and damage to fascia, muscle, tendons and ligaments that happen differently in each woman, all of us have different symptoms. Sherrie urges medical professionals to tune in, use patient-centered care and treat each case individually. POP is also a condition that can be improved with access to physical therapy. Sherrie recognizes the fundamental importance of getting therapists, doctors, and patients to share information and experience. Cross-fertilization of ideas among these three constituencies is the key to innovation, expanding awareness, and proactive prevention.

Most importantly, Sherrie's work inspires us to join forces in order to restore not only our health, but our dignity.

Caitlin Bergin
Washington, DC/USA

One of the greatest challenges as women with POP, is just how isolating it is. That constant 'ache' - that no one understands you or can relate to you; the sense of embarrassment and shame that surfaces even when well-meaning and loving people can inadvertently make an off handed comment that makes you want to retreat back and close off from others even further. Through APOPS, I continue to gain the strength to recognize this health condition for what it is - a part of me, but not all of me. I am more accepting of myself because I know I am not alone. I am forever grateful to Sherrie Palm, for building and nurturing this bridge of compassion, awareness, and advocacy to be listened to and heard.

Karen L. Campbell
Ohio/USA

Through her own heroic efforts and the support of APOPS and Sherrie, I have watched my beautiful wife, Karen, battle from "victim" to "champion" of her own health. As her loving companion, I actively needed to create the safe space to listen to her concerns, learn the language by which we could meaningfully communicate and develop the patience that there are no easy answers. Too few health care providers can truly contribute positive guidance. From watching and supporting Karen, I know that progress can be made and a return to positive health is possible. This comes about through commitment and optimism, a caring community of support, and determined health care professionals who not only have expertise in the field, but the ability to listen to and acknowledge the wide-reaching negative impacts this condition can make in the lives of their patients and those who surround them. Through all the resources and dialogue of the outstanding APOPS organization, led brilliantly by Sherrie Palm, together, we have built capacity and skills to overcome. Sherrie is a true blessing to our community.

John S. Campbell, husband of Karen Campbell
President Clippard Instrument Laboratories
Ohio/USA

Read Sherrie Palm's book, 3rd edition, which will completely explain pelvic organ prolapse. What it is, what to do, where to go, how to repair it, how to be you again. It is a common condition which many women face, and are totally embarrassed to discuss. I don't want other women to suffer, as I did, and neither do you. Bless you, warrior for women!

Ceil LaPorta
Retired social worker
Illinois/USA

I wish to express my sincere appreciation for all that Sherrie Palm has done for women all over the world, but me especially, in my search for answers to POP prior to my surgery Jan 2011. I found her by accident while searching the Internet for answers. Her first edition, "Pelvic Organ Prolapse: The Silent Epidemic" was a godsend. Everything I needed to know before and after my surgery was there at my fingertips with each turn of the page. I consider it my POP Bible and eagerly anticipate the next edition. I feel confident enough now to call myself the "POP Diva" thanks to Sherrie." I consider her my POP angel.

Margaret Forrest, Retired DOD
Supervisory Program Management Analyst
MEDIA AND MORE:

I cannot overstate how important bringing attention to this issue is. Pelvic organ prolapse is something I know has affected so many women close to me, yet it's something we almost never discuss. We need to educate, agitate, and mobilize people on this issue, because women, especially women of color, are most likely not to have adequate healthcare coverage, and therefore less likely to seek medical treatment. Women affected by POP are entitled to their healing, and I'm so glad Sherrie is empowering women with her work. I was so happy to participate in APOPS Stigma Stride Walkathon in 2015, and I look forward to the day when we women can speak loud and proud about our bodies.

Senator Lena C. Taylor
4th Senate District of Wisconsin
Wisconsin/USA

Sherrie Palm brings to light a "hidden" problem that all women and their men should know about. She is warm and engaging and speaks frankly and clearly about this Silent Epidemic. A number of my other medical guests know and respect her work.

Mike Schikman
WSVA Radio
Virginia/USA

Despite progression in women's breast health, little has shifted in vaginal health awareness. Why after all these years does the central source of life remain absurdly stigmatized? Now more than ever we must shine a light on this most significant aspect of women's health, to enable common conditions such as pelvic organ prolapse to become screened for, diagnosed, treated, and most importantly, de-stigmatized. No woman should suffer needlessly. We must demand the right to healthy vaginas as it is equivalent to the demand for a healthy life.

Eve Ensler
The Vagina Monologues

Pelvic Organ Prolapse is a serious problem that I've learned many women are dealing with in silence. With symptoms comparable to puberty or menopause combined with internal injuries, we need to not only be there to support women around us, but to help others become aware of the stigma surrounding pelvic organ prolapse. Tragically few are even aware that this condition exists, or that it causes so much fear and struggle. This is where patients, relatives, activists, neighbors, donors, doctors, and community leaders can come together in agreement and purpose, to ensure that we're doing what we each can to promote awareness of pelvic organ prolapse.

Deanna Alexander
Milwaukee County Supervisor DA
Wisconsin/USA

'Pelvic Organ Prolapse: The Silent Epidemic' is the defining masterpiece of Sherrie Palm's educational mission regarding the origins and concerns surrounding pelvic organ prolapse. Her passion and commitment towards informing women of all ages about this condition is second to none. Being a woman who experienced the symptoms firsthand, Sher has dedicated her life to raising awareness for this often misunderstood and stigmatizing condition, and this book is the number one most informative piece on the market for anyone looking to learn more about this disorder.

Brendan Lee McAvoy, Attorney
McAvoy & Murphy Law Firm LLC
Wisconsin/USA

From personal experience and numerous consultations with experts, Sherrie Palm is committed to help women to improve their quality of life for a stigmatized condition. Her book about pelvic organ prolapse (POP) and related complications addresses the causes, the diagnostic process, treatment options, and preventive strategies. She speaks passionately and advocates to build bridges with diverse stakeholders in addressing POP more openly and effectively.

John Meurer, MD, MBA
Professor and Director of the Institute for Health & Equity
Medical College of Wisconsin, Milwaukee
Wisconsin/USA

DEDICATION

I dedicate this book to women around the world who have suffered with the physical, emotional, social, sexual, fitness, or employment quality of life impact of pelvic organ prolapse, and yet freely share their journey via the APOPS website, support forum, social media, and campaign structures. Patient voice and energy fuel the future of POP awareness, research, and treatment evolution.

"Together we share support; together we manifest strength."
~Sherrie Palm

TABLE OF CONTENTS

ACKNOWLEDGEMENTS   i
FOREWORD BY ROGER DMOCHOWSKI,
  MD, MMHC, FACS   v
INTRODUCTION: THE VAGINA, THE MOST
  STIGMATIZED HEALTH FRONTIER   vii

1. PELVIC ORGAN PROLAPSE: THE BASICS   1
2. CAUSES OF PELVIC ORGAN PROLAPSE   7
    Childbirth   8
    Menopause and Age-Related Muscle Loss   9
    Genetics   10
    Chronic Constipation   11
    Chronic Coughing   12
    Heavy Lifting   12
    Obesity   13
    Hysterectomy   13
    Compounding Health Conditions   15
    Adhesions and Tissue Damage   15
    Diastatis Rectus Abdominus   16
    Fitness Activities   16
3. TYPES OF PELVIC ORGAN PROLAPSE   19
    Cystocele   20
    Rectocele   20
    Uterine   20
    Vaginal Vault   21
    Enterocele   21
4. SYMPTOMS OF PELVIC ORGAN PROLAPSE   25
    Vaginal Tissue Bulge   27

Urinary Incontinence   28
Urine Retention   29
Chronic Constipation   29
Vaginal and/or Rectal Pressure   30
Vaginal and/or Rectal Pain   30
Back or Pelvic Pain   30
Inability to Retain a Tampon   31
Fecal Incontinence   31
Coital Incontinence   31
Painful Intercourse   32
Reduced Intimate Sensation   32
5. WHEN TO SEEK MEDICAL TREATMENT   35
6. MEDICAL EVALUATION: WHAT TO EXPECT   39
The Standing Screen   40
Urodynamic Study   42
Pelvic MRI/Pelvic Ultrasound   43
Hormone Level Testing   43
Cystoscopy   44
Defecography   44
7. NON-SURGICAL TREATMENT OPTIONS   45
Kegel Exercises   47
Kegel Assist Devices   48
Pessary   50
Incostress   51
Impressa   51
Hormone Replacement Therapy   51
Electrical Stimulation   52
Biofeedback   53
Tibial Nerve Stimulation   53
Myofascial Release Therapy   54
Pelvic Floor and Core Exercise Programs   57
Urethral Bulking Agents   58
Support Garments   59
Laser and Radio-Frequency Vaginal Tissue

Restoration Therapy 60
Vaginal Restoration for POP: Round One 66
8. THE PESSARY 71
9. SURGERY 79
10. CHOOSING A HEALTHCARE PROVIDER 87
11. WHAT TO ASK YOUR PHYSICIAN PRIOR
TO SURGERY 89
12. WHAT TO EXPECT WITH POP SURGERY 93
13. WHAT TO HAVE ON HAND PRIOR TO
SURGERY 101
14. IMPACT TO INTIMACY 107
15. THE MESH AGENDA: MISTAKES MADE
AND NEXT STEPS 111
Mesh Presentation to the FDA 117
16. PREVENTION AND MAINTENANCE 121
17. MY POP EXPERIENCE 125
18. HEALTHCARE TUNNEL VISION 133

APPENDIX A: TIPS AND TOOLS 138
APPENDIX B: RESOURCES 142
APPENDIX C: POP-RFQ 144
GLOSSARY 146
BIBLIOGRAPHY 152
INDEX 161

ABOUT APOPS
LETTER FROM APOPS FOUNDER
ABOUT THE AUTHOR

ACKNOWLEDGEMENTS

CONTRIBUTIONS
In warm appreciation for members of the healthcare, advocacy, and academic sectors who so very generously contributed their voices to the third edition, and my heartfelt gratitude to APOPS patient following who contributed to this book, and continue to contribute daily within our patient support spaces.

Red Alinsod, MD/USA *Urogynecologist*
Matthew Barber, MD/USA *Urogynecologist*
Ali Borazjani PhD/USA *Biomedical Engineer*
Sharon De Vries, PA/USA *Physician's Assistant*
Roger Dmochowski, MD/USA *Urologist*
Enrico Finazzi Agro, MD/Italy *Urologist*
Alan Garely, MD/USA *Urogynecologist*
Roger Goldberg, MD/USA *Urogynecologist*
Steven G. Gregg, PhD, *National Association for Continence*
Lennox Hoyte, MD/USA *Urogynecologist*
Mickey Karram, MD/USA *Urogynecologist*
Sumana Koduri, MD/USA *Urogynecologist*
Elizabeth A. LaGro, MLIS/USA *The Simon Foundation for Continence*
Vincent Lucente, MD/USA *Urogynecologist*
John Meuer, MD/USA *Public Health*
Tasha Mulligan, PT, ATC, *Physical Therapist*
Debra Muth, ND, APRN/USA *Naturopathic Doctor, Nurse Practitioner*
Christopher Payne, MD/USA *Urologist*
Holly Richter, MD/USA *Urogynecologist*
Diaa Rizk, MD/Bahrain *Urogynecologist*
Andrew Siegel, MD/USA *Urologist*
Vikas Shah, BSc, MBBS/UK *Radiologist*

Beth Shelly, PT, DPT /USA *Physical Therapist*
Katherine Stevenson, MD/USA *Urogynecologist*
Vivian Sung, MD/USA *Urogynecologist*
Sarah Trunk, PT, DPT *Physical Therapist*
Adrian Wagg, MD/Canada *Geriatrician*
Benjamin Weed, PhD/USA *Biomechanical Engineer*
Jill Wohlfeil, MD/USA *Gynecologist*

PERSONAL
Health evolution and societal change often shift forward slowly
and with great difficulty, particularly when thousands of years of
stigma shroud the reality of a medical condition such as pelvic
organ prolapse. My eternal gratitude to:

- The enlightened, empowered members of the POPS patient
  support community who recognize the significance of
  APOPS's vision and daily share their very personal
  information. Every Voice Matters!
- Gram, my guiding light and source of inspiration.
- My son Erik for his continual, unconditional
  encouragement, and whose faith in my vision has never
  wavered.
- The DBC for the whispers and guidance they provide.
- The dedication of APOPS volunteers who see beyond
  events and projects to the bigger picture.
- Mary, who's positive energy continually lifts me up.
- APOPS dedicated Forum Administrative Team who
  generously volunteer time to keep the ship running
  smoothly behind the curtain.

  ~Larissa Bossaer/USA
  ~Iseult de Burca/Ireland
  ~Cathy Carlin/USA

~Patrizia Clark/USA
~Brynn Cruz/USA
~Valerie Mahon/UK
~Angela Pans/USA
~Mary Pippen/USA

PRO-BONO SERVICES
With warm appreciation to the generous individuals and companies who provided guidance, pro-bono services, and product donations to assist forward evolution of APOPS energy.

~3rd Edition book editing
Andrew Siegel, MD
Urology Attending, Hackensack University Medical Center
Assistant Clinical Professor Surgery, Division of Urology
Rutgers-NJ Medical School
Author: The Kegel Fix: Recharging Female Pelvic, Sexual and Urinary Health
http://www.andrewsiegelmd.com/home.html

~Radio-frequency treatments
Reneu Health & MediSpa
Jill P. Wohlfeil, MD, owner
www.reneuhealth.com

~Diagnostic, hormone, PT and MFR treatments
Balance Within Physical Therapy
Sarah Trunk, PT, DPT, co-owner
www.BalanceWithinPT.com

Serenity Health Care Center
Debra Muth, ND, WHNP, APNP, BAAHP, owner
Wendy Dunbar, LMT

www.serenityhealthcarecenter.com

~Apex M device donations
InControl Medical
Herschel (Buzz) Peddicord, CEO
www.incontrolmedical.com

~POP imagery
Design By Day
Angela Roche, Creative Director
www.designbyday.co.uk

~Branded merchandise donations
First Impressions Promotion
James Warner/Kathy Walker, Owners
kustomkat3@sbcglobal.net

~Legal counsel & services
McAvoy & Murphy Law Firm LLC
Brendan Lee McAvoy, Attorney
www.mcavoyandmurphylaw.com

Additional heartfelt gratitude to those individuals who have
provided services to APOPS and prefer to remain anonymous.

FOREWORD

By Roger Dmochowski, MD, MMHC, FACS*
January 3, 2017

Pelvic organ prolapse (POP) is truly a condition that is disruptive to quality of life, bothersome to women in their most active years as well as later in life. POP is a health concern which connotes almost a "taboo-like" quality related to both interpersonal as well as professional communication, and one that is surrounded by substantial gaps of knowledge and inherently wrong information, much of it imparted by well-meaning but incompletely informed sources.

This book is a sentinel accomplishment, an effort to improve knowledge empowerment and patient awareness of pelvic organ prolapse including the condition's impact on the overall woman, as well as the multi-faceted symptoms associated with this disorder. It has been said previously that "knowledge is power". This tome provides core knowledge which allows women to most importantly, understand POP, as well as consider reasonable options for management of this entity.

I have had the singular pleasure to have professionally worked with and observe Ms. Palm over the last five years. She is an energetic and powerful voice for women with pelvic organ prolapse. Sherrie has traveled the world, understanding cultural adaptations to this condition (given that it affects women of all cultures and geographies). Sherrie's willingness to give of herself to assist her sisters in the management of this condition is exemplary of her commitment and concern for women who experience POP. She has taken a publicly relatively obscure topic and conveyed it in a straight-forward and easy to understand method. Most importantly, she has provided women with the insights to seek intervention and care when appropriate, and to understand the options and choices that are involved in the management of this condition.

Pelvic organ prolapse is a condition that the remedy often offered is surgery. It is important that women understand there are multiple options aside from surgery for the management of this condition and its attendant symptoms, inclusive of a cohesive and global management strategy that includes attention to the urinary, bowel, sexual function, and potential pain components that POP can cause for women.

This is a "must read" for those women who wish to be fully informed in a balanced and reasonable way, and who wish to obtain critical understanding of their condition for purposes of making informed choices.

Sherrie Palm should be recognized for her unwavering commitment to women who suffer with pelvic organ prolapse, and her willingness to give of herself to improve the status of those women.

Roger Dmochowski, MD, MMHC, FACS
Associate Surgeon in Chief
Professor of Urology
Director, Pelvic Medicine and Reconstruction Fellowship
Department of Urology
Professor of Obstetrics and Gynecology
Vice Chair, Section of Surgical Sciences
Vanderbilt University Medical Center
Director of Quality and Safety, Vanderbilt Health System
Executive Director of Risk Prevention for Vanderbilt Health System
Executive Medical Director for Patient Safety and Quality (Surgery)
Associate Chief of Staff
Medical Director of Risk Management
Vanderbilt University Hospital

INTRODUCTION

THE VAGINA: THE MOST STIGMATIZED
HEALTH FRONTIER

The subliminal message women receive from early childhood on is we should not look at, talk about, or explore our vagina or vulva. It's no wonder we have such a difficult time understanding vaginal health. By definition, stigma is a mark of disgrace associated with a particular circumstance or quality. Feeling labeled or defined by a health condition can be devastating.

Women typically have never heard of pelvic organ prolapse (POP) prior to the fateful examination which indicates they are experiencing the condition. Discovery upon diagnosis is unfortunately the end-result of months, sometimes years, with no clue what is causing the painful, awkward, or embarrassing symptoms occurring. Physically incapacitating to varying degrees based on type and grade of severity, POP makes a mess out of nearly every aspect of women's lives. Pelvic organ prolapse stigma often generates feelings of shame, distress, helplessness, anxiety, blame, hopelessness, isolation, embarrassment, and fear. Frequently these stigma symptoms are coupled with shock.

Too often we are reluctant to discuss some of the most intimate of details about our bodies with a physician. Somehow, we think we have done something wrong or have failed somehow to keep our bodies under our control. We self-stigmatize ... and as a result we often miss out on allowing our physicians to help us find a resolution to our problems. We need to realize we have not done something "wrong" and that we have every right to speak up and out about every symptom we have, and seek a physician who is willing to listen and find solutions.

~ Elizabeth A. LaGro, MLIS, The Simon Foundation for Continence

My pelvic health was never optimal, no menstrual flow prior to my 17th year, adenomyosis, fibroids, and polycystic ovaries clearly indicated my female reproductive system had issues. Despite efforts to remain pro-active to maintain my pelvic health throughout my 30s, I was absolutely stunned to be diagnosed with pelvic organ prolapse, a condition that is quite common and yet at the point of my diagnosis, I had never heard of. I had no idea what symptoms the condition displayed. I had no idea what my options for treatment were. I'd always done "the right thing" regarding routine maintenance, and kept up with routine pelvic exams, mammograms, and hormone supplementation. I found it quite unnerving to be told I had a condition that is quite common and yet I knew nothing about.

Even though I had always been pro-active regarding health, I didn't realize that symptoms I started having around the time of my hysterectomy at 40 were cause for concern. Loss of pubococcygeus (PC) muscle strength, inability to keep a tampon in, inability to start my urine stream, feeling of "fullness" in the abdominal area, chronic constipation, and the lump of tissue bulging out of my vagina were all symptoms that, if recognized, might have led me to earlier diagnosis and less aggressive treatment.

I asked multiple clinicians whose paths I crossed during my course of treatment why I'd never heard of POP. I wanted to know why the topic had never come up. I continually received the same response to my query: *women won't talk about it*. I found this both unsettling and unacceptable.

In the course of scouting for answers to address my own needs, I became determined to find a path to enable women to become informed about pelvic organ prolapse prior to diagnosis-not only women seeking treatment, but in essence, all women. The conversation should begin during the first pelvic exam a woman experiences. Women need to be informed and educated about the significance of the PC muscle for pelvic floor health, childbirth health, sexual health, and continence health. This would enable young women to recognize commonly occurring female pelvic health concerns such as POP or incontinence.

It seems absurd that there is so little conversation about pelvic organ prolapse at this stage of women's health evolution. My sincere hope is that this book will generate open dialogue to enable women to recognize symptoms indicating POP, as well as stimulate conversations with clinicians who currently seldom screen for POP during routine pelvic exams. Knowledge of pelvic organ prolapse is a pivotal piece of women's health awareness, whether in modernized societies or in developing zones.

> *Throughout the developing world birthrates remain high and obstetric care suboptimal. Although improvements in health care are reducing the most severe obstetric injuries - maternal death and obstetric fistula - we are starting to see a substantial increase in women presenting with advanced pelvic organ prolapse. This may well become an epidemic over the next decade. There is already a great need for education and training in this area. We and others are broadening our mission to include the care of these women. Prevention, however, will require access to quality obstetric care for all women and broad acceptance of equal rights for women and girls. We have a very long way to go in this regard.*
> ~Christopher Payne, MD

While the statistics behind pelvic organ prolapse are staggering, the reality is we have no accurate data capture on POP prevalence at the current time. Current research often estimates that up to 50% of the female population will experience pelvic organ prolapse, or that half of parous women have POP, or that half of menopausal women have POP. According to a 2009 study, the number of women with at least one pelvic floor disorder will increase significantly between 2010 to 2050, shifting from 28.1 million in 2010 to between 43.8 and 58.2 million in 2050. These figures are inclusive of breakdowns of an increase in prevalence for urinary incontinence by 55%, fecal incontinence by 59%, and pelvic organ prolapse by 46%. Both urinary and fecal incontinence frequently occur with POP. The current number of women in the US estimated in this study to have POP is 3.3 million. Considering lack of POP screening that currently exists, I ponder what accurate POP prevalence figures are at the current time and will become when we add routine POP screening into the mix.

Considering many women do not disclose or discuss embarrassing POP symptoms with their physicians, and standardized POP screening currently does not occur, it is not surprising that accurate figures for pelvic organ prolapse prevalence do not exist. As recognition of pelvic organ prolapse goes main stream and global POP initiatives shift, women will take comfort in the knowledge that they are not alone. Currently women shy away from disclosing signs and symptoms of POP to others because of the stigma attached to vaginal tissue bulge, urinary or fecal incontinence, and sexual dysfunction. Awareness is key to reduce stigma and generate comfortable open dialogue.

Along my journey, I have been incredibly fortunate to meet many progressive healthcare professionals, individuals who recognize change is coming in the pelvic organ prolapse arena.

Biomedical engineering has revolutionized medicine from the implantation of artificial organs to the optimization of complex surgeries in many fields, but has only begun to scratch the surface in women's health. Pelvic organ prolapse is a disorder that encompasses the entire field of biomedical engineering including mechanics, physiology, and clinical treatment. Every aspect of understanding, treating, and managing POP from the birth trauma (mechanics) to the progressive weakening (physiology) to the reconstructive mesh surgeries (clinical treatment) can benefit from the unique, interdisciplinary insights biomedical engineering provides.

A small number of exceptionally dedicated researchers have made incredible progress in POP and incontinence research, but they can only do so much. Because of the code of silence surrounding POP, few researchers and fewer research dollars are applied to solving these far-reaching problems. It is absolutely imperative that our society breaks from this trend.
~Benjamin Weed, PhD
~Ali Borazjani, PhD

I encourage all women to take control of their pelvic health and to recognize that each of us has the power to search for the answers. Pelvic organ prolapse is one of the most significant challenges women will address in the on-going struggle to attain health balance for our gender, no matter what barriers we face. For a female health condition to be shrouded in silence because of embarrassment at this point in history, after all we have achieved as women, is unacceptable. Women need to recognize that POP is a health concern, not a roadblock. As we push forward to raise POP awareness for the betterment of women's collective health, individual women will become familiar with this common, cryptic health concern, recognize the symptoms, and seek appropriate medical intervention.

Life teaches us that the lessons that cause the greatest pain, whether physical or emotional, are the lessons that remain most firmly planted in our brains. I've had the great fortune to watch countless women come into the support structures Association for

Pelvic Organ Prolapse Support (APOPS) provides. Devastated by what was occurring in their bodies, these women slowly morph, strong, empowered, and in control, upon securing the information and guidance needed in their unique and very individual journeys to recapture health balance. I can't begin to express the pride in womanhood I feel each and every time I see the transformation occur. Equally uplifting is watching women continue on in our space after finding info to help themselves, choosing to stay in order to pay the support forward to additional women.

As we continue to advance pelvic organ prolapse directives, generating awareness, providing patient support and guidance, defining patient needs, clarifying misconceptions, and sharing insights within medical, academic, research, policy, and industry sectors to enable evolution in POP treatment, we will spawn a new era in women's vaginal health, speaking out loud unabashedly about this last forbidden health frontier. The vagina is after all, far more than a vessel of intimacy-it is a vessel of life.

PELVIC ORGAN PROLAPSE: THE BASICS

POPS Patient Perspective: *"It is amazing to watch women enter APOPS 'POPS' support forum scared, angry, powerless, and lost, and over time as they gain support and knowledge, they become strong, confident, empowered women. Priceless."*
~MP, Kentucky/USA

In this time of enlightened self-help, it is hard to imagine a health condition that is widespread, yet for the most part unheard of.

Today's women are educated, self-reliant, pro-active individuals who seek answers. When a health concern of any nature arises, we immediately jump online, searching for answers. I find it frustrating that an extremely common female condition exists that has been documented in medical records for nearly 4000 years and causes significant physical, emotional, social, sexual, fitness, and employment quality of life impact, can be corrected, and yet the majority of women have no knowledge of the condition prior to diagnosis.

Being told at the age of 54 that I had pelvic organ prolapse was a shock. I wasn't concerned about the need to address a health condition; that was clear from my symptoms. To learn that I had a common condition that *I'd never heard* of, the progression of which I possibly could have prevented or reduced severity of with awareness, screening, and routine maintenance had I known about it earlier, infuriated me. We frequently see pharmaceutical television ads for erectile dysfunction (ED), a condition where erection of the penis is difficult or impossible to achieve, obviously very personal, and potentially embarrassing. The breast health movement is robust; despite the stigma attached to this campaign in it's infancy, the indignity has all but disappeared. Yet meaningful discussion about or reference to pelvic organ prolapse remains nearly nonexistent. Vaginal health is without a doubt currently the most stigmatized health frontier.

Many of the factors that contribute to POP occurrence were as prevalent in the days of early man as they are now. Pelvic organ prolapse documentation goes back to the Kahun Papyrus in Egyptian times circa 1835 BC. The word prolapse is Latin in origin, meaning "to fall". Hippocrates wrote about inserting a pomegranate into the vagina as a treatment for prolapse (hmmm, fruit in the vagina, that's a conversation starter…).

In general, pelvic organ prolapse in its entirety is not openly discussed. This needs to change. POP needs to be brought out into the open to enable women suffering in embarrassed silence with symptoms they don't understand access to diagnosis and treatment. If the importance of Kegel exercises was emphasized to young women during routine pelvic exams - and repeated on a regular basis to all women during those routine exams as well as during childbirth classes - recognition of pelvic floor issues and the reason for pelvic health maintenance would become common knowledge. Pelvic health education could enable women to recognize POP at an earlier, more treatable stage. As POP awareness becomes mainstream, the field will continue to evolve and the most beneficial management tools and treatments clarified.

Pelvic organ prolapse is a highly viable condition, and includes 5 types and 4 grades of severity. When pelvic organ prolapse occurs, an organ or organs in the pelvic cavity shift downward out of their normal position (multiple organs are often involved). The uterus, bladder, vagina, urethra, rectum, or intestines bulge out of their normal position, pushing down into the vaginal canal and/or outside of the vagina.

The complex support structure within a woman's pelvic cavity includes ligaments, muscles, fascia, and soft connective tissues, enabling the organs to maintain their positions within the pelvic cavity. The two most important structures that provide support for pelvic organs are ligaments and the pubococcygeus muscle (PC) or pelvic floor muscle, which is a trampoline like band of muscle which sits below the pelvic organs. When any part of the pelvic organ support system is torn, damaged, or weakened, the structural integrity of the system as a whole is reduced, enabling organs to shift position. Pelvic organ prolapse typically worsens over time. Eventually many women choose surgical repair to reduce symptoms and restore quality of life.

Displaced pelvic organs can create a wide variety of symptoms. When in supine position during a pelvic exam with speculum inserted (lying down on your back), POP may not be recognized. POP is typically more pronounced when standing or straining, as occurs with heavy lifting. Unless tissues are clearly bulging from the vaginal canal during examination, pelvic organ prolapse may go misdiagnosed or undiagnosed.

Woman's bodies are as unique on the inside as they are on the outside. This individuality makes it difficult to wrap a single set of boundaries around woman's treatment options, which include both surgical and non-surgical choices. Undoubtedly POP is one of the most awkward health concerns women will address. As POP awareness increases, the field will continue to evolve and the most beneficial tools will become evident.

Accurate statistics for pelvic organ prolapse are sorely lacking. Additional figures I find eye opening include:

- 13-57% of women suffer from some level of incontinence (stats vary by study).
- There are more than 300,000 surgeries for POP annually in the U.S. alone.
- Childbearing and menopause are the leading causes of POP, but multiple additional causes increase risk factor for women of all ages.
- Up to 35% of women suffer sphincter damage during childbirth.
- 21% of patients who have POP have some loss of

bowel control.

- 30% of women with urinary leakage suffer from loss of bowel control.
- 30% of women will undergo multiple surgeries for pelvic floor disorders.
- In 2001, the estimated annual cost of surgical treatment for pelvic organ prolapse in the U.S. surpassed $1 billion.
- The number of women who will undergo surgery for POP is predicted to increase by 46% by 2050.
- POP is a common, global women's health concern.

While pelvic organ prolapse is seldom life-threatening, it is nearly always life altering. POP ultimately causes considerable distress, impacting multiple facets of a woman's life - physical, emotional, social, sexual, financial, fitness, and employment. When you don't feel well, it is difficult to enjoy any aspect of life. When health concerns impact a woman's capacity to care for her family, it creates an emotional burden. Continuing to generate income becomes a serious challenge when you are in pain at work, especially if your job involves heavy lifting or standing for long periods of time. At times, pelvic organ prolapse can generate significant difficulty fulfilling employment responsibilities, and generate conflict in the workplace. Knowledge of pelvic organ prolapse is a pivotal piece of women's health awareness, whether in modernized societies or in developing zones.

> *If we are truly going to advance the treatment for women with pelvic organ prolapse, we need to better understand the experiences, feelings, emotions and goals of the women suffering from this condition. Research using patient-centered outcomes is the key.*
> ~Matthew Barber, MD

Many assume that POP is a "little old lady" syndrome, but POP does not discriminate by age, race, nationality, country, employment, or socio-economic status. It is unfortunate that many women live their lives tolerating symptoms they don't understand.

CAUSES OF PELVIC ORGAN PROLAPSE

POPS Patient Perspective: *"Finding POPS was like finding thousands of other women who understood everything I was going through, their stories, voices, and support shining light through some of my darkest nights."*

~AMK, Florida/USA

I f there was only a single cause of POP, it would be considerably easier to diagnose and treat; unfortunately, there are many potential causes. Each case of POP is as unique as the woman experiencing it, and every woman with POP will have her own distinct set of causal factors. Some of the symptoms of POP overlap with other health conditions. By its very multifaceted nature, POP often goes unrecognized or misdiagnosed. Multiple factors or an isolated incident (such as a difficult vaginal delivery) may initiate POP.

> *The lifestyle and childbirth decisions of today's thirty-year-old may impact key aspects of her physical function at age forty, fifty, or sixty; and incontinence, prolapse, or sexual dysfunction in a fifty-year-old may relate to childbirth and lifestyle decisions she made years before. Knowledge is the most powerful compass with which to navigate your health most wisely.*
> *~Roger Goldberg, MD*

Many different types of clinicians including gynecologists, physical therapists, urologic and women's health nurse practitioners, myofascial release therapists, and biofeedback therapists, provide POP evaluation and treatment.

The primary causes of POP are:

- Childbirth
- Menopause and other causes of estrogen loss
- Genetics
- Chronic constipation
- Chronic coughing
- Heavy lifting
- Hysterectomy

In addition, there are other factors which may contribute to POP such as neuromuscular conditions, tissue damage from prior surgeries, obesity, high impact athletic activities (marathon running, jogging, aerobics, gymnastics), and diastatis rectus abdominus (DRA), a split in the abdominal muscle related to pregnancy. Most women will have one significant causal factor along with additional less pronounced risk factors.

CHILDBIRTH

Childbirth is the leading cause of POP. Childbirth can be stressful and potentially damaging to the pelvic floor muscles, nerves, and surrounding support tissues. Hormone levels fluctuate radically throughout pregnancy as well as post-partum, impacting tissue integrity. Carrying extra weight and bulk stretches soft tissues that support the organs in the pelvic cavity. Each additional pregnancy magnifies the tissue stress and damage of the previous pregnancies.

Tissues that are damaged during delivery seldom completely recapture original elasticity. The nature of childbirth is pushing to deliver the baby. When a woman has two of more pregnancies close together and tissues haven't healed completely or properly from a prior delivery, additional damage may be sustained. Studies indicate the risk of POP increases with every vaginal delivery. Despite a period of rest between deliveries, additional vaginal deliveries may cause further tissue damage whether stretching structural tissues or tearing them.

Cesarean section (C-section) deliveries come with risk of POP as well. Research indicates elective C-section (no labor) results in less POP; however emergency C-section carries similar risk of POP related to labor trauma that has already occurred. Surgical procedures that involve cutting into core tissues of the body may impact the structural integrity of those tissues.

Delivery factors that impact the likelihood of damage are prolonged labor and/or a large birth weight baby. Use of instruments to assist a difficult delivery (forceps, vacuum) may compound damage. When a woman gives birth, damage may occur to the levator ani muscle group (PC or pelvic floor muscle). This trampoline shaped muscle layer supports the uterus, bladder, and rectum. Sustained pressure from the baby's head on delicate tissues and nerve fibers in the vaginal canal during a lengthy 2nd stage labor may cause long term damage. Vacuum or suction delivery may also injure soft tissue structures. Damage may be obvious a short time after delivery; other times the impact might not be recognized for years, sometimes decades. Damage to the tissues and nerves in this area impact the ability of the PC to contract making it difficult to sustain support for the organs and the structural tissues that surround them. Additionally, nerve damage may contribute to urinary or fecal incontinence.

One study indicated the likelihood of developing POP may increase eight-fold after two vaginal deliveries, and increased by twelve times after the delivery of four or more vaginal deliveries. Women who experience vaginal childbirth have an increased risk of developing POP over women who have not delivered babies. However, women who have never been pregnant may also develop POP since there are multiple causes.

MENOPAUSE AND AGE-RELATED MUSCLE LOSS

A decrease in women's estrogen levels from the onset of menopause can contribute to further loss of muscle tissue strength, elasticity, and density. HRT (hormone replacement therapy), whether traditional or bio-identical hormone replacement, can be helpful in maintaining balance. However, women who have experienced cancer are unlikely to be able to use this kind of therapy. Hormone levels should be evaluated to assist diagnosis regarding estrogen loss impact to pelvic floor tissues.

All muscles (both internal and external) weaken as we age, pelvic floor and core muscles are no exception. It is extremely important to have good structural support in the core and pelvic floor to support the organs within the pelvic cavity. When muscles, ligaments, and tendons have lost density or strength, they can no longer effectively support the organs within the abdominal cavity.

Exercising the abdominal and PC muscles helps build and sustain core and pelvic floor support structures. Both muscle groups can be strengthened to some degree any time or place by randomly contracting them repetitively or contracting and holding for a count of 10. Of greater benefit is engaging in a core and pelvic floor muscle training program. Refer to chapter 16, *Prevention and Maintenance,* for additional information.

GENETICS

As with other medical conditions, a genetic link may impact your risk of developing POP. Research indicates the possibility of a gene that predisposes women to POP. Discussing POP with your mother, grandmothers, sisters, aunts, and cousins may provide insights into whether you have a predisposition to POP. If one or more of your relatives has experienced pelvic organ prolapse or related surgery, there is a chance you may have inherited a structural or genetic predisposition to POP. Recognition of POP symptoms is pivotal to early diagnosis and less aggressive treatment.

If someone in your family has had POP or incontinence surgery, it would be beneficial to inquire what kind of repair they required.

It is quite possible that someone you are related to has had a POP procedure, but as is common with prolapse issues, it simply wasn't talked about. All information you gather is helpful to finding answers for yourself, particularly if you may require surgery.

Additional genetic factors that may come into play are specific hereditary diseases that impact muscle, soft tissue, or nerve tissue integrity. Hypermobility, a condition more commonly known as double-jointed as occurs in Ehlers Danlos Syndrome (EDS), increases the risk of POP occurring. Women with more flexible bodies experience additional risk of structural tissues not being able to support organs properly. Women who are "double-jointed" should pay attention to their pelvic floor whether or not they have given birth.

Marfan Syndrome is another genetic disease evidenced by collagen deficiency. Collagen is a protein that contributes to the elasticity and integrity of tissues; without sufficient levels of this protein, the pelvic floor muscles may become weak. Women with EDS or Marfan will find it valuable to seek counsel with genetic specialists as well as female pelvic medicine reconstructive surgeons (FPMRS) prior to surgery to discuss potential complications regarding lack of tissue integrity, which increases risk of surgical failure.

CHRONIC CONSTIPATION

Constipation is both a cause and symptom of pelvic organ prolapse. Chronic constipation can have a significant impact on general health balance as well as pelvic organ and soft tissue placement within the pelvic cavity. When you repetitively bear down to have a bowel movement, recurring downward pressure on the organs in your pelvic cavity may cause POP or may compound other POP risk factors. While pushing to have a bowel movement, you not only put pressure on your rectum (which can cause hemorrhoids), you also generate pressure on other organs in the pelvic cavity.

Irritable bowel syndrome (IBS) is a relatively common condition related to stress. IBS often bounces back and forth between constipation and diarrhea. For those who suffer more from IBS constipation (or even those that do not have IBS but simply have constipation issues because of poor diet), it is important to recognize that this can have a major impact on the state of your abdominal organs.

IBS constipation may contribute to POP. Considering the hectic lifestyle and chronic stress most people experience, it is not surprising how common IBS is in the general population. We no longer eat properly, we are often sleep deprived, we don't take the time to exercise, we have little free time to relax after we take care of the family and household concerns, all on top of punching out forty plus hour work weeks.

CHRONIC COUGHING

Smoking can lead to multiple health issues. Smoking or living in a house with a smoker can lead to chronic coughing. Coughing can also be the result of allergies, emphysema, bronchitis or other lung diseases, poor air ventilation, or a poor working environment. Chronic coughing causes repetitive pressure on the abdominal and pelvic organs. The strain from chronic coughing may weaken support structures in the pelvic area. The repetitive jerking and downward displacement of organs may lead to POP.

HEAVY LIFTING

Everyone needs to lift heavy objects occasionally, but for some people, heavy lifting is continual or repetitive. Many occupations require heavy manual lifting; nursing, some factory jobs, daycare workers, retirement home and rehabilitation facility staff, and farm workers are prime examples. Nearly all women who have children also subject themselves to heavy lifting over and over. When our children hurt themselves and need comforting, we lift them. When we are rushed and the kids are taking too long to walk to where we want them to go, we lift them. When they are in trouble and we want to remove them from the scene of their activity, we lift them. When we put them into their car seats, in shopping carts, or bath-tubs, we lift them. For women who have more than one small child, the motion is repeated continuously. Every time a woman lifts something heavy, downward pressure is exerted on everything within the pelvic cavity. Typically, women do not contract their pelvic floor or abdominal muscles when lifting children, so the pressure directly impacts internal pelvic organs and tissues.

This is also true for women who weight train, whether for health, muscle strength, or professional reasons. The repetitive motion of lifting heavy hand held weights creates that same downward pressure on the pelvic region. Women who are competitive weight training athletes are particularly prone to POP issues because of the substantial weight they lift repetitively.

OBESITY

Obesity has hit epidemic proportions in our country, and can significantly impact POP. Excess weight may compound POP issues because of the constant additional pressure exerted on abdominal and pelvic tissues, including the pelvic floor muscles. Maintaining a healthy weight may help slow progression of POP.

HYSTERECTOMY

Hysterectomy is a procedure that at times cannot be avoided. There are approximately 600,000 hysterectomies annually in the US. Some women feel a strong emotional attachment to their uterus; others have so much pain and dysfunction with their reproductive anatomy that they are thrilled to explore surgical removal. I had a hysterectomy on my 40th birthday. I suffered a great deal of pain and looked 5 months pregnant the entire year prior to my hysterectomy. I had several large fibroids on my uterus, one ovary covered with cysts, and aggressive adenomyosis (benign growth of tissue that embeds into the uterus). Despite an abdominal incision, I felt better 2 weeks' post-surgery than I'd felt the entire year prior. To say I was delighted to have my uterus and one ovary removed is a bit of an understatement.

Women need to know however that hysterectomy may result in vaginal vault prolapse if the apex (top) of vagina is not properly secured. As is true of all surgery, technique utilized during hysterectomy plays a role as does the skill of the physician performing the procedure. But for women who are suffering and want to recapture quality of life, a hysterectomy can often provide a path to health balance.

The "cave in" effect can occur after a centrally located organ like the uterus is removed. Since organs in the core and pelvic cavity are all in close proximity, it stands to reason that when you remove one, the others will shift around the empty pocket to some degree. If the organs in the pelvic cavity collapse into each other, this can increase the risk for POP. If the uterus is removed, it is not uncommon for the small intestine to become displaced into that space, despite efforts by surgeons to establish structural attachment points. This herniation of small intestine through the apex of the vagina at the site formerly occupied by the uterus is called an enterocele. The potential for an enterocele occurring post hysterectomy is a concern of significance worth discussing with your surgeon.

Hysterectomy can also lead to vaginal vault prolapse, a condition in which the top of the vagina caves in on itself if the apex (top) of the vagina is not secured properly. I had asked my gynecologist prior to my hysterectomy "what stops stuff from falling out?" Although I had no idea that POP existed at this point in my life, I did not experience vaginal vault prolapse but did have an enterocele. There is increased risk of both vaginal vault prolapse and enterocele after a hysterectomy. It would have been great if after I opened the door to prolapse concerns with my gynecologist (albeit blindly), my physician would have taken the initiative to have a conversation explaining potential POP concerns. If I had known pelvic organ prolapse was a common condition, I'd have started digging right away for more information.

I experienced a symptom of POP prior to my hysterectomy at the age of 40; I had difficulty keeping a tampon in. I did not mention it to my gynecologist prior to my hysterectomy; perhaps if I had, our conversation would have gone in an additional direction. It is important to ask the right questions when discussing pelvic health with your physician.

COMPOUNDING HEALTH CONDITIONS

Neuromuscular diseases like multiple sclerosis increase risk of POP. MS (multiple schlerosis) can contribute to muscle weakness. When nerves can't fire properly, muscles tissues won't fully engage. Diabetes may be a factor as well since diabetics often suffer from neuropathy, which impacts how well nerves fire to initiate muscle contraction. 60 to 70% of diabetics have some level of neuropathy. When diseases cause paralysis or restriction of muscle or nerve tissue, the muscle tissue can waste away. The pelvic floor is deeply innervated muscle tissue; deterioration will prevent it from supporting the pelvic organs properly.

ADHESIONS AND TISSUE DAMAGE

Pelvic or abdominal surgery, whether hysterectomy, tubal ligation, removal of one or both ovaries, rectal surgery, or any other surgery in the pelvic vicinity, may compound POP risk. Scar tissue restricts organ and structural tissue movement. Failure to repair structural support during childbirth or gynecologic surgery can lead to tissue defects that may later contribute to POP.

Tissues torn during childbirth might not get repaired because the damage is not visible, and inadequate support of organs or scar tissue and adhesions may contribute to POP. Damage may also occur to the nerves during long 2nd stage labor, which may cause improper function of the muscle tissues, compounding the risk of

POP. It is important to remember that there is seldom one cause only for POP, more typically a combination of factors coming into play.

DIASTASIS RECTUS ABDOMINUS

Another potential POP risk factor is diastasis rectus abdominus (DRA), a widening or separation between the 2 bellies of the long abdominal muscle during pregnancy. While few studies validate that DRA increases risk of urinary or fecal incontinence, myofascial pelvic pain, and pelvic organ prolapse, anecdotal feedback from women experiencing pelvic organ prolapse indicates this is an area in need of additional research exploration.

FITNESS ACTIVITIES

There is notable potential for women who are joggers or marathon runners, or who participate in aggressive aerobics or gymnastics which 'stick the landing', to experience POP. 30-40% of women experience urinary leakage while exercising; the main complaint of female marathon runners is not joint pain, it is incontinence. According to Running USA, in 2015 57% of runners were women, and 9,755,500 females finished road races.

Utilizing internal support while engaging in any aggressive exercise regimen is a valuable proactive step women need to utilize. Inserting an internal support device such as a pessary prior to high impact athletic activities may provide internal structural support and decrease impact of repetitive downward jerking of pelvic structural tissues and organs. It should also eliminate incontinence concerns while participating in athletic activities. Millions of women participate in fitness and sport activities; it is crucial that POP awareness is addressed in this pocket of women. Exercise is key to maintaining health balance. It is pivotal women recognize the need for internal support when participating in fitness activities to avoid trading one health concern for another.

Jogging for heart health resulting in POP issues is not a desired direction.

TYPES OF PELVIC ORGAN PROLAPSE

POPS Patient Perspective: *"APOPS taught me that having POP is a journey, a process that often begins with anger, grief and disbelief, followed by acceptance, discovery of knowledge, and ultimately advocacy and empowerment to make surgical and/or nonsurgical decisions uniquely suited to me."*
~AP, New Jersey/USA

There are many combinations of pelvic organ prolapse. Since the organs and tissues in the pelvic cavity are tightly grouped, and since the functions of these organs and tissues are interrelated, it makes sense that women may experience multiple types of POP at the same time. It is important that the physician you choose to treat pelvic organ prolapse is thorough and take each kind of prolapse into consideration when guiding treatment; clearly a POP specialist is the best choice.

It is imperative that docs, nurses, patients, trainees all work together to understand the impact of these disorders on women and help to optimize treatment outcomes in an individualized manner.
~Holly Richter, MD

POP does not occur because of a defect in pelvic organs, it occurs because there is a weakness in the organ supportive tissues such as ligaments, muscles, and tendons. There are five types of pelvic organ prolapse.
- Cystocele
- Rectocele
- Uterine Prolapse

  • Vaginal vault prolapse
  • Enterocele

CYSTOCELE

A cystocele occurs when the bladder bulges into the front vaginal wall, pushing through the vagina to the outside of the body. The bladder and urethra prolapse together. (The urethra is the tube that urine flows through from the bladder to the outside of the body.) Cystocele symptoms are frequent or urgent need to urinate, general urinary leakage, urinary leakage during sexual activity (coital incontinence), pressure, and discomfort. In advanced grades of cystocele, it will become difficult to urinate. Incomplete emptying of the bladder may result, and the potential for urinary tract infections (UTI) increases.

RECTOCELE

Rectocele occurs when the rectum pushes into the rear vaginal wall. A hernia or bulge may occur in the large bowel; stool typically gets trapped in the bulge, resulting in chronic constipation. Along with constipation, hemorrhoids, incomplete stool emptying, rectal pressure, general pelvic discomfort, or impacted stool may occur. Splinting, inserting a finger/fingers into their vagina to push the bulge back into place, may be necessary to assist bowel emptying.

UTERINE

Uterine prolapse occurs when the uterus pushes downward through the vaginal canal toward or to the outside of the vagina. The uterus may rest partially inside of the vagina, completely within the vaginal walls, or push out of the vagina far enough for the cervix to be viewed outside of the vaginal opening. The most severe level of uterine prolapse occurs when the uterus has pushed completely through the vaginal opening to the outside of the body, a condition called procidentia.

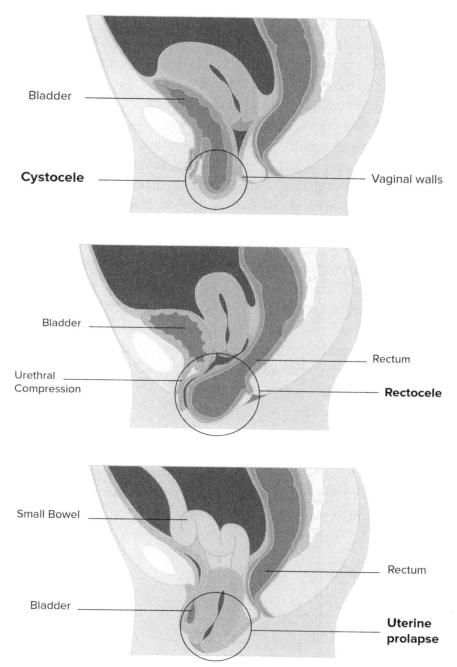

Cystocele (top), Rectocele (center), Uterine prolapse (bottom).

VAGINAL VAULT

The vaginal vault area is located at the apex or top of the vagina. If the top of the vagina is not properly secured during hysterectomy, the vaginal walls may cave in on themselves and the vagina may invert like a pants pocket turned inside out. Vaginal tissue bulge and pressure are the most common symptoms. Studies indicate vaginal vault prolapse prevalence as a result of hysterectomy vary between 15-43%, however techniques have evolved considerably and although accurate data is scarce, this risk factor likely falls somewhere in the middle of those 2 figures.

ENTEROCELE

An enterocele is a prolapse of the small intestine. An enterocele characteristically occurs following a hysterectomy. The intestine can push through any area of weakness, most commonly in the apex (top of the vagina) where the uterus was formerly positioned. Intestines may push down between the rectum and the back wall of the vagina, but may also push down along the front vaginal wall as well. An enterocele often occurs simultaneously with a rectocele or vaginal vault prolapse.

As POP progresses and the organs and tissues shift and push against each other, the severity or complexity may be compounded. Early POP diagnosis is advantageous to contain the degree of severity and enable less aggressive treatment. Paying close attention to your body and knowing what is normal for you is normal is key to early awareness, diagnosis, and treatment.

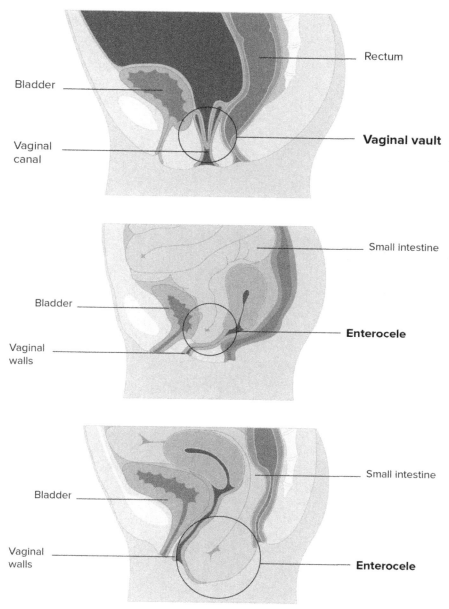

Rectum

Bladder

Vaginal vault

Vaginal canal

Small intestine

Bladder

Enterocele

Vaginal walls

Small intestine

Bladder

Vaginal walls

Enterocele

Vaginal vault (top), Enterocele front (center), Enterocele back (bottom).

SYMPTOMS OF PELVIC ORGAN PROLAPSE

POPS Patient Perspective: *I felt like my 30-year-old soul was trapped in an*
80-year-old body, but the POPS group has provided much needed empathy, support, and guidance to both me and my partner that even my doctors couldn't provide.
~RK, Australia

Many women with POP are simply not aware that there is a name for the symptoms they feel. Some are too embarrassed by the symptoms they are experiencing to describe them to their physicians. Some women are simply not in tune with their bodies, and are unable to recognize that the symptoms they are experiencing are abnormal until the level of discomfort becomes too great to ignore. Some women assume the symptoms they are experiencing are part of menopause or aging and because of that, are not concerned enough to approach a physician. Others are simply too busy to take the time to address these concerns.

There is still a lack of awareness amongst women of the range of symptoms caused by prolapse, but likewise, many women do not recognise the term. There is much to be gained by increasing education and awareness of prolapse and the range and extent of available treatments.
~Adrian Wagg, MD/Canada

POP symptoms typically progress if the underlying condition is not addressed; it is important to seek the advice of the clinician who provides your pelvic exams and request POP screening if you experience symptoms. When POP is diagnosed, most diagnostic physicians refer their patients to a specialist for further evaluation. Frequently women experiencing POP symptoms will request their physicians provide a pelvic exam, but if POP symptoms are not clarified by the patient, the condition often remains unrecognized, unacknowledged, and is not addressed. Pelvic organ prolapse is not typically screened for during routine pelvic exams. POP symptoms come and go for many women, varying by activity level and body position. When lying down in supine position with feet in the stirrups (standard pelvic exam position), the condition may not be clearly visible. Even if POP is apparent, the degree of severity is significantly reduced when lying down because organs slide back into their normal position. A specialist often uses a screening technique called POP-Q, but primary care and gynecologists will more typically ask patients to perform a Valsalva maneuver (bare down) to demonstrate the degree of POP.

There are five types of POP and because the combinations of those types vary, symptoms can be unique from woman to woman. The degree of prolapse severity varies from individual to individual as well; some women with a very mild degree of prolapse may not recognize symptoms at all. Some women find symptoms very pronounced and embarrassing, and at times are not comfortable discussing them with their physicians. POP symptoms may masquerade as other conditions. The most common symptoms of POP are:

- Vaginal tissue bulge
- Urinary incontinence
- Urine retention
- Chronic constipation
- Vaginal and/or rectal pressure
- Vaginal and/or rectal pain
- Back or pelvic pain
- Inability to retain a tampon
- Fecal incontinence
- Coital incontinence
- Painful intercourse
- Reduced intimate sensation

The symptoms of POP vary considerably from woman to woman and can masquerade as or intersect with other disorders such as irritable bowel, PMS, or general incontinence. It is extremely important that you share a complete list of symptoms with your physician so if signs indicate POP, a specialist referral can be initiated to control POP progression. The POP Risk Factor Questionnaire (POP-RFQ) is a document that will help clarify if symptoms being experienced indicate pelvic organ prolapse, and is available for download on the Association for Pelvic Organ Prolapse Support (APOPS) website. This checklist of questions may enable you to recognize POP as well as initiate a dialogue about POP with your clinician. You can download the POP-RFQ on the APOPS website at www.pelvicorganprolapsesupport.org/pop-risk-factor-questionnaire.

VAGINAL TISSUE BULGE

The vaginal pressure that occurs with POP is difficult to imagine without experiencing it. Some women describe it as the sensation of their insides falling out, others indicate it feels like sitting on a ball.

You may notice a "bulge" in the vaginal canal or outside of the vaginal canal.

This bulge may be the cervix (the opening to the uterus), the uterus pushing out of the vaginal canal, the vaginal wall with the bladder behind it, the vaginal wall with the rectum behind it, the vaginal wall with intestines behind it, or if you've had a hysterectomy, the top of the vaginal walls themselves. This sensation may come and go for some women because prolapsed organs may recede back into the pelvic cavity. For women who are on their feet all day because of their jobs or childcare, POP may not be recognizable for some time because they are distracted by everyday activities. Since pelvic organs can retract into their normal position when a woman lies down in bed at night, she may no longer feel any pain or discomfort.

When organs or tissues have shifted into the vaginal canal to the point that they are literally bulging out, some women will push the "lump" back up into the vaginal canal. This is a very short-term fix at best; the only purpose it serves is to temporarily relieve the sensation, enable urination, or assist defecation.

URINARY INCONTINENCE

Urinary incontinence (UI) is one of the most common symptoms of POP, particularly with cystocele. Not all incontinence is POP, but there is frequently a POP connection. Millions of women suffer with UI and most do not seek medical evaluation; often women with UI believe it is a normal part of aging and don't recognize incontinence is a symptom of a health condition which needs to be addressed. Americans annually spend about $19.5 billion managing urinary incontinence, along with an additional $12.6 billion for urinary urgency and frequency.

Urinary incontinence comes in different forms including the need to urinate immediately (urge incontinence), or leakage with coughing/sneezing/running and other fitness activities (stress urinary incontinence). Some women experience both types of urinary incontinence (mixed incontinence). Women who have neuromuscular diseases such as multiple sclerosis may be predisposed to leakage related to bladder over-activity (OAB). Women who have diabetic neuropathy may have leakage because the nerves that cause the bladder to contract do not function properly. Multiple health conditions create additional risk for POP.

UI is more typical of early stages of prolapse; as POP advances to a more pronounced stage, voiding difficulties and incomplete emptying become more pronounced. Not all incontinence is due to prolapse however, so it is important to get an accurate diagnosis. Urinary incontinence occurs frequently in women after childbirth because of obstetrical trauma to the pelvic floor structural support tissues and/or nerves in this area. If urinary incontinence does not resolve after childbirth (especially if you experienced a difficult labor), it is important to request appropriate evaluation.

URINE RETENTION

Often women who have incontinence in early stages of prolapse have difficulty voiding effectively later in the more progressive stages of prolapse. When POP has progressed to an advanced stage, urine retention, a weak urine stream, or difficulty emptying the bladder completely is likely to occur. With advanced cystocele, the urethra may kink (the tube through which urine passes from the bladder to the outside of the body), which makes it difficult for the bladder to empty. If urine cannot flow from the body effectively or fully, there is an increased risk for urinary tract infections (UTI).

A study indicates obstruction of the urethra occurred in 58% of women with grades 3 & 4 prolapse, as opposed to only 4% of women with grade 1 or 2 prolapse. As the degree of prolapse advances, it is more likely that a woman will have difficulty initiating the stream, and may even have to manually reduce the prolapse (with finger/hand pressure on abdomen or in vagina) to void urine.

CHRONIC CONSTIPATION

Although constipation has many causes, chronic constipation is frequently an indicator of POP in women. When the rectum balloons against the rear vaginal wall, it prevents stool from passing normally down the bowel. Constipation may occur on a regular basis or it can be an on again off again scenario. There may be a need to "splint" to enable defecation (inserting fingers into the vagina to push stool out). Often this change in bowel habits is confused with IBS. Sometimes stool incontinence may occur simultaneously. Since the constipation is caused by this hernia-like bulge in the rectum, the use of high fiber diet may not ease it. Increasing water intake, supplementing with probiotics, and using fruit rather than grain fiber sources sometimes helps, but typically POP treatments need to be utilized to relieve POP related constipation.

VAGINAL AND/OR RECTAL PRESSURE

It is extremely difficult to explain the sensation of vaginal or rectal pressure to someone who has not experienced it. The feeling of "fullness" that accompanies the pressure sensation can easily lead to an incorrect diagnosis. Women who are used to the bloated feeling that accompanies PMS may misinterpret this sensation. POP pressure sensation is truly in the rectum or vagina.

Nearly everyone is familiar with the sensation of rectal pressure that is felt when a bowel movement is coming on; however, for a woman with a rectocele, a bowel movement may only minimally relieve the pressure sensation. Because a woman with POP typically cannot have a complete bowel movement, the sensation of pressure occurs nearly all the time. Women with rectoceles frequently navigate on-going constipation or incomplete defecation that no amount of fiber will fix. Some women find they can assist the bowel movement by inserting a finger into their vagina to push the bowel back into place; this enables them to empty their bowels.

VAGINAL AND/OR RECTAL PAIN

Since the sensation of pain is unique from person to person, it is important to note that one woman may perceive a rectal or vaginal fullness as pressure, another may perceive it as pain. The level of discomfort that grows with each day of not being able to properly empty your bowels can be very stressful. If a woman assumes she has IBS or simple constipation, and tries several remedies to no avail, it would be worthwhile to explore whether other POP symptoms are occurring, and if so, explore appropriate POP diagnosis and treatment.

BACK OR PELVIC PAIN

Because there can be multiple combinations of organs and tissues involved with POP, the type and degree of pain will differ from woman to woman. In general, there can be lower back pain, pressure type pain of the rectum or vagina, generalized pelvic or distention related pain, pain similar to a urinary tract infection, pain with intercourse, as well as a general heaviness in the pelvic region. Often with POP, the pain and discomfort eases when lying down. Not all pelvic pain is related to POP, so it is important to keep track of all symptoms to clarify if the pain you feel is truly related to POP.

INABILITY TO RETAIN A TAMPON

One indicator of POP that may occur before any other symptom is recognized is the inability to keep a tampon in place. Normally when a tampon is inserted into the vagina, soft tissues and muscular structures naturally hold it in position. When POP occurs, the tissues will literally push the tampon out. If this is something being experienced, it makes sense to watch for other symptoms of POP listed on APOPS POP Risk Factor Questionnaire and question your physician about the possibility of POP. Early diagnosis of POP may enable less aggressive treatment.

FECAL INCONTINENCE

It is estimated that up to 40% of women will sustain some damage to the sphincter muscle or it's nerve supply during childbirth. After obstetrical anal injury and repair, 50% of women will still have some element of fecal incontinence. Fecal incontinence may not show up for decades after childbirth; women seldom recognize that there is a connection between the two.

COITAL INCONTINENCE

Incontinence is enough to put the skids on romance completely-talk about taking the spontaneity out of intimacy. Most people aren't comfortable talking about incontinence; it's even more difficult to approach the topic of intimacy related incontinence, particularly fecal incontinence. Any woman who must worry if she is "clean enough" to engage in sex at a moment's notice will walk away from being spontaneous nearly all the time.

Since there is a possibility of stool or urine leakage with different types of POP, women may refrain from sexual relations for fear of either of these issues occurring. It can be extremely uncomfortable to talk about stool or urine leakage with the closest of partners, which can create an awkward gap in a relationship. The resulting dynamic is one partner thinks the other partner is not interested in sex, when it is simply a medical condition that has not been recognized, diagnosed, or treated.

PAINFUL INTERCOURSE

The displacement of organs may also create sexual pain or discomfort for some women. Rather than reveal that intercourse is painful, a woman may choose to just say she is not interested in sex. Others share that intercourse is painful, but their partners may not always believe them.

Sometimes struggles with intimacy are what bring POP to the front page. When a woman who has enjoyed sex her entire adult life suddenly finds intimacy painful, confusion and frustration can result. Since POP often presents itself at the time of life when a woman may be going through peri-menopause or menopause, she may assume the changes are due to those body changes rather than something more significant. While vaginal atrophy (drying of vaginal tissues occuring during menopause) is very real, not all pain with intimacy is related to atrophy. A clinician may check your hormone levels to determine whether estrogen replacement may address pain with intimacy. If pain continues after atrophy has been addressed, the pressure of POP organ displacement or rectocele related abdominal bloat may be the source of discomfort.

REDUCED INTIMATE SENSATION

For some women, nerve damage may block sensation from reaching areas that were previously sensitive. If there is little or no sensation during foreplay or intercourse, a woman may lose interest in intimacy. This loss of intimacy can absolutely have an impact on a relationship.

Most women have a difficult time discussing intimate sensations with their physicians or their sexual partners. Intimacy conversations are often awkward to initiate, making it difficult to explore concerns freely, whether they have medical, physical, or emotional roots. However, these concerns can and should be examined.

These last four symptoms, fecal incontinence, coital incontinence, painful intercourse, and loss of sensation, along with vaginal tissue bulge, can radically impact an intimate relationship for the sexually active woman. Open communication between two intimate partners is ideal, but truly not common when it comes to concerns of this delicate nature.

This change in the sexual dynamic may create tension in the relationship with your intimate partner. Telling your partner about any of the above concerns is difficult enough, but having your partner assume you are making excuses to get out of having sex can be both hurtful and frustrating, and it does nothing to enhance the relationship. Initiating a conversation, as difficult as it may be, may ease tensions. Lack of information can often lead an intimate partner to assume there is no interest in intimacy at all.

~ 5 ~
# WHEN TO SEEK MEDICAL TREATMENT

POPS Patient Perspective: *"From this group, I have found more reliable information than any place else, including from doctors, and more support and understanding, and hope for the future.*
~MFC, Virginia/USA

How can we seek medical treatment for a condition that we aren't aware exists? One of the reasons for writing this book is to generate awareness of POP so that when women experience symp-toms, they will go to their physicians with questions in hand.

Early stage POP often doesn't initiate symptoms pronounced enough or continuous enough to generate concern. POP screening seldom occurs during routine pelvic exams. The best method of finding out if you have POP (or any other medical condition for that matter) is to pay close attention to your body and the changes you are experiencing. Recognizing what is normal for you, rather than what media indicates is normal, is a good starting point. Whenever you have a condition that makes you head to your physician, and tests come back negative, and if the symptoms persist or worsen, continue to dig until you find answers.

To self-screen for POP, take a hand-held mirror and look for tissues bulging from the vagina while standing. It is best to perform this self-test later in the day, because POP tends to become most pronounced when pelvic floor muscles become fatigued.

If you see tissues bulging from the vagina, consult your primary care clinician, gynecologist, or Ob/Gyn with your discovery. Initially, the person that diagnoses POP will likely be your gynecologist or family physician. Once a preliminary diagnosis is made, you will likely be referred to a specialist. Although women are often referred to many different types of specialists, a FPMRS urogynecologist or urologist is the specialty trained physician for pelvic organ prolapse. A FPMRS specialist can address and repair any of the five types of POP.

Since POP isn't a condition routinely screened for, it is possible that your physician will not recognize it. If Kegel exercises and POP awareness education were initiated during the first pelvic exam and during childbirth classes, and women were continually re-educated about pelvic organ prolapse in their early 20's during routine PAP smears and gynecologic checkups, we would be more likely to recognize which symptoms to report to our physicians.

The optimal time to seek treatment for POP is when experiencing symptoms on a repetitive basis or in a pronounced way, such as vaginal tissue bulge, incontinence, or vaginal and/or rectal pressure. If POP is caught in early stage, non-surgical treatments can be fairly effective.

> *Conservative management of POP is related to forces. Ideally the forces from below the organ are greater than the forces from above, enabling the organs to stay in proper position. If the forces from above are too great (bearing down, poor lifting technique, constipation, weak abdominals and more) or the forces from below aren't strong or stable enough (weak pelvic floor muscles, torn ligaments), organs will shift downward. Women's health physical therapy teaches women to understand how to decrease the forces from above and increase the forces from below.*
> ~Beth Shelly, PT, DPT

However, when POP continues to progress to an advanced stage without diagnosis, there is a strong possibility that surgery may become a likely consideration for repair. If a mild prolapse is diagnosed, it can be monitored while using any of multiple less aggressive non-surgical treatment options. Seek additional medical attention when:

- Symptoms become more pronounced.
- New symptoms occur.
- New pain or discomfort arises.
- Unusual vaginal or rectal bleeding or discharge occurs.

It is difficult to judge how often you should see your physician when first diagnosed with mild POP. If additional symptoms occur or if your symptoms worsen, the degree of POP severity should be checked again. If the treatments you are using are not effective, your POP may have progressed to the point where you need to consider additional treatments or surgery.

If prolapse has already progressed to a moderate or severe level, you should consult with a POP specialist, particularly if you have pain or discomfort. You should be referred to a Female Pelvic Medicine Reconstructive Surgeon (FPMRS) urogynecologist, urologist, or a women's health physical therapist. A FPMRS urogynecologist or urologist can provide both surgical and nonsurgical treatment options. Physical therapists who specialize in women's health can provide assessment and multiple types of nonsurgical treatments as well. These specialists are the experts in pelvic medicine, and typically treat any of the five types of POP.

It is in your best interest to have one surgeon who specializes in all aspects of POP complete all surgical procedures rather than have two different surgeons repairing individual types of POP. Ask your referring physician whom she would use if she needed to have POP surgery. There is often value in seeking a 2nd opinion with an additional specialist. Because POP can impact urinary, bowel, and sexual anatomy, it is a good idea to check references and do your homework before deciding which surgeon will provide your repair.

MEDICAL EVALUATION: WHAT TO EXPECT

POPS Patient Perspective: *"After a diagnosis of POP at 29 years old, I was devastated and alone; this group has helped me to realize that I am not alone and I feel more empowered as a woman, wife, mother, nurse, and human being."*
~RF, IA/USA

P rior to getting a specific pelvic organ prolapse diagnosis, you will likely need to have at least one, and possibly several tests done to distinguish what kinds of POP you are experiencing. It won't be possible for your physician or surgeon to recommend treatment options until he or she knows exactly which organs are prolapsed.

The diagnostic process of a woman with POP is not just to execute some examinations taken from a list: one should consider the anatomical defects and the correlated symptoms, keep in mind the possible pathophysiology together with the patient's real aims and expectations and make all the evaluations needed. Sometimes take the history and make a physical examination may be enough, sometimes instrumental examinations may be needed. The patient's needs should rule this process, always.
~Enrico Finazzi-Agro, MD

The starting point for a POP evaluation is a pelvic examination by your gynecologist or primary care physician. This will reveal what type of POP you are experiencing and possibly the degree of severity. Besides visually inspecting the vagina, a clinician may check the level of muscle control a woman has with her pc (pelvic floor) muscle and sphincter muscles. During this basic test, the physician will insert fingers manually and ask you to squeeze down. There are additional tests that may or may not be performed, depending on the discretion of your physician. Some of the tests that may be performed are:

- Standing exam
- Urodynamic Study
- Pelvic MRI
- Pelvic Ultrasound
- Hormone level testing
- Cystoscopy
- Defecography

Once it has been determined that you are experiencing POP, you will likely be referred to a specialist. Bring your list of symptoms and questions to this exam. Bring a notebook along as well to take notes to review later.

After discussing the reason for your visit and reviewing your symptoms, a FPMRS urogynecologist or urologist will most likely perform both a pelvic and rectal exam to make an initial determination about the kinds of prolapse you have and their degree of severity. The initial inspection will be similar to any other pelvic exam, feet in the stirrups, legs spread, speculum inserted. By visually inspecting each wall of the vagina while you cough and bear down (Valsalva maneuver) in addition to palpating the abdominal area, your specialist can determine which organs are prolapsing and the degree of prolapse severity.

Your physician will also likely perform a rectal exam if he/she suspects a rectocele. For this exam, the physician will insert a lubricated, gloved finger into the rectum, and possibly a finger into the vagina, then ask you to push or bear down to better palpate the area. It is a relatively quick check, so the discomfort only lasts short time.

THE STANDING EXAM

It is possible for some prolapse symptoms to disappear when

lying down, so in addition to being examined lying down your physician may additionally examine you while you are standing. If your clinician performs the screening lying down and indicates the degree of POP severity is mild, but your symptoms tell you otherwise, request the standing screen if it is not offered to you.

A good physician will explain what he/she is doing before performing each part of the exam. If at any point you feel your physician is not explaining in advance what is going to be done, speak up! If you experience pain during any part of the exam, speak up! If you do not have a good comfort level with your physician during this exam, it will surely not get any better once you get to the point of surgery. If your physician is gentle and concerned about the sensitive nature of this exam, it is a good sign that you have a compassionate specialist. If at any point during this exam you have a question, again, speak up! Patients often hesitate to ask questions because they feel the physician is busy and they don't want to bother him/her, but the more knowledge you have, the fewer surprises you will get. Remember, you are paying for this medical service, whether out of your own pocket or paying for the insurance coverage - view it like any other service provider, expect and seek the best.

There grading system used to describe the severity of prolapse, 1, 2, 3, or 4, with grade1 being the mildest prolapse, grade 4 being the most severe. A grade 1 prolapse may not generate symptoms. By grade 2 there are often symptoms, and it can be usually be seen by a physician familiar with POP. At this point, there will likely be the characteristic tissue bulging out of the vagina. By grade 3, the physical characteristics are not only felt by the patient, they are typically quite significant. At the point of grade 4, symptoms and vaginal tissue bulge are substantial. Despite obvious symptoms, women often go undiagnosed with POP for years, often decades, because they are either too embarrassed to share their symptoms with their clinicians or diagnostic practitioners are not adequately educated to screen appropriately.

Once the initial pelvic exam has been completed, and your physician has made a preliminary diagnosis about what type/types of POP he/she thinks you have, you may need to have additional diagnostic tests done to find out more conclusively what needs to be repaired. If your POP is not too severe, typically if it is still stage 1 or 2, your physician may recommend that you try a combination of non-surgical treatments instead of surgery, such as a pessary, Kegel or pelvic floor strengthening exercises, hormone replacement, electrical stimulation, biofeedback, myofascial release therapy, support garments, tibial nerve stimulation, or core strengthening exercises. At this stage, it is valuable to recognize and address behaviors that may be making POP worse, such as heavy lifting or downward pounding fitness activities such as jogging or marathon running.

URODYNAMIC STUDY

Your physician may give you a series of bladder tests prior to surgery even if you don't have leakage problems. In more advanced cases of POP, the POP itself may mask urinary incontinence because the prolapsed organs or tissues which press against the urethra may create a kink in it (the tube through which urine flows from the bladder to the outside of the body), and prevent the urine from leaking out. Once the POP issues are repaired, and the urethra is no longer kinked, you may find out that you now have a urine leakage problem. Since urinary incontinence is common in women, it makes sense to test for incontinence concerns prior to surgery so in the event you have leakage that you aren't aware of, it can be addressed at the time of POP surgery. The urodynamic study is a test to determine how well the bladder can store and empty urine. The amount and force of the urine stream will be measured in the first portion of the test. A catheter will be inserted for the second part of the test and the bladder will be filled with sterile water. A measurement will be taken for the volume at which the patient feels the need to urinate. The patient is then asked to bear down and cough to see if urine leaks out. This test also determines bladder flow and bladder pressure at the time of urinating to treat bladder function. The results of this test help the surgeon determine the best type of surgical repair.

PELVIC MRI/PELVIC ULTRASOUND

A pelvic MRI or pelvic ultrasound provides an image of the soft tissues inside the body. The pelvic MRI provides a detailed three-dimensional image of the pelvis and its contents. A pelvic ultrasound will image the bladder or kidneys in women that are having problems with urinary incontinence or urine retention in the bladder, or can be used to visualize muscles around the anus for evaluating fecal incontinence.

> *It is important to have a high quality diagnostic test such as an MRI or an x-ray defecogram for several reasons. It objectively confirms the degree of POP during evacuation, which provides a better measure than during just straining. In my experience, for many patients, seeing their own imaging provides some welcome relief that their symptoms have a real physical cause and aren't "just in their heads". It provides one more step to empowering women to take ownership of their health and well-being."*
> ~Vikas Shah, MBBS

HORMONE LEVEL TESTING

Hormone level testing is a blood test. All female hormone levels can be checked, but if a woman is already on hormone replacement therapy, this test may not be a necessary. Women who have not used hormone therapies and are in menopause should request a check of hormone levels since loss of estrogen can impact tissue strength and integrity in the vaginal canal as well as the PC (pubococcygeus or pelvic floor) muscle which is the structural base for the organs in the pelvic cavity. Physicians may recommend hormone supplementation for women in peri-menopause or menopause temporarily for a prior to and post-surgery to enhance the healing of the vaginal and pelvic floor tissues.

CYSTOSCOPY

Cystoscopy is a test used for viewing the bladder and urethra. It is used to help evaluate problems with urinary frequency and urgency, as well as problems with bladder pain or blood in the urine. A small tube with a light and camera are lubricated with an anesthetic gel and inserted into the urethra; images are then projected onto a screen for viewing.

DEFECOGRAM

Defecography is an x-ray test which shows the rectum and anal canal in action while having a bowel movement. It will indicate where weak walls bulge out as a hernia as occurs with rectocele.

Upon completion of testing, your physician will determine the treatment which will provide the best options, whether surgical or non-surgical. The significance of these tests is they enable specialists to precisely determine the types and severity of your POP, allowing all prolapsed organs to be repaired in one procedure. Find a physician you are comfortable with and trust, ask tons of questions, and then feel confident that the path you choose to address your POP issues will be the best one for you.

Since POP has similar symptoms to many other conditions, it is often misdiagnosed or undiagnosed during primary care and gynecologic exams. For example, if you have been diagnosed with irritable bowel syndrome (IBS), and are being treated for it, and the constipation/loose stool issues continue, it would be worth reviewing the symptoms caused by POP to see if there is a possibility that there are prolapsed organs creating the problem or additionally aggravating the problem.

NON-SURGICAL TREATMENT OPTIONS

POPS Patient Perspective: *"One of the greatest challenges as a woman with POP, is how isolating it is. That constant 'ache' - that no one understands you or can relate to you. Through APOPS, I continue to gain the strength to recognize this health condition for what it is - a part of me, but not all of me. I am more accepting of myself because I know I am not alone. I am forever grateful to Sherrie Palm - for building and nurturing this bridge of compassion, awareness, and advocacy to be listened to and heard."* ~KC, OH/USA

There are two treatment paths for POP, surgical or non-surgical. Once your primary care physician or gynecologist has diagnosed pelvic organ prolapse, a FPMRS urogynecologist or urologist or a women's health physical therapist can guide your choice. Each choice has its benefits and the choice you make will be influenced by your type and degree of POP, whether or not you choose to have additional children, (or have a child if you haven't had onemSyet), the length of time you have been suffering with symptoms, the intensity of your symptoms, any complications your unique medical conditions may pose to complicate surgery, your age, your desire to continue to have normal sexual relations, and medical in-surance coverage considerations.

Once you have been screened for and diagnosed with POP, what type or types you have, and the degree of severity, you will need to analyze treatment choices. POP specialists will guide you through these options. These treatments may be administered by a urogynecologist, a physical therapist, an occupational therapist, a urologic nurse practitioner, a biofeedback clinician, or a myofascial release therapist. Treatments utilized by therapists can provide POP management instead of surgery, and these therapies

are additionally beneficial for maintenance post-surgery as well as in place of surgery. Make sure the therapists you choose are certified in women's pelvic health. Links to multiple clinician locator pages are listed on the APOPS website Practitioner Locator page.
http://www.pelvicorganprolapsesupport.org/healthcareconnections/

Becoming aware of your body and the sensations that are created by POP will be of great value in monitoring your path to pelvic floor health. Many women with grades 1 or 2 POP find combinations of the following treatments effective to control POP symptoms. Additionally, these treatments are valuable to use for long-term maintenance post-surgery should the surgical route be your treatment choice.

- Kegel exercises
- Kegel assist devices
- Pessary
- Incostress
- Impressa
- Hormone replacement therapy
- Electrical stimulation
- Biofeedback
- Tibial nerve stimulation
- Myofascial release therapy
- Pelvic floor and core exercise programs
- Urethral bulking agents
- Support Garments

Laser and radio-frequency vaginal tissue restoration therapy.

Any combination of these approaches may be used, depending on the type or types of prolapse being experienced. Your healthcare professionals can assist your exploration of a combination of therapies to attempt to improve the strength of the PC muscle, which in turn may help stabilize the degree of POP. These therapies may improve your POP or at least prevent worsening of the POP level of severity and may also reduce symptoms such as pain, discomfort, or incontinence. It will generally take a few months for these types of therapies to be beneficial.

KEGEL EXERCISES

Kegel exercises were developed in 1948 by Dr. Arnold Kegel and can be beneficial for general pelvic floor health and maintenance, for POP treatment, and for maintenance post-surgery for nearly all women. Dr. Kegel was light years ahead of his peers, recognizing the significance of exercising the pelvic floor muscle, also known as the pubococcygeus or PC muscle. This important support structure is a part of the levator ani muscle, which stretches from the pubic bone to the tailbone like a trampoline, supporting the organs above. Kegels should not be viewed as a "quick-fix"; they should be utilized for long term preservation of the PC muscle much like brushing your teeth maintains oral health. If practiced prior to and throughout pregnancy (check with your physician first to make sure there aren't any contraindications, particularly if you have miscarriage concerns), the pelvic floor remains more elastic and resistant to damage during childbirth. If practiced following childbirth, they can help restore tone to the muscles of the pelvic floor. Kegel exercises can be performed anywhere, in any position, standing, sitting, or lying down, although when first learning proper Kegel technique it is a good idea to perform them lying down until you easily recognize contraction sensations.

A Kegel contraction is the same contraction that is used to stop the flow of urine. Once a woman recognizes this sensation, she can repeat it throughout the day, no matter where she is or what she is doing. It can and should be repeated multiple times throughout the day until it becomes second nature, because the more often it is practiced, the more it becomes a habit. It can be helpful to establish a ritual time or way to perform Kegel exercises. While you will achieve the strongest contraction while lying down, some advantageous times to practice Kegels are while cooking, using your phone, brushing your teeth, standing in line at the store, or while watching TV (Kegel throughout the commercials). There are conflicting schools of thought regarding Kegel contractions when in a sitting position; I find this position a valuable variation because I spend so much time on the computer and the position targets the muscle tissue differently. Once your pattern is established, it will become second nature to spontaneously contract without thought. Even if additional treatments need to be used for POP, it is always a good idea to continue to practice Kegel exercises because they help prevent urine leakage and increase sexual sensation. Kegels can and should be practiced by all adult women-there is no such thing as being too young or too old to Kegel.

To locate the PC muscle in order to get familiar with Kegel contractions, you can insert one or two fingers (wash first please!) into the vagina, and squeeze your PC muscle until you can feel the contraction around your fingers. Another way to locate the PC muscle and get familiar with what you are trying to strengthen is to stop and restart the flow of urine a while urinating (once only please to recognize the sensation, do not stop/start the flow repetitively).

Individuals who want to take Kegeling to the next level can incorporate Kegel breathing into their daily ritual, or utilize a Kegel exercise tool. To Kegel breath, keep your belly relaxed as you breath in and as you let the air out contract your PC muscle and hold the contraction for as long as possible. This can be done any time throughout the day.

KEGEL ASSIST DEVICES

There are numerous devices available to help strengthen the PC muscle, including vaginal cones, ceramic eggs, and others. Some of these are devices are inserted vaginally and left in place for a specific period of time, others are designed to be inserted only while doing Kegel exercises. I've tried several types of Kegel assist devices over the past years and as a woman post-surgery, I've found the devices currently most user friendly for me are the type that are relatively compact and easily kept clean which makes them convenient for travel.

I use my Kegel assist device while standing up although most women should start off using them lying down. As you build up your PC muscle strength, you may be able to advance to a more upright position adding gravity resistance. When you feel you have reached a degree of PC strength lying down that you feel needs to be bumped up a notch, you may want to try a more advanced sitting position and then on to a standing position. PC strength will fluctuate from day to day. I can tell as soon as I insert the device if my PC muscle is strong enough to hold the device in without assistance from my hand. I do a series of 10 contractions holding each for a count of 10, plus 10 quick grab/release contractions. Doing multiple sets of Kegels may over-fatigue the pelvic floor. I stick to one set and focus on quality.

Women who have had multiple vaginal births or a single rough delivery may find the PC muscle so weak that it can barely contract at all. These devices, if used properly and consistently, truly can help recapture former PC muscle strength and integrity. PC muscle assist devices are extremely beneficial for treatment of many levels and types of POP. They can be used prior to surgery to optimize the tissue health. They can be used post-surgery to help rebuild and maintain tissue strength. They can be used in place of surgery for women in earlier stages of POP. They may be helpful for stress incontinence, urge incontinence, lack of vaginal tightness, or unsatisfactory orgasm.

Women who have a good understanding of their PC contraction may want to add a weighted Kegel device, which may provide the same benefit as you would get by adding hand held dumbbells to your upper body exercise routine. Creating weighted resistance will make your PC muscle work harder during contraction. Make sure you have good control and recognition of your PC muscle contraction prior to adding a Kegel device to your treatment path however. If you use Kegel tools before you are ready for them you will further weaken the muscle.

If you have a high grade of POP severity, you might not be able to do a Kegel contraction. A physical therapist can be very beneficial to assist women unable to identify a PC contraction. Once you can recognize the contraction sensation, repeat Kegel contractions whenever you think about it during the day. Make sure you are not confusing contracting your PC muscle with your abdominal, thigh, or butt muscles; remember the PC is the muscle that stops the flow of urine.

It is important to recognize that even if you have POP surgery, you should continue with Kegel exercises after you have healed up from surgery. These exercises will help maintain and possibly increase the PC muscle strength for continued support of your POP repair.

PESSARY

A pessary is a latex or silicone device similar to a contraceptive diaphragm that comes in many shapes and sizes; the most common style used is a ring pessary. The pessary is inserted into the vagina to support prolapsed organs. A pessary can decrease the symptoms of POP, be used temporarily to delay or avoid surgery, and may even help prevent POP from getting worse. Pessaries come in many different shapes and sizes, and should be fitted to the individual by a clinician. The particular type of pessary used will depend on the type(s) of prolapse and grade of severity; a ring pessary is the most commonly used type. A pessary may be recommended for women whose POP has not progressed to a grade 4 (the most severe level of POP), for women who want to be comfortable while they are waiting to have surgery, for women who are pregnant and need additional internal support, or for women who are not surgical candidates. Some women simply choose to not have surgery; a pessary may provide some beneficial internal structure along with external support garments. For additional information on pessaries, see the chapter, "The Pessary."

INCOSTRESS

Incostress is a reusable medical grade silicone device for treatment of urinary incontinence, the most common symptom of POP. Incostress provides internal support for the urethra, bladder neck, and pelvic floor; it is inserted vaginally and is reusable for 6 months after which time it should be replaced. It can be purchased without prescription and has received favorable reviews in UK clinical trials. A reusable apparatus, Incostress enables women to recapture control of their normal daily routine by removing the stress of worrying about leakage in public.

IMPRESSA

Impressa is a disposable, internal device designed for temporary control of stress urinary incontinence. While this non-absorbent, removal product is designed for incontinence, it may also have value for women in early stages of POP by providing internal support during activities that create pressure on the pelvic floor such as during exercising.

HORMONE REPLACEMENT THERAPY

Hormone replacement therapy (HRT) is an option for POP treatment in peri-menopausal and menopausal women. Hormone replacement can increase the estrogen level in the body which may reinforce the natural tissue integrity in the vaginal walls and pelvic floor. Hormone replacement may be of value in conjunction with other treatments. Although hormone replacement therapy alone will not be of huge benefit for women with advanced POP, it can be helpful for women experiencing low hormone levels who are in early stages of POP. Most women who have experienced or are in treatment of some types of cancer will not be able to utilize this treatment option, so it is important to make the clinician providing hormone therapy aware of previous or current cancer treatment.

Hormone replacement therapy can be provided with pills or hormone creams which are applied externally on various parts of the body such as the neck or chest, or inserted into the vagina. The cream preparations can help avoid many of the side effects caused by oral therapy. There are two kinds of hormone replacement therapy. The most commonly known hormone replacement therapy is traditional HRT which is manufactured synthetically by pharmaceutical companies. The other choice is bio-identical hormone replacement therapy, which is an exact replica of the hormones already in your body. You may have to search a bit for a physician who leans on the holistic side or is a naturopath to get a prescription for bio-identical hormone therapy. You can usually find a physician who provides natural hormone therapy by Googling bio-identical hormone replacement or by going to a local health food/vitamin store and asking who they recommend in the area. A good book to read on bio-identical hormone therapy is Natural Hormone Balance for Women by Dr. Uzzi Reiss, MD. It is not a good idea to randomly buy bio-identical hormone supplements over the internet. It is imperative to optimize hormone balance by having hormone levels monitored by a physician. Let your physician guide you on where to get bio-identicals in the correct strength to suit your body.

ELECTRICAL STIMULATION

Your physician or physical therapist may feel that electrical stimulation will be of benefit to improve POP. During electrical stimulation, a small probe is inserted into the vagina or electrodes are placed around the anus and a slight electrical current is applied to the tissues in these areas. A mild electrical impulse generates a contraction that can strengthen muscle fibers, allowing the PC muscle to once again regenerate the support needed for the organs and tissues in the area. Electrical stimulation can also fire nerves related to proper function of urge sensations. Women who have little sensation or muscle strength in their pelvic floor at times can't tell if they are contracting, making it nearly impossible to do a Kegel contraction properly or effectively. Electrical stimulation may improve sensation and the ability to contract.

There are also home versions of electrical stimulation available for purchase online without a prescription. There may be benefit to using these devices for long-term maintenance post-surgery or possibly for prevention of POP progression. There may additionally be value for women who have lost intimate sensation due to nerve damage related to childbirth or surgery.

BIOFEEDBACK

Biofeedback may be used to determine how well your pelvic floor muscles can contract, how well they relax post contraction, and how long you can sustain a contraction, all beneficial information to have prior to establishing a POP treatment plan. Biofeedback can be used in conjunction with other treatments to monitor improvement of the contractions of the PC muscle. A sensor will measure the contractions of the muscle tissue; it can then be determined if electric stimulation, Kegel exercises or other treatment modalities are improving the strength of the targeted muscles. ApexM is portable device available online with an inflatable probe that utilizes both electrical stimulation and biofeedback to strengthen a woman's pelvic floor.

TIBIAL NERVE STIMULATION

Posterior tibial nerve stimulation (PTNS) is a method of treatment worth exploring for incontinence. Research indicates an intimate connection between incontinence (both urinary and fecal) and the tibial nerve, a branch of the sciatic nerve. Treatments are typically once a week for a 12-week period to see if any improvement to urinary leakage occurs. Statistics vary by study, but indications are that 50-79.5% of women have a reduction in urinary incontinence of at least 50%. This treatment is also utilized with a surgically implanted nerve stimulator for fecal incontinence with some success.

MYOFASCIAL RELEASE THERAPY

Several years ago, I learned about myofascial release therapy (MFR) while participating in a local business meeting that included clinicians from multiple fields of practice. While the meeting had nothing to do with my personal healthcare, conversations that occurred included info share by a therapist who specializes in treating women's pelvic floor dysfunction with MFR. My curiosity led to me to explore more deeply to better understand the treatment, but also to share it with APOPS following. To say I was shocked at the difference in my capacity to contract my PC muscle post internal MFR treatment during my first exploration with this treatment is an understatement. I was equally shocked during my second MFR exploration at how many internal sore spots existed in my vaginal canal. Much gets lost in translation when describing MFR; you simply have to experience it to better understand the sensations that occur upon release of bunched up fascial tissue.

MFR can be a valuable tool for treating women's pelvic health issues. Whether exploring MFR as a non-surgical treatment, to maintain post-surgical pelvic health stability, or to level issues with the complex combination of a hypertonic pelvic floor and POP, this is a treatment worth educating yourself about. Following is a series of questions I asked the therapist who provided my most recent MFR treatments, Sarah Trunk PT, DPT.

What is the theory behind the John F. Barnes approach to Myofascial Release?
This approach takes into account the fact that our body is surrounded by and made up of fascia (our connective tissue which is similar to a 3-dimensional webbing). This

structure is full of collagen and weaves in and out of our entire body, head to toe, to provide support. *Trauma, surgical scars, and inflammation can cause our fascia to tighten up and solidify, placing up to 2,000 pounds of pressure per square inch on sensitive structures. Myofascial release gently releases the pressures this system exerts on our bodies, including our joints and organs, which can be life changing in improving our function.*

How does the John F. Barnes approach differ from other types of MFR?
John F. Barnes has been teaching this method for more than 40 years. His method has continued to be characterized by gentle hands-on soft tissue release with prolonged holding times of several minutes. Since that time, other approaches also deemed 'myofascial release' have arisen which often use a more aggressive pressure over a shorter time frame. Any massage therapist or physical therapist could tell you they practice 'myofascial release' which can be confusing as they are typically referring to many other styles of soft tissue mobilization. After practicing physical therapy for many years in various settings, I almost exclusively practice the John F. Barnes approach due to its gentle nature with much more effective and long-lasting results.

Explain MFR treatments for the pelvis:
Your practitioner will meet with you to take a thorough health history then begin an exam both externally and internally. It's important to assess and work both internally and externally to gently restore proper alignment to the pelvis and coccyx, and to decompress any areas of tension along the organs of the pelvis.

How can MFR be helpful as a non-surgical POP treatment?
Tightness in our fascial system can exert up to 2,000 pounds per square inch of pressure on various tissues and organs. These forces can push and/or pull the pelvic organs out of place. Gently releasing tight tissues throughout the lower abdomen, pelvis and even the thighs can help the organs return to their natural resting place and reduce or eliminate the pressure. For example, I've worked with several patients where I am able to feel the bladder ascending back where it belongs as we perform the gentle myofascial release work, hugely helpful with their urinary incontinence symptoms.

Are there any types of POP or degrees of POP severity in which MFR would be contraindicated?
Mild forms of POP are more easily treated than severe prolapses which have progressed quite significantly. I would recommend talking with your physician about this, especially with moderate to severe cases. In any instance, this type of therapy is extremely gentle and the risks are quite low.

How many MFR treatments or how soon after an MFR treatment will I experience symptom relief?
Most patients will notice some sort of change in their body with three sessions. Every person is different however; some may experience relief in a few sessions while with others it may take months. The severity of your symptoms and how much strength you have in your pelvic floor muscles will also be important factors. I would recommend asking this question of your therapist after the first session once they have evaluated your condition and can give you a more exact idea. It's a great idea to work with a John Barnes' myofascial release therapist who is also a physical

therapist, as they will be able to address strengthening with you as well.

Can MFR help with both POP pain and pressure?
Yes, the extreme amount of pressure exerted by the fascial system on nerves, organs and other structures in the pelvis can cause significant feelings of pain and pressure in our bodies. Gently releasing this 'vice grip' of the fascial system can provide significant relief.

Is MFR beneficial for women for long term maintenance post POP surgery?
In recovering from surgery, it's important to first regain the strength of your pelvic floor and abdominals. Following this, myofascial release can be especially helpful as well to gently balance the pelvis and the contents within. You will want to get your physician's approval to start physical therapy and/or MFR after surgery, often 6-8 weeks following. Long term after surgery, it's important for you to know your body and what feels normal to you. Physical therapy and myofascial release can be wonderful tools to utilize as needed to keep you functioning optimally as the years go on.

PELVIC FLOOR AND CORE EXERCISE PROGRAMS

All women should attempt to optimize pelvic floor health. It's beneficial to women prior to pregnancy; a healthy pelvic floor translates to an easier delivery and speedier recovery. It's beneficial for women post-partum to recover former pelvic floor muscle tone to prevent POP from progressing. It's beneficial to women post hysterectomy and POP surgery to maintain the benefit of repairs. As women, we must recognize the value in pulling the belly button "in and up" and contracting the pelvic floor randomly throughout the day every day. Pelvic floor and core maintenance is essential much like brushing your teeth is for good oral health- daily attention is key.

There are many exercise regimens available for pelvic floor strengthening. An exercise regimen is only beneficial if it is one you will continue to utilize. Some women prefer a condensed program because they have little free time; others prefer a diverse, detailed format. What worked for me was taking the specific exercises that worked well for my body from different programs and adding them to the exercise routine I already had in place. It is truly a matter of personal choice. Pay attention to the impact a regimen has on all areas of your body rather than just the pelvic floor; if you feel a program is causing pain or problems in areas of your body, it probably is. Back or knee pain are indicators that the program might not be appropriate for you. The same can be said for programs or particular core or floor exercises that generate vaginal or rectal pressure.

The exercise program I feel is most beneficial is Hab-it. Hab-it is a pelvic floor strengthening program developed by physical therapist Tasha Mulligan, a triathlete who experienced pelvic floor weakness after giving birth. This program focuses on both pelvic floor and core muscle strengthening. Hab-it has multiple workouts to choose from and is based on physical therapy treatment for pelvic floor disorders.

URETHRAL BULKING AGENTS

Bulking agents can be injected into the wall of the urethra to reduce the space and decrease urinary incontinence. This outpatient treatment is best suited for women who have a urethra that is weak but has good support. Women who have a weak urethra or poorly supported urethra are less suitable for this procedure.

Additionally, although this procedure is a quick one (only takes a few minutes), the results typically last 6 months to 2 years and then have to be repeated. If considering this procedure, request specific details from your clinician about how many of the procedures he/she has performed, what the success rate is, whether urine retention may occur and if so, for how long, and if there may be an allergic response to the materials used.

SUPPORT GARMENTS

Support garments are often beneficial for women who are experiencing discomfort with POP; supporting your core from the outside may relieve the pain on the inside. Women with POP who have occupations which require being on their feet all day often have considerable pain or discomfort. POP support garments are girdle like undergarments that have 'V' shaped support bands to push organs and tissues upward. These support garments are much more comfortable and attractive than old style girdles used to be. Most of them are adjustable in support and can be washed like other undergarments. While support garments developed specifically for POP can be purchased online, it is a good idea to first purchase them locally in local lingerie departments to determine if you can tolerate the pressure on your abdomen; some women find abdominal pressure uncomfortable. It is of value to experiment with a department store support garment to see if it helps prior to purchasing the more expensive online versions which can be located with a search engine for pelvic organ prolapse + support garments.

Support garments may provide comfort for women who are suffering from back pain, urinary frequency, abdominal strain, and that "falling out" feeling while they are waiting for surgery. They also are beneficial for women who choose to not have corrective surgery for more advanced POP. To use a support garment, wash your hands, lay on the bed or other flat surface, and gently push protruding tissues back inside. While still lying down, slip the support garment on. The compression provided by the support garment may help contain tissues inside the pelvic cavity until the garment is removed.

LASER AND RADIO FREQUENCY VAGINAL TISSUE RESTORATION THERAPY

The most recent non-surgical treatment generating buzz for pelvic organ prolapse (POP) is vaginal tissue restoration (VTR) therapy. Both radio frequency and laser treatments have become available in the US (these treatments have been studied in Europe since 2008), and both research and patient feedback are extremely positive. While developed for incontinence and atrophy, these treatments may additionally have value for overactive bladder (OAB) atrophy related pain with intimacy, urinary tract infections (UTI), or loss of intimate sensation. These devices are not FDA approved for additional uses at this time, but patient feedback pretty much tells us what we need to know about the extra value these treatments may provide. VTR therapy is available in 2 forms, laser and radio frequency.

VTR therapy may be of value to address symptoms of pelvic organ prolapse. Radio frequency projects heat deep into tissues, improving tissue structural integrity; laser treatment makes microscopic perforations in vaginal tissue, generating a wound/healing process. VTR therapy strengthens mucosal tissues (both vaginal and rectal) by stimulating production of collagen and elastin, important connective structural tissues in the pelvic cavity. Documented benefits are a reduction in incontinence (stress, urge, and overactive bladder urinary incontinence, and possibly some benefit for fecal incontinence), and reduced vaginal atrophy (dried vaginal tissues). Additional benefits that may occur are a tightening of the vaginal space (less vaginal space could translate to better organ support), and increased intimate sensation. Research additionally indicates a tightening of sagging labia lip tissue for those interested in the aesthetic value.

Studies are in progress by companies who provide these treatment devices; there will be considerably more validated research over the next several years. Insurance currently does not cover them and will not until additional research validates their value, so treatment can be cost-prohibitive. VTR therapy is not of value for uterine prolapse, enterocele, or vaginal vault prolapse.

Women of childbearing age should have a negative pregnancy test prior to receiving VTR therapy, as well as a normal PAP smear for the prior few years and a recent pelvic exam. Currently there are more dermatologists and plastic surgeons than gynecologists providing these procedures in the US; women with POP should locate a gynecologist or a POP specialist (FPMRS) or gynecologist to provide VTR therapy if possible because multiple women's pelvic and vaginal health conditions can occur simultaneously that non-gynecologic clinicians might not recognize. Safety first!

Treatments typically take place every 4-6 weeks for the series of three treatments in year one, followed by annual maintenance. Information women should share with clinicians prior to VTR therapy is IUD use, implanted Interstim device, herpes or other sexually transmitted conditions, implanted mesh (treatments can be provided to mesh patients, but until research validates laser use is appropriate for mesh patients, I recommend that group of women explore radio frequency), mesh complications, chronic vaginal or pelvic pain, or pregnancy. Fully inform your clinician of any/all of these aspects of impact to vaginal tissue balance.

Menopause is the second leading cause of POP; VTR therapy may provide a beneficial alternative to hormone treatment in women who have had cancer and can't utilize hormone therapy. Treatments are typically avoided in women actively under-going treatment for cancer, but may be used in women post cancer treatment.

As a women's pelvic health advocate, I'd be failing in my responsibilities if I didn't explore new avenues of treatment available for POP. That being said, as a woman very pro-active with my health, particularly pelvic health, I am extremely cognizant of shifts in my body. While I for the most part do the right stuff regarding my pelvic health, my body gets a bit sassy from time to time. I'm as human as anyone else-upon occasion I slip up. I'd noticed a bit of advancing atrophy. Despite having effectively balanced my hormones with prescribed bio-identicals for 20 years, I was a bit disillusioned that I couldn't seem to get the atrophy under control despite modifying my regimen. Time for the big guns-I decided to explore VTR therapy myself to better understand the treatment and share insights.

I reviewed multiple vaginal tissue restoration research papers and engaged in conversations with a few companies that provide these services. To say I wanted more information is an understatement. I had the opportunity as a patient advocate to question a patient immediately following a training session which made me all the more intrigued. I went on the table to experiment with radio frequency VTR therapy up close and personal. Nothing like playing guinea pig to better find out exactly what the treatment is like and how effective it can be. I met with Jill Wohlfeil, MD, to better understand the radio frequency procedure I would receive from her clinic. Sharon De Vries, PA, who administered my radio frequency treatments, also provided valuable insights. The following information is a blend of feedback provided by several VTR therapy gynecologic and urogynecologic clinicians regarding both types of procedures, in response to questions I asked during in-depth discussions.

Who can provide ThermiVa treatments?
While many in plastic surgery and aesthetics are advancing their knowledge and skillset in vaginal restoration procedures, it makes sense for women with pelvic organ prolapse to locate a gynecologist or other clinician who specializes in women's pelvic health to provide this procedure if possible. POP is complicated and you want someone who is very familiar with female anatomy providing these kinds of pelvic procedures - whether radio frequency or laser. Multiple conditions can exist at the

same time in a woman's pelvic zone.

How do these treatments work?
Heat is the source of these treatments; radio frequency generates heat, fractional laser therapy in which thousands of tiny, deep perforations are made in tissue is the alternate option. These kinds of treatments stimulate collagen and elastin production which strengthens tissues in the vaginal canal. Explore how many treatments your clinician has done-you want someone with experience); too much heat in one area during a laser procedure may cause blistering-this can cause some temporary discomfort. However, both treatment types are considered very safe procedures.

What do the treatments cost?
Cost varies significantly from clinician to clinician with both of these procedures, from a few hundred dollars per procedure to a few thousand. The individual medical practice sets the price; it tends to be more expensive on the coasts than in the Midwest.

What if I've had mesh surgery?
Use of laser in women who have mesh, IUD, any kind of internal devices is not validated by research at this stage. Radio frequency generates less heat, which may be more appropriate for use in women with mesh. As always, take your questions to your consultation and reveal all devices and procedures you've had to your clinician for the best outcome.

Can these treatments be of value for conditions beyond pelvic organ prolapse or incontinence?
These treatments may be worth exploring for treatment of Lichen Schlerosis and Ehlers-Danlos Syndrome (EDS).

There aren't completed studies in the US at this time for these conditions, but they have been minimally explored in Europe and show promise. It will take time to capture data.

Will I need more than one treatment?
Both laser and radio frequency treatments require three treatments the first year, with an annual treatment suggested after that to maintain. Women may be happy with results after the first treatment and cancel the others-not a good idea for long term value. There will be swelling from first treatment which can simulate success, but it takes 3 treatments to properly jump-start collagen building process, which is what brings results that continue over the next year related to the symptom(s) being treated. Long term results are currently unknown and are believed to start to fade about a year post treatment, thus the annual reboot.

Do I need to continue my core/floor exercises if I have a vaginal restoration procedure?
It is important that women recognize engaging in additional forms of maintenance (pelvic floor and core strengthening) prior to and post treatments will bring them the greatest value in achieving and maintaining results. It is important to remain proactive with pelvic health, whether utilizing non-surgical or surgical treatments.

Will results be different for a woman in her 40's than a woman in her 60s?
Results are reported to be similar regardless the age of a woman, however length of time to achieve these results during active treatment may vary a bit. Success is based on patient feedback; results are related to quality of life impact. There is no standardized test analyzing vaginal

tissue post procedure. If the patient recognizes she has less incontinence, or discomfort from atrophy, or sensation is increased, the procedure has done what it is supposed to do. Impact to a patient's quality of life is the target.

Do I need to have any tests prior to the treatment?
A pelvic exam is required prior to the procedure to ensure an undiagnosed condition or health concern does not exist; it can be provided by your gynecologist or primary health clinician. On site treatment evaluation should also include info about other pelvic surgeries you've had which may cause concerns regarding whether the procedure can move forward (for example, complications from hysterectomy or bowel resection that may cause organ shift or have created excessive scar tissue, or the patient has considerable undiagnosed pain). It may be necessary to go through other treatments such as estrogen therapy or dilators to balance your pelvic tissues prior to moving forward with vaginal restoration. These treatments are not a miracle cure to fix all vaginal health conditions.

Will these treatments fix failed POP surgery?
Vaginal restoration procedures will not address prior POP surgical failure related to incompetent surgeon or complications beyond the surgeons control. These procedures may have some value related to longer success of mesh free surgeries, or age/menopause related vaginal health concerns, but research lags beyond atrophy and incontinence value. Multiple aspects of these procedures are uncertain because women have multiple lifestyle, behavioral, and coexisting condition causal factors.

Will there be any discomfort with my procedure?
Typically, there is very little discomfort, if any. Some

*women may experience warmth or redness, and some
women may have a little vaginal discharge or bleeding
after a treatment.*

Do I need to completely shave my pubic area before
treatment?
*We recommend shaving or closely trim the hair in the pubic
area; this is for better contact with the skin to achieve
therapeutic temperatures.*

I shared information about my personal exploration with radio
frequency from November 2016 through January 2017 via
LinkedIn and other social media. Here's an instant replay:

VAGINAL RESTORATION FOR POP: ROUND ONE

Heading into a medical procedure you've not previously
experienced can be a bit nerve wracking, I don't care who you are
or what your area of expertise is. There is no such thing as a
worry-free procedure with first-time health treatments. As a pelvic
organ prolapse advocate, I intersect with clinicians daily, have
witnessed some relatively invasive procedures, and have watched
more than my fair share of surgical videos. But being the body on
the table…let's just say the analytical brain takes the day off and
anxiety comes up a tad. Did I have concerns about having a radio-
frequency vaginal procedure - absolutely! Vaginal procedures in
general raise anxiety for most women no matter what concern is
being addressed or what procedure is being utilized. There's
something about being naked from the waist down with legs spread
wide and people or machines poking at your nether regions that
brings out the angst in the strongest of us.

To clarify my backdrop, in 2008 I had transvaginal mesh repair
for rectocele and cystocele, along with a mesh free enterocele
repair. Over the years, I'd noticed symptoms I was not sure were

related to a return of POP or to the aging process. An appointment with my FPMRS urogynecologist the summer of 2015 confirmed that my repairs were all intact, no mesh erosion, all was well in that camp. That undoubtedly meant symptoms I was noticing were related to the aging process. As a POP advocate, rest assured I do the right stuff most of the time regarding floor and core exercises, body stature, and diet. But despite daily efforts, I didn't feel being pro-active was turning out as successful at maintaining pelvic health as I wanted, based on symptoms I was experiencing.

In line of duty, I explore POP avenues and read research nearly every day, so I was very excited when I first learned about new vaginal restoration POP treatments that improve symptoms without cutting into the abdominal cavity. These procedures are currently becoming more popular to address some of the symptoms of pelvic organ prolapse (they have been explored in Europe since 2008), enabling women to postpone or avoid surgery. After a year of exploration into research and brain-picking several clinicians and industry reps about radio-frequency and laser vaginal restorative treatments, I was happy to have an opportunity to experience radio-frequency vaginal restoration up close and personal. My curiosity was specifically related to the value of these treatments as a long-term post maintenance tool after POP surgical procedures. Neither POP surgery nor non-surgical treatment will *prevent* the aging of vaginal and pelvic tissues.

On the morning of my first of three radio-frequency procedures, I shared with a friend that I was a bit anxious. I was of course concerned that despite being told and reading in multiple studies that these procedures are not painful, that mine would be. Radio frequency produces heat to generate collagen and elastin production, while laser treatment causes microscopic punctures in vaginal tissue, stimulating the same result. I totally freak out about needle stuff, no matter if it is a simple blood test or pin prick - I'm a needle wienie - so was thrilled upon exploration to discover that both types of vaginal procedures were supposed to be painless and needle free. I'd been in the room when a woman had radio frequency treatment, and she didn't even bat an eyelash.

Beyond pain, other treatment concerns I was anxious about were similar to those women with pelvic organ prolapse worry about, the issues that come with aging. Am I going to leak gas when someone is poking around down there? Will my shaven pubic patch look as ridiculous to the clinician as it does to me and make her laugh? What if I experience spillage? Will I be clean enough? I don't care where you hail from or what your background is, these are concerns that most women experience in like circumstances. To compound my anxiety, there would be a clinician audience observing, learning the procedure. I wasn't concerned about being a model to educate clinicians, but was a bit nervous not knowing if they would be male or female. A male gyne working down below is one thing, a room full of them looking - yikes, even though they see female anatomy every day. On my way to the clinic, I felt naked despite being fully clothed, and envisioned a room full of clinicians chuckling to themselves about my pubic haircut. Obviously it did not occur; in this arena, clinicians see every pubic hair style, piercing, and tattoo you could possibly imagine-my look was hardly radical.

On the day of procedure, the treatment itself very comfortable on the inside, but did get uncomfortably warm in a couple of spots on external labial tissues. As soon as I informed the physician assistant providing my treatment that I was feeling uncomfortable (my procedure took place at a gynecologist's office) she added more gel, and I was again comfortable. The PA and I chatted comfortably throughout the procedure. I left the office with vulva red and a bit swollen, but with no discomfort whatsoever.

The day after the procedure I recognized relatively quickly that I needed to urinate less frequently. To say I was intrigued is a bit of an understatement. I was not expecting this kind of result to manifest so quickly. I am not usually placebo impacted, but I had to wonder if this treatment was working well for me because I wanted it to after listening to difficulties women deal with all day every day, ever hopeful better POP treatments will come along.

Two days' post-procedure, my overactive bladder (OAB) was gone-completely eliminated. Let me express that I did not realize I had OAB, likely because running to the bathroom 97 times a day was my normal. The next day I noticed that I'd only had to get up once in the middle of the night prior to urinate, and in days to follow my overnight pattern became urination once between 4 to 6 hours after I went to bed, depending on how much water I drank before bedtime. This little perk alone had me doing cartwheels. Labial tissues returned to their normal color as well and swelling subsided.

At five days, I noticed there was no fecal "residue" when defecating (no need to wipe and wipe and wipe to get clean), stool was more formed instead of my usual gravel shaped stress stool, and I absolutely noticed less rectal pressure. I no longer needed to run to the bathroom when urge hit whether for urination or defecation, I could take my time getting there. I also noticed less gas buildup.

At eight days, I absolutely noticed more vaginal moisture. In the past six months, I'd been experiencing advancing atrophy despite having balanced my hormones for over 20 years with bio-identical hormones. My external tissues would become very irritated by soap when I showered - this was no longer an issue after radio-frequency.

I had no interest in these treatments from the aesthetic angle; I'm perfectly comfortable with the way my bottom end presents (as opposed to my neck skin sag…geez don't get me started on that).

Over the course of the month, the positive effects of my first treatment waned, as I was told and read in research would occur if I completed one treatment only. Three treatments are recommended for both radio frequency and laser vaginal restoration, with annual renewal for continued most effective benefit. I am currently two weeks post my second treatment, and the benefits I received from the first returned. I am pleased to share my experience.

- Elimination of overactive bladder (urinary urge and frequency).
- Radical reduction in overnight urination to one time.
- Radical reduction in fecal urge and need to get to bathroom immediately.
- Elimination of rectal pressure.
- Radical improvement in atrophy.
- Reduction in gas, better able to control passing gas.
- Reduction in fecal residue when wiping.
- Better formed stool.
- Urine stream radically stronger.
- More normal and regular bowel movements.

The one symptom I was hoping would be improved that I have not noticed much change in is intimate sensation. I've read reports of women becoming multi-orgasmic (who doesn't want that, sign me up!), and over the years I've noticed a reduction in sensation which may or may not be related to surgical scar tissue/adhesions or possibly nerve damage from childbirth. I'm obviously thrilled at the other symptoms that have improved however, the outcome without a doubt being significantly improved quality of life.

I give these treatments a big thumb's up. Based on what I experienced, the improved internal tissue support normalized multiple body functions. My continuing journey has never been about how I look down below, it's about how I feel down below. When we feel healthy, we stand a little taller, walk a little prouder. We clearly need additional research to better understand the value as well as spark approval by Medicare, enabling the cascade to insurance coverage so more women can have access. Once in a blue moon a treatment gives me hope-file VTR therapy under that category. There is zero doubt in my mind, VTR therapy is a valuable treatment to improve POP symptoms and restore quality of life.

~ 8 ~
THE PESSARY

POPS Patient Perspective: "*I have seen four urogynaecologists. This forum has been more informative. I wouldn't have gotten a diagnosis without knowing the information that I was offered here. There seems to be no support elsewhere.*"
~MO, Australia

P rior to being diagnosed with pelvic organ prolapse, I had never even heard of a pessary. Once again, I was amazed that despite researching various women's health issues, asking questions when something cropped up that I didn't understand, and openly discussing health topics with my clinicians, I had not only never heard of pelvic organ prolapse, but I'd also never heard of a pessary. I wondered how I could be so in the dark, it's not like I live in a cave.

Prolapse can present in many ways. Sometimes it is easiest when it occurs suddenly; then the patient sees it, feels it and they know that something is not right! More often though, prolapse creeps up on us. Something feels different, there might be discomfort, or pressure, or a change in bladder or bowel function, but it's not clear what is happening.
~Katherine Stevenson, MD

While I started gathering survey data to capture insights on whether women I knew had heard of pelvic organ prolapse, I also regularly asked women I engaged in casual conversation if they had ever heard of a pessary. I pretty much discovered that the two subjects went hand in hand, those who knew about POP, knew about pessaries; those that hadn't heard of POP, were not familiar with pessaries.

A pessary is a device that can be inserted into the vagina to provide support for a woman's pelvic organs. These man-made devices have Latin and Greek origins, and the mechanical devices from ancient times are very unlike like the modern versions. The first pessaries were tampon-like devices, similar to a ball of wool or lint soaked in drugs. Hippocrates was a bit more creative and utilized natural items close at hand, such as pomegranates. The pessaries currently in use are made of plastic, silicone, or medical grade rubber. (If you intend to use a pessary, it is important to inform your physician about latex allergies.) Silicone pessaries have the advantage of being non-allergic, they do not absorb secretions or odors, stay pliable and soft, and retain their integrity after repeated cleanings.

A pessary is a conservative means of controlling the symptoms of POP and is one of several non-surgical tools that can be especially beneficial in the early stages of POP, although different types can be used with any stage. Pessaries can help reduce urinary incontinence, back pain, abdominal pain, vaginal or rectal pressure, and vaginal tissue bulge.

A pessary can also be a beneficial tool to prevent progression of early stage POP. Some of the reasons for using a pessary are:
• Maintenance while waiting for a surgical repair.
• Surgical delay for financial reasons, lack of childcare assistance, work conflicts, waiting for health insurance deductible to be reached, etc.
• Guidance on whether to proceed with surgery.
• When there is high risk of surgical complications because of advanced age, medical co-morbidities, etc.
• To help control incontinence during fitness activities.

Some women prefer to avoid surgery and a pessary will address invasive POP symptoms. Sometimes a pessary is used prior to surgery to determine if surgery will bring relief of symptoms that do not match the physical findings, such as severe pain with mild prolapse which may in reality be pain caused by something besides POP. It is relatively common for women who start POP treatment utilizing a pessary to eventually shift to surgical resolution. We live in an extremely active society, and although pessaries are relatively easy to use, the more maintenance free we become, the less complicated our lives are.

The type of pessary used for prolapse treatment will depend on the type and degree of POP. The most commonly used pessaries are ring shaped. Similar to a diaphragm, holes allow secretions to pass through since the pessary may be left in place for extended periods of time. There are also many other types of pessaries, very specific to different types and degrees of prolapse as well as other medical conditions. Pessaries can be divided into two categories, support and space filling. Support pessaries are typically used for stage II and III POP; while a space-filling pessary is more typically used for stage IV prolapse.

Women come in all shapes and sizes, and their internal organs and tissues are no different. Pessaries need to be fitted to the individual woman. If a pessary is too small, it will not provide adequate support or it may pop out. If it is too large it will be uncomfortable. You may need to try a few different sizes or types of pessaries in your physician's office before you find one with the correct fit that feels comfortable and stays in place. For the fitting itself, your physician will initially insert a pessary based on what the type and size he/she thinks you may need. You will be asked to squat, sit, walk around, cough, and bear down to see if the pessary is the correct fit for you. Do no hesitate to let your physician know if the pessary feels uncomfortable or causes pain, even if it is the second, third, or fourth pessary tried; it is important to get the correct pessary so you can continue to use it comfortably. When a pessary fits correctly, you should not be able to feel it, much like a tampon. Pessaries that do not fit properly will either not adequately support or will cause tissue irritation as well as possible tissue erosion.

Once you and your physician find the appropriate fit for your needs, you will be asked to make a follow up appointment within a few days to a month so your physician can check to see if it still feels ok and to make sure it is not creating any irritations, allergic reactions, or pressure sores. If prior to your appointment you experience tissue irritation, vaginal discharge, pain, if the pessary pops out, if you can't empty your bladder, if bleeding occurs, or if the pessary you have been given no longer feels "right", contact your physician's office immediately to have the pessary checked as you may either need a different size or different type of pessary. Do not wait for your follow up appointment if this occurs, do it right away or the irritation will progress and you may have to go without pessary use until the tissues in the area heal up. The most common complaint with pessary use is discomfort. If this occurs, contact your physician's office right away.

Some pessaries can be inserted, removed, cleaned, and reinserted by the patient themselves, others must be maintained by the clinician. I highly recommend that your physician instruct you how to insert and remove your pessary if at all possible. It will enable you to be pro-active in controlling prolapse. It will also make it easier for you to decide whether you will be able to tolerate using a pessary long term, or if you will want surgery for a more permanent fix.

Your physician will teach you how to insert and remove your pessary while you are being fitted. It takes a bit of practice to get comfortable using a pessary, similar to the learning curve necessary to get comfortable with contact lenses for vision correction. In the beginning, it seems to take forever to get them inserted and feel comfortable, but in a very short time, the insertion and removal process goes quickly.

It is important to follow your physician's instructions in regard to the care of your pessary. Some may be worn for days to weeks at a time, but from personal experience I recommend taking the pessary out nightly, cleaning it with soap and water, then reinserting it in the morning. Leaving a pessary in 24 hours a day increases risk of tissue erosion.

Some women may not be comfortable with the idea of inserting their own pessary; others simply don't want to be bothered. If this is the case, let your physician know at your fitting, as this may impact the type of pessary he/she chooses for you. If you won't be removing your own pessary, your clinician will need to remove it for cleaning minimally once every three months. At that time, your clinician can also check for any ulcerations or irritations.

There is a possibility that you may need to use a vaginal estrogen cream to prevent erosions of the vaginal tissues from the pressure of your pessary against vaginal tissues. Even though the pessary is an extremely safe device to use, it is still a foreign object in your body. If a pessary does not fit properly or does not get removed and cleaned regularly, it may cause irritation to the vaginal walls and ulcers may occur. If this happens, the pessary will need to be removed until the sores are healed. Under these circumstances, the use of a vaginal estrogen cream will facilitate the healing process.

If you notice a foul-smelling discharge, the vaginal acid balance needs to be restored. An acidic vaginal gel such as Trimo-San will reduce vaginal irritation and odor. Women who are post-menopausal whose vaginal tissues are thinner and dryer may need to use both an estrogen cream and the acidic vaginal gel.

There are a few contraindications for using a pessary. Some women will have more problems than others with infections or irritations of the vaginal tissues. Women who suffer from pelvic inflammatory disease will not be able to use a pessary. Women who are not willing or are unable to perform the necessary maintenance, whether doing the maintenance themselves or having it done at the physician's office, are not good candidates for a pessary. Women not willing or able to get to the physician's office for routine checkups should also not use one. Women who have an allergy to latex may have problems with an allergic reaction to a pessary. Women with advanced POP that have persistent or extensive vaginal erosions will be unable to use one. Occasionally, the vagina and its outlet are so dilated (enlarged) that the pessary will not stay in position.

The following are additional tips that may be helpful to know about the use of a pessary:

- Sexual intercourse is possible with certain kinds of pessaries in place. Check with your physician to see if the pessary you will be using will interfere and need to be re-moved prior to intercourse. Some women find it uncomfortable to have sex with their pessary in. Some men find it enhances sensation for them, while others find it uncomfortable. If you have a pessary that can be left in during intercourse, you will have to experiment to see how it will work for you as a couple.

- A pessary can be "pushed out" when you bear down to have a bowel movement. It is helpful to "bridge" the labia (the vaginal lips) with your fingers while pushing down to pass bowel movement.

- The vagina is a closed pocket, the pessary can *not* shift or get lost anywhere else inside of the body. It can pop out of the vagina if it is too small or if you bear down to have a bowel movement. If it pops out without bearing down, contact your physician, as you probably need a different size or type.

- A pessary will not set off a metal detector at an airport, but there may be metal components in some of them so they may need to be removed prior to an x-ray or MRI scan.

- A pessary may need to be occasionally resized with weight gain or loss. A pessary will typically last two to three years before needing to be replaced.

- Some patients who use pessaries over an extended period may find it necessary to switch to a smaller pessary. There is some evidence to indicate that POP status may improve over time with extended pessary use.

• Pessaries may be beneficial for elderly patients with POP who are not candidates for surgery because of compromised health; these women will need to go to their physicians to have the pessary inserted, cleaned or removed.

• Patients that can't be fitted for a pessary, feel uncomfortable with a pessary in, or have problems with a pessary popping out are potential candidates for surgery.

• Women with severe POP that are advised against having surgery or who don't want to go through surgery may be able to use two ring pessaries together for additional support.

Pessaries play an important role in POP treatment for temporary control of symptoms and for permanent use in those women who can not or do not want to have surgery. No matter what or stage of POP you have, there is a strong possibility that at some point you will be introduced to the use of a pessary.

~ 9 ~
# SURGERY

POPS Patient Perspective: "*I and my husband, are amazed
that so little importance is placed on rehabilitation after
childbirth in the UK and the US. Our physical and mental
health, the success of our relationships and the happiness of
our families are all dependent on this.*
~SC, UK

Studies indicate that 1 in 5 women will have surgery to repair
POP at some point in their lifetime. As POP awareness goes
mainstream, and women recognize symptoms and request
screening, this figure will undoubtedly increase considerably. As
the extent of prolapse progresses to the point of continuous discomfort or pain, women may consider more aggressive treatment
measures to recapture quality of life. Women who hesitate to have
surgery and utilize non-surgical treatments but can no longer
tolerate classic symptoms including vaginal tissue bulge, urinary or
fecal incontinence, urine retention, chronic constipation, pelvic or
back pressure or pain, vaginal or rectal pressure, pain with
intercourse, lack of sexual sensation, or vaginal ulcerations from
pessary use, have one additional treatment option-surgical repair.
Women who are extremely active may choose to have surgery
relatively quickly after diagnosis; they simply can't tolerate the
negative impact POP symptoms have on their lives.

*Sherrie Palm has written a beautiful chapter which
discusses some of the hardest decisions a woman will have
to make about her body. Addressing the need for vaginal
surgery, she has sensitively outlined the options and
approaches that an informed patient should take. This is
must read for anyone considering surgery.*
~Alan Garely, MD

POP surgery can improve the anatomical position and function of the pelvic organs, but more importantly, it can improve the quality of life for women who have been in pain or discomfort, or embarrassed to go out in public for fear of having an "accident". It can reconnect women with their sexuality once they have allowed sufficient time for post-surgical healing.

The pelvic cavity is an extremely intricate interrelated arrangement of organs, muscles, nerves, and structural tissue. Many surgeons address specific types of POP, but if a non-specializing surgeon is repairing a cystocele and finds a rectocele or other type of POP during surgery, will it be repaired, or if it is will it be repaired in the best way possible? It is important that the physician who performs your POP surgery is a specialist to ensure the best outcome. The potential for mesh and other types of complications is very real when proper surgical technique is not utilized. A FPMRS urogynecologist or urologist can address all POP issues, providing a 'one-stop-shop'. This does not mean other types of physicians are not qualified surgeons; you simply want to utilize the most qualified specialist for POP, an extremely complex, diverse condition.

During the period between 2007 through 2011, mesh was repeatedly utilized for POP surgical repairs by surgeons not specialty trained in pelvic organ prolapse, resulting in transvaginal mesh complications. Multiple stakeholders gathered in September 2011 for the Food and Drug Administration (FDA) Obstetrics and Gynecology Devices Panel meeting to discuss and determine which surgeons should use transvaginal mesh, as well as to develop appropriate guidelines. In the interests of achieving the most positive surgical outcome, ask your surgeon if he/she is specialty trained to provide mesh procedures prior to agreeing to surgery that includes mesh.

One third of POP patients require additional prolapse surgeries for a variety of reasons. A non-specialist may not recognize prolapses occurring in additional compartments beyond those displaying distinct symptoms; frequently two or more types of POP occur at the same time. Native tissue repairs (repairs stitching your own tissues rather than using mesh) may fail in 1-5 years, requiring repeat surgery. Patients who are extremely active may not modify their behaviors or utilize pelvic floor strengthening techniques or devices to maintain their native tissue repairs long term. Women may return to lifting heavy weight such as picking up their children too soon after surgery, vacuuming, or exercising too soon post POP repair. What occurs post-surgery has a significant impact on long term surgical results.

The uterus may be removed during POP repair if the uterus if it is significantly prolapsed, and there is no interest in having additional children. Undergoing a hysterectomy however, may predispose you to other types of prolapse. The removal of the uterus creates an empty space within the abdominal cavity that other organs - particularly the small intestine - can occupy. Vaginal vault prolapse (the vagina caves in on itself) is a possibility as well if the top of the vagina is not properly anchored during hysterectomy. Like all types of POP, this too can be corrected, but it is important to discuss the possibility of this occurring if your surgeon plans on providing a hysterectomy to address uterine prolapse. If your gynecologist is providing the hysterectomy, inquire whether steps will be taken to secure the top of the vagina to prevent vaginal vault prolapse.

Some women feel a sense of loss when their uterus is removed. Other women are thrilled to not have to deal with having a period anymore. For those women who hesitate to "give up their uterus", it would be practical to discuss your concerns with your physician or seek counsel on this concern prior to deciding whether to have a hysterectomy as part of your POP repair, to assure you are making the best decision for your needs. Uterus preserving procedures for uterine prolapse are becoming more commonly practiced in the field of urogynecology.

Women are typically informed that POP surgical recovery time is 6-12 weeks. Plan on 12 weeks; while women with less aggressive stages of POP may feel better at 6 weeks, but assuming you'll be ready to rock at 6 weeks is a mistake. Often as we heal and become more active, inflammation can reoccur, generating significant pressure sensations. Many women fear POP has returned, when it is simply the body telling you to slow down.

POP surgeries may be vaginal, abdominal, or laparoscopic (which often utilizes robotic technology). The type of procedure provided will vary by surgeon; it is in your best interest to inquire about the type of procedure being utilized for your repair. Ask your surgeon to explain any questions you have about your procedure. A list of potential questions is available on the APOPS website, including how much experience your physician has performing your procedure. Being an informed patient is in your best interest: www.pelvicorganprolapsesupport.org/pop-questions-to-ask-your-physician.

Colpocleisis is a surgical procedure available for women who no longer have a desire or interest in engaging in sexual intercourse. In this procedure; the vaginal opening is literally sealed off, with a small opening to enable secretions to escape. Some women are medically fragile and cannot tolerate POP surgery, and may find this procedure the easiest to recover from. Other women choose to have this procedure because they recognize that the vagina is not the core of their sexuality, the brain is, and understand that this procedure may eliminate their discomfort and improve their quality of life in multiple ways beyond being able to engage in intercourse. Intimacy and sexuality can be expressed in many alternative ways. Upon healing, women having colpocleisis can resume a full life in every respect excluding the ability to have intercourse.

Colpocleisis can be performed using general, regional (spinal or epidural), or local anesthetic. The cure rate for uterine prolapse or vaginal vault prolapse with this procedure is 90-95%. For the woman who has no interest or desire for intercourse and who is experiencing pain and discomfort from POP symptoms, or for the woman secure in her sexuality who recognizes that she can still maintain her sense of sexual self without the use of her vagina, this is an option to consider. It bears repeating, that this procedure will permanently close the vagina. It will no longer be possible to have vaginal intercourse after this surgery.

Throughout my journey, I have been continually amazed by the deeply personal stories women have shared with me; to say I am grateful is an understatement. One of those women approached me about her journey with colpocleisis. Typically considered a treatment for women who are no longer sexually active and who have significant health as well as pronounced prolapse issues, K, a forward-thinking woman, opened my mind to the potential for copocleisis to be utilized by women beyond traditional reasons. Women who are in close relationships with their partners but no longer have the need or capacity for intercourse, and who have concerns that other POP procedures might lead to complications, should explore this option.

At the time she first reached out to me, K was a vibrant 70+ years young woman. She presented with both cycstocele and rectocele issues; K's history was one that included 2 vaginal births, hysterectomy at the age of 35, weight fluctuation, and an occupation including years of being on her feet as a hairdresser.

After discussions with both her husband and her physician, K made the decision to move forward with copocleisis as her POP surgical treatment choice. Her relationship with her husband was a close and loving one, but because of health issues they were no longer engaging in intercourse. After discussing the surgical options with her physician as well as her husband, K decided that colpocleisis was the most logical choice. The procedure closed off the top 2/3 of her vagina; no mesh was needed to address her cystocele or rectocele. K was very happy with the outcome of her procedure. She maintains an active lifestyle and her surgical choice has not changed how she views her sexuality or her intimate relationship. My hat is off to this amazing, intelligent woman for recognizing the value in a procedure many would hesitate to consider.

C is another amazing, intelligent, articulate woman in her 70's, who decided on exploring colpocleisis to address her cystocele. Her initial procedure was a hysterectomy and sling for incontinence, but because the sling caused her pain, it was cut, releasing the tension and disabling it from serving its purpose. Soon after this procedure, her bladder dropped, as can occur after a hysterectomy, particularly in women who are menopausal or post-menopausal, since the supportive tissues in the pelvic cavity loose strength and integrity with the drop in estrogen that occurs during menopause. C consulted with a urogynecologist and moved forward with a procedure which included lifting the bladder and closing the vagina to provide mesh free support. While C has experienced incontinence post procedure (it is imperative incontinence issues are explored by clinicians prior to colpocleisis procedures to prevent this occurrence, ask your clinician if this concern will be addressed), she remains very satisfied with her procedure because she no longer must deal with tissue bulge or pain.

K and C and other women I've met over the years who chose copocleisis as an option are warriors, exploring treatments that few will consider simply because they simply 'aren't done' in women of relatively good health beyond their POP concerns. Colpocleisis is simply another tool in the POP surgical toolbox to be considered as a mesh-free alternative for those who are no longer engaging in intercourse.

Lack of intercourse clearly does not have to mean lack of intimacy. The bottom line is as women, we should never let the vagina define our sexuality or who we are. Our sexual energy is the sum of all of our parts.

Since the incidence of a second surgical procedure for POP is statistically alarming, it is in your best interest to research your surgeon. The incidence of a second surgical procedure for POP is statistically alarming. Studies indicate up to 30% of women will undergo a second POP operation. Getting references is helpful. You can also check physician watchdog websites on-line, there are listings in the resources section in the back of the book, but be mindful that happy patients seldom report results online, they simply get on with their lives. Check with your state medical board for complaints. For all intents and purposes, you want your repair to be a one-time fix if possible. POP surgery is typically major surgery, (depending on procedure chosen).

Most POP surgeries are performed under general anesthesia. There was a time when you would probably have been in the hospital for a week after POP surgery, but that is no longer the case. It is much more likely that you will have a short hospital stay or your procedure will be performed on an outpatient basis. This means you will go home still feeling pretty rough around the edges. It is imperative you have backup support at home if possible and prep your home prior to surgery with all the post-surgical items you will need. For more information, reference chapter 13, *What to Have on Hand Prior to Surgery.*

Surgical outcome will depend on the skillset of the individual surgeon, as is the case with any surgery. Most FPMRS surgeons have a preference for specific types of procedures (robotic vs nonrobotic, vaginal vs abdominal, etc.). Your surgeon will discuss your options with you prior to surgery. It is important to do your homework and ask the proper questions regarding types of procedures your surgeon provides, how many he/she has done, and what the long-term success rate is.

Procedures can be done either vaginally or abdominally. Post-surgical pain may be less with a transvaginal procedure. Sometimes there is no choice but to have an abdominal procedure if it will provide the best outcome. The most important thing to keep in mind is that the surgeon will choose the type of incision that best suits your POP damage. Once again, it is important to realize that you want the repair done properly so there will be no issues that require a second surgery.

> *If you are contemplating surgery for pelvic organ prolapse, try your best to find a surgeon who does a lot of prolapse repairs, and don't assume that all of your functional symptoms (problems with your bladder, bowel, or sex) will be addressed as the correlation between functional derangements and pelvic organ prolapse is very poorly understood.*
> ~Mickey Karram, M.D.

Take as much time locating the best surgeon for your needs as you require; there is seldom a need to rush into POP surgery. Women at times choose to seek a second and third opinion in order to find a clinician that most appropriately fits their needs. Once you select the most suitable surgeon based on your needs, discuss the benefits and risks of each treatment option to enable you to make the most fitting and informed choice.

CHOOSING A HEALTH CARE PROVIDER

POPS Patient Perspective: *I found my prolapse at 6 weeks post-partum and started to go down a really dark hole. My OB disregarded this, as this was my new vagina and I had to become my own advocate. I found this group and I wouldn't have been able to survive my first year of motherhood without it.*
~DO, NJ/USA

Using the services of someone who specializes in pelvic organ prolapse or is at least certified in the field makes sense, as opposed to seeing a primary care practitioner, gynecologist, Ob/Gyn, or gastroenterologist. You wouldn't trust the care of your teeth to a nose specialist just because both areas of the body are in close proximity on your head. A specialist is most likely to provide services that will result in a successful outcome.

Finding the best provider is key when it comes to dealing with POP, whether minimally invasive solutions or surgical options for managing your condition.
~Debra Muth, ND, WHNP

Pelvic organ prolapse is typically diagnosed by your primary care clinician or gynecologist. Often, they will make recommendations for treatments and may fit you for a pessary. Although many specialists can address aspects of pelvic organ prolapse, FPMRS urogynecologists and urologists are specialty trained in all five types of POP. It makes sense to consult with a specialist in this field.

Women's health physical therapists (PT) are on the front lines for non-surgical treatment of POP. Often physicians refer patients with POP to physical therapists. It is important to make sure the PT you are being treated by is specifically women's health sanctioned (ask if you are not sure), because a women's pelvic floor PT will optimize your treatment. Additionally, urologic nurse practitioners, occupational therapists, myofascial release therapists, and biofeedback therapists specialize in pelvic floor treatment.

The Practitioner Locator page of the APOPS website has links to each of these women's pelvic floor health specialists to assist in finding clinicians in your area. Do your homework prior to surgical procedures. POP surgery is intricate and the ideal is a one-time procedure with no complications: www.pelvicorganprolapsesup port.org/healthcareconnections.

WHAT TO ASK YOUR PHYSICIAN PRIOR TO SURGERY

POPS Patient Perspective: *I was 36 when I first realised something was wrong. Typically, I self-diagnosed on the internet first – I then went to an NHS GP who examined me and agreed I may have a cystocele. I was referred to a specialist who told me that I did not have one. I asked him if he said he was sure – as I had all the symptoms. He replied with "you have not had any children, you cannot have a prolapse. Believe me this is what i do every day." Needless to say, he was wrong. A few months later I got diagnosed privately and fitted with a pessary. That was more than two years ago.*
~AR, UK

Once you make the decision to move forward with surgery to repair POP, a pre-surgical appointment will be scheduled. Prior to this appointment, write down your questions and take them along to your consultation. Make sure your surgeon answers all of the questions you have; at the very least, the surgeon should have a physician's assistant or nurse practitioner available that can address your concerns. If your surgeon or the PA/NP will not take the time to answer your questions, seriously consider finding a different surgeon. A surgeon who will not take the time to answer questions about the surgical procedure and heal curve is not the best provider of quality healthcare.

With a good understanding of the problem and their options, women can make good informed choices regarding their care. As a surgeon, I spend a lot of time explaining pelvic organ prolapse to my patients.

~Lennox Hoyte, MD

Here is a list of suggested questions to consider asking your surgeon. Do not hesitate to ask all questions you have; the more knowledge you have going into POP surgery, the less surprised you will be by events that occur afterward.

1. What grade of severity is my prolapse?
2. What type of POP surgical repairs are recommended, rectocele, cystocele, enterocele, uterine, or vaginal vault prolapse repair?
3. Is my prolapse minimal enough that I can maintain it at the same level by doing Kegel exercises and using a pessary?
4. What are the pros and cons of using a pessary as opposed to having surgery?
5. What are the odds of a repeat POP occurrence after I have surgery.
6. What are the surgical risks or potential complications?
7. What type of anesthesia will you use for my procedure?
8. Will I need to stay overnight in the hospital after my procedure?
9. Will the surgery be done vaginally, robotically, or abdominally? Will there be laparoscopic incisions as well? How many laparoscopic incisions will there be?
10. Will mesh be used for my procedure? Which repairs will mesh be utilized for?
11. What are the risks of erosion if mesh is used to repair my prolapse?
12. How many of these types of procedures have you provided? How often do you provide them? What is the success rate?
13. What are other potential complications?
14. How successful is this procedure at repairing POP long

term?

15. Will this procedure relieve all of my symptoms? If not, which symptoms are likely to remain?
16. Will one surgery treat all my POP issues?
17. Will this surgery eliminate my incontinence?
18. What are other treatment options if I choose to not have surgery?
19. Will I need to wear a pessary after surgery?
20. Will I need to wear an abdominal support belt after surgery if I normally lift heavy objects?
21. How long will I need to be on strong pain medication after surgery?
22. If you find any problems with my ovaries or uterus during surgery, is there a chance that they will be removed?
23. How will this surgery affect my sex life?
24. Will this surgery have an impact on my ability to have an orgasm?
25. How long will it take for sexual sensations to return?
26. Will sex be painful after my surgical repair has healed?
27. How long will I need to wait before I can have intercourse after surgery?
28. How long will it take to get my normal urinary sensations back?
29. How long will it take to get normal defecatory sensations back?
30. How long will I need to wait to return to my normal activities after surgery, including work?
31. What kind of maintenance should I do after I am through healing from surgery?

Always ask all of your questions! There are no bad questions; any concerns you have should be addressed prior to surgery. It bears repeating; a physician who won't take the time to answer all of your questions or tries to rush you through a pre-surgical appointment is a red flag. Search for a surgeon who is willing to address your needs.

WHAT TO EXPECT WITH POP SURGERY

POPS Patient Perspective: *I've learned more from the women in the POPS group than the three specialists I saw combined; the knowledge here is invaluable and I thank you for that.*
~EC, CA/USA

S urgery of any type can be frightening and stressful; surgery for a condition that is seldom talked about even more so. Many women with pelvic organ prolapse are often so embarrassed to bring it to the attention of their physicians that by the time they do, it has progressed beyond the point of effective management with Kegel exercises or other non-surgical treatment options. Most of us have multiple resources including friends, family, and work colleagues that we can brain pick about experiences regarding a

C-section, appendectomy, tubal ligation, or hysterectomy, but since women seldom share pelvic organ prolapse experiences, few know who to reach out to regarding POP surgery.

If you're considering surgery for pelvic organ prolapse, be sure that you are comfortable with your surgeon and that she or he specializes in the type of surgery you are thinking about. It might also be helpful to talk to other patients to understand what to expect during the recovery period.
~Vivian Sung, MD

The amount of time surgery will take depends on what repairs need to be addressed, the technique, and skill of the surgeon. The typical POP surgery will take between one and three hours, but since some POP procedures address one type of POP and others include multiple repairs, it is best to discuss with your physician the time frame anticipated with your individual surgery.

POP surgeries may include vaginal or abdominal incisions, and may include laparoscopic or robotic portals. Heal time with vaginal, laparoscopic, or robotic procedures will be faster than with abdominal procedures which involves healing of multiple layers of abdominal muscle. Take the time to find a physician you feel you can trust to perform the least invasive procedure for your POP repair. In some cases, there is no choice but to have abdominal surgery. When in doubt, get a second opinion.

After your surgery, it is important to start assisted walking as quickly as the medical staff allows. If you feel your pain is too intense to get out of bed, make the nursing staff aware that you need more medication prior to walking. The sooner you can get out of bed and get the blood pumping in your body, the sooner the healing process will progress. Your first walking should be prompted and assisted by nursing staff; never try to get out of bed without calling your nurse until you are told you are able to. The one thing you don't want to do is fall; injury to a freshly repaired site could be a significant setback. Sitting up in bed and walking around may be quite uncomfortable at first. The hardest aspect will be getting into walking position the first time. Once you are moving around, it gets easier.

Women often have a catheter placed after POP surgery, so don't be alarmed if this occurs. You may be sent home with the catheter, or alternatively, the catheter will be removed when you are awake and alert, and you will need to urinate after it is taken out before the hospital will allow you to go home without one. If swelling prevents an adequate amount of urine from being released, the catheter will be re-inserted. It is quite common go home with a catheter that needs to stay in place for a couple of additional days to a couple of weeks, varying by the complexity of your procedure and degree of swelling. Once internal swelling goes down and tissues start to heal, it will be easier to urinate. You will be instructed on how to use the catheter at home before you are released from the hospital. You will also be told when to make an appointment to come back to your surgeon's office for catheter removal. It is a good idea to wear loose fitting clothing like jogging pants a size too large or bring a beltless robe to the hospital for POP surgery; loose clothing feels better around a swollen surgical site. It will also make the catheter collection bag less noticeable for the trip home. (It will likely be strapped to your leg underneath your pants).

It is common after POP surgery to be sent home with vaginal packing. Packing the vaginal cavity controls bleeding post-surgery and reduces swelling. The packing is typically removed in three to five days at your surgeon's office. Instructions on when to make an appointment with your surgeon to have packing removed will be given prior to leaving the hospital.

It is likely that both the vaginal packing and the catheter will be removed during the same appointment at your surgeon's office. Catheter removal and packing removal only takes a few minutes and typically neither procedure is painful, usually just a bit uncomfortable. At the point both of these procedures are done, you will likely still be on pain medication which will help buffer discomfort.

You will likely be on pain medications for about a week after POP surgery; the type and length of time will of vary of course, depending on the type of POP surgery you have. Pain is a very individual thing, it is important to discuss pain concerns with your surgeon *prior* to surgery, sharing any concerns you have about pain control. Make your physician aware of your level of pain tolerance. If you have any allergic reactions to pain medications, be sure to discuss this with your surgeon prior to your procedure. Icing the surgical sites the first week post-surgery helps reduce both pain and swelling. If you feel a sneeze coming on, do not panic, simply grab a pillow and hold it to your abdominal/vaginal area with gentle pressure while you sneeze. Continual coughing as may occur with a cold may cause discomfort however. If continual coughing occurs, be sure to contact your surgeon.

Expect considerable bruising and swelling to the entire vaginal area post-surgery. Whether you have a vaginal incision, a vaginal incision plus laparoscopic incisions, or an abdominal incision, this is a major surgery and with it comes an expected amount of discomfort. Bruising and swelling may last for a few weeks. Like any other major surgical procedure, the amount of discomfort, swelling, or bruising will vary based on the particulars of your surgical procedure.

Towards the end of the first week following your surgery, the swelling and irritation to the entire surgical area may increase. This is not cause for alarm, it is occurring simply because you are up and moving around more.

Difficulty urinating and moving your bowels may occur after surgery. I found that if I urinated a little, then defecated, then tried to urinate again, it gave my bladder time to relax enough to empty completely. The entire pelvic area becomes swollen and sensitive, so do not rush elimination. I felt more comfortable after bowel movements by cleaning the entire region with baby wipes and then lubricating with KY Ultra Liquid after every defecation. A peri-bottle (a bottle to squirt water onto the area), is helpful as well.

It is very likely that you will need at least 6 weeks off work following POP surgery. Since it is relatively common to have more than one POP repair done simultaneously, and since POP repair is in a region of your body that is impacted by standing, sitting, bending over, and walking, it is extremely important that you discuss how much time you will need off from employment when making your surgical plans. The type of job you have will have a definite impact on the length of time you need to take off before returning to employment.

It is also likely that your surgeon will ask you to refrain from exercise for six to eight weeks after surgery, and with more complex repairs, it may extend to three months. Aerobic exercise, weight training, weight machine, and floor exercises have the potential to damage the surgical repairs. Follow physician guidelines, but pay close attention to body signals when you resume exercising. Pushing into pain post-surgery is never a good idea. At some point, more active women will want to get back to routine exercise regimens, but resuming exercise too soon is truly a mistake. In order to avoid a repeat POP repair, you will want to abstain from any form of exercise for the full amount of time your surgeon has designated.

It will take about 12 weeks to recuperate from POP surgery. Within 3 weeks you will start to feel a great deal better, but it is important to adhere to your surgeon's instructions. In order to reduce the risk of re-injury, avoiding any type of pushing, pulling or lifting motion is essential. There are many household-cleaning chores that should be eliminated throughout your heal curve. If you have no one living with you who can help out with chores, consider alternate ways to accomplish the things that absolutely have to get handled. Carrying a few items of clothing to put into the washer is acceptable; carrying a laundry basket full of clothes is not. Consider getting a wagon or plastic sled to move items from one end of the house to the other. Your surgeon will give you a weight limit for lifting things around the house, and it is in your best interest to stick to what your surgeon recommends.

There will likely be a bloody vaginal discharge after surgery. It may increase in volume after the packing is pulled out. For those women who haven't had a menstrual period in years, it will seem a little unsettling to wear sanitary pads again. After 2 to 3 weeks, you should be able to use a panty liner. If you still need a full pad after this length of time, inform your physician. You should not wear tampons. You truly won't want to; the vaginal area will likely be too tender to even think about using them. You will be able to resume using tampons again, but not until the area is completely healed. This could take three months, possibly more.

You will need to refrain from intercourse for a period of time as well, likely six to twelve weeks depending on your procedure. Most women will not want to engage in sexual activity for at least that length of time anyway, the area will simply be too tender.

If the vaginal area seems very dry and tender to the touch, there are two options to ease the discomfort. For those women who are of menopausal age or past menopause, applying vaginal estrogen cream to the area helps. If you normally use a vaginal applicator to insert the cream, do not use the applicator until the area is healed enough to feel comfortable with its insertion; this will probably be around six weeks. During this period, you can put the cream on the tip of a finger and insert it a short distance into the vaginal canal. It also helps to apply estrogen cream to the external vaginal tissues. Women who are too young to use estrogen therapy can apply KY Ultra Liquid to the entryway to the vaginal canal and to the internal areas of the labial folds and the rectal area (the liquid works better than the gel for this purpose). Lubricating the entire area after urinating or defecating will truly help maintain your comfort level. KY Ultra liquid will also be helpful for the post-menopausal population. Remember when applying topical substances to this area, first cleanse the area after urinating or defecating, and then apply estrogen or KY from the front of the body towards the back to avoid any fecal contamination to the vaginal area.

If you've had a rectocele repair, you may continue to feel pressure and pain in the anal sphincter area until these tissues are completely healed. Unless there are distinct feelings of great discomfort or pain, the discomfort is likely the normal tissue healing sensation. During the healing process, the internal tissues will become a bit hard and rough, but in time, they will soften again.

It is important to maintain soft stools while healing from a rectocele repair. Straining to have a bowel movement impedes the healing process and can damage the repair. Make sure to eat plenty of fresh fruit fiber, especially apples, (fruit fiber works better than grain fiber unless you are experiencing diarrhea). Use a stool-softener to keep the stool soft enough to evacuate easily; your physician will likely recommend one prior to your release from the hospital. Make sure to take the stool softener every day while on narcotic pain meds. Narcotic pain medication prescribed post-surgery are extremely binding, and for this reason it is best to get off of them as soon as possible. However, stopping narcotic pain meds too soon is not a good idea. Muscle tissue contracts with pain, which can impede the healing process.

When you feel a bowel movement coming on, lubricate the anus with the KY Jelly, (not the Ultra Liquid, in this case KY Jelly will work better). Lubrication will enable the stool come out more easily, especially beneficial during your first bowel movement. Trust me, you'd rather insert something the size of your finger into your anus to lubricate it than to suffer through a hard, regular sized stool slowly pushing out. Remember to try to not bear down to force stool out.

There may be some blood loss from surgery, which may cause iron-deficiency anemia. If you are already taking a supplement with iron, resist the temptation to take an additional iron supplement unless your physician tells you to. Excess iron can cause constipation, compounding post-surgical defecation difficulties. Try to supplement iron from food sources like eggs, red meat, dark green leafy vegetables, or Malt-O-Meal cereal.

It is extremely beneficial to go into surgery with all your questions answered; knowing what to expect reduces fear of the unknown. For guidance in what questions to ask your surgeon prior to repair of POP, refer to Chapter 11, *What to Ask Your Physician Prior to Surgery.*

~ 13 ~
# WHAT TO HAVE ON HAND PRIOR
# TO SURGERY

POPS Patient Perspective: *The POPS group was my safe place to ask all the questions I had no one else to ask; it was empowering and compassionate and the reason I found my solution.*
~JB, PA/USA

I t's of great value to purchase post-surgical care items prior to your hospital visit so they are readily accessible when you come home from surgery. Since the length of a hospital stay has shortened immensely in recent years, it is important to have a family member willing to take care of the duties that would normally be handled by hospital nursing staff. You will want your in-home recuperation area set up prior to your trip to the hospital. Aside from the traditional items to have on hand for comfort, there are many additional supplies that will be helpful to make your initial days of healing more comfortable.

Awareness of pelvic organ prolapse will only occur when we share what we know with others. Women keep their symptoms, treatments, and avenues of self-help for pelvic organ to themselves because of embarrassment. As POP becomes common knowledge, they will feel more comfortable sharing information with the world at large. Knowledge is power. It is my hope that as we continue to do what women do best - network, guide, and provide support for each other - POP will soon become common knowledge.
~Sherrie Palm, APOPS Founder

The first thing you will want to do is set up your "bedroom" area, whether that will be in your actual bedroom, a spare bedroom, or on the couch. Take into consideration the mid-body/lower body discomfort you will have after surgery. Check how easily you can get up from a lying position in your couch, bed, or other furniture you plan to recuperate in. Find which seems to be the best height for getting into an upright position to go to the bathroom. If you need to contract your abdominal muscles to stand up from your resting position, it is likely going to be a bit uncomfortable to get up for a bathroom run post- surgery. Your physician may not want you to contract your abdominal muscles when you are first home from surgery, even if you don't have an abdominal incision. The pelvic floor and abdominal area should be allowed to heal for six to eight weeks before you start intentionally contracting so the tissues have time to rebuild properly. Any pushing/pulling motions will be counter-productive to the healing process.

An end table or portable TV tray of some kind is useful to put items on that you need close at hand. This may seem obvious, but since you will need several items on that table the first week after you get home from surgery, you will want to make sure it is large enough to hold everything you need close at hand. An inverted plastic milk crate works out well if you put a towel or oblong cake pan on top to catch the spills and keep things from falling through the holes. You can usually find these in the school supply section of any chain retail store.

There are many other items that you can consider to make your first days at home more comfortable. Give some thought to whether any of the following items may be helpful to you:

- Preemie baby diapers make great icepacks; open one end and fill it with ice cubes and then reseal it with the sticky tabs. It is extremely beneficial to use one on your abdomen and one in your vaginal area post-surgery to help control pain and swelling. Since they are absorbent baby diapers, there is no water leakage and the soft side feels comfortable against the skin. They are very small and fit quite comfortably in the crotch area and their natural curve makes them stay in place on the abdomen. They are sold in bags of twenty; you may want to purchase a couple bags. Use icepacks on and off around the clock for the first 4-7 days after you get home from the hospital, as they will have a tremendous impact on reducing your pain. I made up two extra icepacks every evening so when I woke up in the middle of the night needing a fresh one, I just had to grab it out of the freezer.

- Beanbag style heating pad can be squished comfortably into the vaginal area. It can be heated in the microwave repeatedly and there are no electrical cords to get caught on anything. I used these in the crotch area and on the abdomen; it felt great in both places. Once I was past the initial four days of icing, I continued with the beanbag heat pad for a few weeks.

- Hydrocortisone 1% cream or a hemorrhoid cream for rectal discomfort after your bowels start moving again. Typically, it will be several days after surgery before your bowels become active, and if you've had a rectocele repair, you will want to do everything you can to make the first bowel movements easier. You will not be able to get into a bath to soak for some time, so you'll want to do whatever is necessary to keep rectal discomfort under control.

- Colace stool softener to make sure the first bowel movement is as easy to pass as possible. Typically, narcotics are used for pain management after POP surgery and they will constipate you. Surgical blood loss may cause anemia so try to supplement iron from natural food sources like spinach, meat, fish, liver, Maltomeal and other enriched cereals rather than an iron supplement because iron is constipating. A stool softener will make that first movement more tolerable.

- Apples for their fiber will also help make that first bowel movement easier. If you do not care for apples, at least have some apple juice available. The fiber in apples is more effective as a gentle bulking agent than grain fiber, especially for women who have IBS issues.

- <u>KY Jelly</u> to lubricate the anal canal prior to bowel movements will make evacuation easier.
- <u>KY Ultra Liquid or Liquid Silk</u> will keep the external tissues on the bottom end more comfortable. Check with your physician about how soon you can use these products, as there may be incisions that they should not be used near. I found putting KY Ultra Liquid on the entire labial area made me quite a bit more comfortable and eliminated any "pulling" when I changed sitting or lying positions.
- <u>Foam or inflatable donut</u> will take the pressure off the bottom when sitting for a long time.
- <u>Baby sippee cup</u> or a cup with an attached straw (like the ones children use) comes in handy at bedside. It is much less likely to spill if it gets tipped over.
- <u>Cranberry juice</u> is a good liquid to drink after any surgery, as it contains a compound that can inhibit bacteria from attaching to the lining of the bladder and causing a urinary infection. Drinking a lot of water is essential too.
- <u>Sanitary pads and panty-liners</u>, even if you haven't had a period in years. It is normal to have vaginal bleeding after this type of surgery. If you have vaginal packing, there will be extra bleeding after this is removed, and you will want a pad absorbent enough to handle the flow. After a couple of weeks, you may be able to use panty-liners instead.
- <u>Baby wipes</u> are one of the best inventions around, handy for so many things. Once you start having bowel movements, you will want to keep the area very clean to expedite the healing process. I found the easiest way to stay comfortable on my bottom end was to clean up using toilet paper, then grab a baby wipe to thoroughly cleanse the area, then follow up with hydrocortisone cream or hemorrhoid cream. I also

asked my doctor to prescribe a prescription hemorrhoid cream that had lidocaine in it to numb the area a bit as well as help it heal.

- <u>Loose jogging pants or dresses</u> for clothing, any friction in the vaginal area will create discomfort. I experimented with wearing loose dress slacks and then jeans several times before I was actually able to tolerate them. Women going back to work at six to eight weeks should experiment at home before wearing pants to work.

- <u>Pain medication</u> will be prescribed by your physician. I recommend that you drop off your prescriptions at a pharmacy on your way home from the hospital. Once you are home and situated, the individual who drove you home from the hospital can pick up your medications. By the time you need your next dose of pain medication, you will have it on hand. It is also a good idea to have whatever over-the-counter anti-inflammatory pain medications you use on hand (check with your surgeon whether to use ibuprofen, naproxen, or acetaminophen), so when you are ready to wean off the prescription pain medication, you have an alternative accessible. I was given naproxen at the hospital along with the narcotic pain medication and continued to use this at home since it stays in your system longer than ibuprofen does. Since aspirin may cause bleeding issues, it is best to avoid it to reduce risk of bleeding post-surgery.

If you are only reading sections in this book instead of the entire book, I would recommend that anyone having surgery also refer to Chapter 12, *What to Expect With POP Surgery.*

IMPACT TO INTIMACY

POPS Patient Perspective: *APOPS has given more information than all of my doctors' visits combined! And I have searched hard for good doctors! Sad, but true...* ~MM, CA/USA

The aspect of POP that I get the strongest reaction to when speaking at conferences or public events or while being interviewed by the media, is the impact POP has on intimacy. Both coital incontinence (leakage of urine or stool during acts of intimacy) and pain with intercourse can have a significant impact to intimacy and relationships. Women may avoid intimacy out of fear that their vaginal tissue bulge or leakage will be discovered by their partner. Pain with intimacy is another reason women may avoid intimate relations.

Coital incontinence (CI) occurs relatively frequently; most studies indicate it occurs in 10-27% of women with 1 international, cross-sectional study indicating it may occur in up to 40% of women. Accurate statistics are difficult to come by because women underreport CI out of embarrassment. Leakage during intercourse can include leakage during the act of vaginal penetration or during orgasm. Women unfamiliar with pelvic organ prolapse typically have no idea that coital incontinence might be related to POP. Many women struggle to find a way to balance the intimate aspects of relationships while dealing with the other signs and symptoms of POP. As with other areas of the POP dynamic, women dealing with the impact POP has on intimacy need to know they are not alone and there is help available. Coital incontinence and pain with intercourse are aspects of POP that can be addressed with treatment.

The physical act of intimacy is often a pivotal piece of maintaining a close connection with our partners; without it women may experience a disconnect in the bond that cements their relationships. Awareness of a pelvic health issue that needs to be addressed may help intimate partners recognize that it is not for lack of wanting intimacy that women hold back - it is a matter of discomfort, embarrassment, or both. Treatment often helps intimate partners reconnect.

> *POP is a health concern which connotes almost a "taboo-like" quality related to both interpersonal as well as professional communication, and one that is surrounded by substantial gaps of knowledge and inherently wrong information, much of it imparted by well-meaning but incompletely informed sources.*
> ~Roger Dmochowski, MD

As I engaged more deeply in POP advocacy, more and more women came forward, some looking for emotional support, some needing to share baggage, some confused where to find the specialists to treat POP, some simply looking for basic POP info. Multiple common themes emerged. These women were angry that they were not informed about POP until after they were diagnosed. Many were fearful of losing their husbands or boyfriends because having sex was painful and their partners didn't understand their pain or believe them.

D was extremely distraught when she first approached me, her life had completely unraveled before she was able to figure out what was happening to her body. At the age of 45, she was newly divorced. The prior four years she'd had significant pain while engaging in intercourse. While she also had on-going problems with stomach bloat and distention, the multiple tests her physician ran all came back negative and he recommended she consider utilizing anti-anxiety medications. D did not want to take medications that would alter her state of mind, she was still raising two teenagers and wanted to be as clear headed as possible to address their needs. Her relationship with her husband started to deteriorate when she found intercourse so painful, she started to find excuses to avoid it. She tried to tell her husband it hurt to have sex; initially he believed her, the second time he accepted it but was quite disgruntled. After the third refusal, he stopped attempting intimacy. He started working late at night and going to the office on the weekend.

When her husband asked for a divorce D was devastated. How on earth was she supposed to pick up the pieces of her life and start a new relationship when intimacy was painful? What man would want her? D felt like damaged goods that no man would want. It was difficult enough meeting someone new, how on earth do you explain to someone of the opposite sex that intercourse is painful? Fortunately, the change in her insurance coverage related to her divorce led to a new gynecologist who diagnosed D's symptoms as pelvic organ prolapse. Once she was referred to a specialist and diagnosed with a grade 3 rectocele and cystocele, she went online looking for answers and found APOPS support forum. Being able to share her story with other women helped her get through the steps she needed to make treatment decisions as well as helped her gain the confidence to move on with her personal life.

N experienced coital incontinence. She was not aware that coital incontinence was "a thing"; all she knew was every time she attempted to be intimate with her partner, she leaked urine. The day she leaked stool, sex was over for her - talk about a mood breaker. She found it unbearable to be intimate for fear of a repeat episode. She could not bring herself to disclose the issue to her physician, and she couldn't bear the thought of asking other women about her symptoms. She suffered in silence as often occurs. Fortunately for N, her husband loved her greatly and kept prodding her about the reasons for lack of intimacy and encouraged her to speak with her physician, which led to a POP diagnosis and treatment.

T was a young woman in her 20's who experienced traumatic

forceps delivery along with considerable damage to her pelvic floor. She never recovered from the birth trauma, and within months of her delivery, noticed tissues bulging out of her vagina Horrified her husband would see them and be turned off, she also started refusing intimacy, and figured her sex life was over. Luckily for T, someone in her inner circle who was also experiencing pelvic organ prolapse shared that information and this empowered T to start asking questions and digging online for information.

All the women I have mentioned had one thing in common - none of them knew about pelvic organ prolapse prior to being diagnosed. Because of that, none of them recognized warning signs or symptoms, none of them knew causes, none of them knew of measures they should be taking, none of them knew how to address intimate quality of life issues, none of them knew where to get information when they first realized they had pelvic organ prolapse, because so little open dialogue about POP occurs.

15

THE MESH AGENDA: MISTAKES MADE AND NEXT STEPS

POPS Patient Perspective: *Don't treat me like I'm some kind of web-browsing-self-diagnosing-wackadoo-hypochondriac. I know my own body, I've had it my whole life!*
~LL, PA/USA

You've finally taken the steps to approach your Ob/Gyn or primary care physician about your incontinence concerns, the pain you experience with intercourse, and/or the bulge coming out of your vagina. You've been referred to a FPMRS urogynecologist or urologist and have a definitive diagnosis of one or more types of pelvic organ prolapse. Your journey to health balance is now shifting forward. But when the dialogue starts to flow toward whether or not to utilize mesh for repair, you are frozen in fear. What to do?

Controversy abounds regarding the use of mesh for surgical treatment of pelvic organ prolapse. The FDA issued a press release in July of 2011 regarding concerns about transvaginal mesh procedure complications. We all need to know our options; there are choices with POP surgical procedures just as there are options whether or not to utilize surgical procedures at all.

I have yet to meet an individual who was not nervous heading into surgery. We all hope our health concerns will be addressed and resolved when having surgical repair; we all hope procedures will be complication free. Every surgical procedure comes with risk, thus the importance of looking for the best surgeon for your unique surgical needs and the most appropriate type of surgery to optimize results.

Success for one woman may not be the same for another.
~Roger Dmochowski, MD

A common topic in APOPS support forum is the safety of mesh procedures for pelvic organ prolapse repair. Much has been addressed to improve the outcomes of mesh procedures, yet fear factor remains high for many women who read stories of mesh complications online or see litigation commercials on television, in magazines, or in newspapers. Seldom do women who've had successful mesh procedures talk about them, they simply get on with their lives. Every week women newly diagnosed with pelvic organ prolapse find the APOPS forum; frequently they reach out for guidance on mesh. Let's revisit the purpose and value of mesh treatment for pelvic organ prolapse, as well as share insights on best practice techniques utilized by female pelvic medicine urogynecologists and urologists.

Every woman navigating POP would like to have a magic list of "the best of the best" when it comes to pelvic floor clinicians. Unfortunately, it is not that simple because needs differ significantly from woman to woman. Some women prefer a practitioner who's the most qualified surgeon, with little concern about bedside manner. Some women prefer great bedside manner, but may be disappointed that the surgical outcome is not perfect or the healing took longer than expected. Surgeons are as individual as the patients they treat, they are human after all. The skill set of clinicians will vary with time, experience, continuing education, and new innovations and tooling.

It truly takes a specialist to repair the intricate female pelvic cavity, a diverse mass of organs, soft tissues, muscles, ligaments, tendons, boney structures, and nerves pushing against each other in a very compact space. To complicate matters, women with POP typically have more than one type of prolapse in need of repair and each POP type shifts organs from their normal positions. It is kind of like putting an assortment of large cooked vegetables into a Ziploc bag lying flat on the cupboard-when you hold the bag upright or shake it around, everything squishes together and shifts position. As much as you love your gynecologist, it is imperative that you see a specialist for POP repair.

> *Urogynaecology is a sub-specialty in its own right- the literature and clinical experience have both clearly shown that the best results of POP surgery are obtained when the attending surgeon is a urogynaecologist rather than a general gynaecologist/obstetrician.*
> ~Diaa Rizk, MD

If considering mesh surgery, it is important to find a clinician with extensive mesh experience. Write down the questions you want to ask your doctor before your appointment to make sure you don't forget any. Let your practitioner know you have mesh/surgery fear if that is the case. Ask your surgeon what he/she does to avoid mesh complications. Small incisions, proper mesh insertion location, preparation of mesh insertion site, use of estrogen cream pre and post-surgery, degree of mesh tension, and an appropriate closure are important considerations for a quality mesh procedure, whether your doctor performs mesh surgery through a transvaginal, laparoscopic, robotic, or abdominal approach.

> *Mesh surgery is not a magic cure. Proper pre-operative evaluation of women with POP who need surgery will dictate the best surgical approach whether mesh or native tissue repair.*
> ~Roger Dmochowski, MD

It is a red flag when clinicians or industry magnify the benefits only of only one a product or procedure. You should hear both sides of the story, risks and benefits, in order to be fully informed and better enabled to make the most appropriate decision whether to move forward with surgery. My POP procedure in February 2008 was transvaginal, and a consultation with my urogynecologist in 2015 at 7 years past that surgery confirmed that my tissues remained healthy, the mesh was in proper position, and there was no erosion. By the time this edition is published, I will have reached the 9-year post mesh procedure point with no complications that I am aware of. I am grateful mesh was an option for my surgery; the value of finding the right specialist is priceless. Obviously, there is never a 100% guarantee of success with any surgery, but if all of your questions are answered, it will give you peace of mind heading into a procedure.

> *It is important to counsel women pre-operatively about the efficacy and complications of mesh repair to enable them to make an informed choice.*
> ~Roger Dmochowski, MD

It is important to understand that in the hands of a qualified practitioner, mesh is typically used to prevent additional POP surgery down the road. Without mesh, surgery often fails in one to five years if our own tissues are not strong enough to maintain the repair long term. Considering the multitude of POP causes, it is no shock that lifestyle and the aging process increase the risk of surgical failure when mesh is not used. While childbirth is absolutely the most common POP cause, most women have a multitude of additional risk factors. Menopause is the second leading cause of POP (estrogen loss impacts muscle tissue strength and integrity), heavy lifting (every mom and grandma I know loves picking up babies and toddlers can get pretty heavy), athletic activities with downward pounding (many women like to run and jog but a water filled balloon jerked up and down gives you an idea what you organs are going through), chronic constipation (we seldom know which comes first, constipation causing rectocele, or rectocele causing constipation).

Additional causes adding to the risk factor list are chronic coughing, diastatis rectus abdominus or DRA (the long abdominal muscle splits down the middle during pregnancy), genetics, hysterectomy, neuromuscular and connective tissue conditions such as hypermobility Ehlers-Danlos (EDS, different degrees of hypermobility and weak tissue integrity), multiple sclerosis (MS), Marfan Syndrome, spinal cord injury, the list goes on and on. Show me a woman with one cause alone and I'll show you a woman who is the exception to the rule.

> *Obesity is also an important risk factor for failure of mesh repair because the accumulation of fat in the abdomen increases the intra-abdominal pressure similar to straining.*
> ~Diaa Rizk, MD

> *Know your symptoms and be able to identify the most bothersome.*
> ~Roger Dmochowski, MD

The diagnosis and management of pelvic organ prolapse will evolve considerably over the coming years. While APOPS pushes the envelope behind the scenes to generate broad-spectrum awareness, research is exploring every flavor of the POP dynamic and practitioners evolve skill-set and treatments. There is little doubt, pelvic organ prolapse awareness, screening, and treatment will generate the next significant shift in women's health. Women, clinicians, and research are all learning side by side.

> *With aging of the female population, the prevalence of POP will significantly increase creating a greater demand for services worldwide.*

> ~Diaa Rizk, MD

There are multiple links to clinicians who specialize in surgical and nonsurgical POP treatment on the APOPS website Practitioner

Locator page. Try to find a few practitioners in your area and Google them individually to see what information you can capture regarding experience, location, length of time in practice, etc. Physician review websites will give you basic information to start with, but are not a 100% guarantee of practitioner quality. It is in your best interest to meet clinicians in person to decide if your unique needs will be met. Pelvic organ prolapse is a condition that absolutely warrants a second opinion if you are not comfortable with the first specialist you see. Surgical skill should be a top priority. A practitioner who answers your questions and understands your specific needs is priceless. Some women prefer a doctor with top surgical skill, some prefer good bedside manner- the ideal is a mixture of both.

> *The health care providers responsible for treatment of POP besides urogynaecologists, include pelvic floor physiotherapists, nurse continence advisors and female pelvic health urologists.*
> ~Diaa Rizk, MD

An informed patient will have less anxiety and greater opportunity for the best outcome. Important mesh questions to consider asking your physicians prior to POP surgery are:

1. Do you plan to use mesh for my POP repairs?
2. How many mesh procedures like mine have you provided?
3. What surgical alternatives do I have to mesh for repair?
4. Is there any reason I would be a bad candidate for mesh?
5. Will my POP repair be successful long term without mesh?
6. How long has the mesh product you use been on the market?

7. How long have you been using this particular mesh product?
8. Is there a chance mesh surgery won't fix my POP?
9. What side effects should I be concerned about after mesh surgery?
10. Will my partner be able to feel mesh during intimacy?
11. What are the chances mesh will erode through my vaginal wall?
12. If I have mesh complications, will you be able to address them?
13. How will you repair mesh erosion?

As patients, it is our responsibility to do our homework. Check references, get referrals, and consider obtaining second opinions. Pelvic organ treatment is diverse, complex, and continually evolving. Get all your questions answered and do not move forward with surgery until you are sure you are ready.

At the time of the following FDA presentation in 2011, the estimated prevalence of POP was 3.3 million women in the US alone. Current studies indicate prevalence may be closer to 50% of the female population.

MESH PRESENTATION TO THE FDA OB-GYN ADVISORY PANEL

The following speech was given in Washington, DC by Sherrie Palm to the FDA OB/Gyn Advisory Panel Addressing Transvaginal Mesh Protocol on September 8, 2011, in representation of APOPS position on the value of transvaginal mesh procedures for repair of pelvic organ prolapse.

I'm Sherrie Palm, the founder and president of the Association for Pelvic Organ Prolapse Support. Neither me nor APOPS has any financial relationship with any person or group involved in any POP mesh agenda. I am simply a woman who's had transvaginal mesh surgery to repair pelvic organ prolapse; I had 3 of the 5 types of POP. I am a success story and would like to share some insights with the committee members. Like most women, I'd never heard of POP prior to my diagnosis. My urogynecologist utilized a transvaginal mesh procedure for my surgical repair. I had concerns about repeat surgery if mesh was not utilized, an all too common occurrence. I've been extremely pleased with the outcome of my surgery for pelvic organ prolapse and I guide others daily how to investigate the benefits of locating a specialist in POP procedures.

As a women's pelvic floor health advocate, I truly felt the need to weigh in on this topic. It's vital that committee members recognize that the common denominator for all women is the desire to return their bodies to normal. This is what drives women to seek treatment including surgery for POP. All women with POP have symptoms, ALL WOMEN WITH POP HAVE SYMPTOMS; they just don't talk about it with their physicians, husbands, even their friends, they are simply too embarrassed - but they talk to me. I speak with women daily regarding the baggage that comes with pelvic organ prolapse.

I'll admit that I'm a bit more proactive than the average woman; I networked to find the best urogynecologist in my area, I checked her credentials, I went to my appointment with my questions in hand with no intentions of leaving until all of my concerns were addressed. My physician is an expert in her field; she took her time with me and my successful transvaginal mesh procedure substantiates that this treatment option does have great merit.

I recognize that few women do their homework when

approaching POP treatment; because of that some women have transvaginal mesh procedures performed by physicians without the proper training and expertise for this procedure. With so many organs, muscles, and connective tissues coming together in a tightly compacted area, it truly takes an expert to get it right. A urogynecologist or urologist should be the physician of choice.

When the efficacy of a medical procedure is questioned, the catalyst typically comes from complaints filed by individuals who suffer complications after having procedures by physicians with inadequate training or experience. My heart goes out to the women suffering with these complications; it truly does. I've spent time discussing their histories with them and it is vital that we listen to their voices. These are women who had pain and dysfunction, opted for surgery to correct it, and now their pain and dysfunction is compounded. However, eliminating this beneficial procedure from POP treatment options is not the answer-monitoring who can perform procedures is a more practical direction. Advancement of any medical pathway will always be littered with the "yikes" factor of those who add procedures to their itinerary as though picking up a tool at Home Depot. It has always been this way; it probably always will. Thankfully we have the FDA to monitor and create ballast.

I feel strongly that transvaginal mesh procedures should be recognized as a valuable option in the choices for pelvic organ prolapse treatment. I also feel strongly that these procedures should only be utilized by physicians who are specialists and have gone through the intensive training necessary to perform them. I am hopeful the FDA will consider monitoring the training protocol rather than preventing urogynecologists and urologists from performing transvaginal mesh procedures. It's likely that the majority of the complications that occur are the result of inadequate training and experience - POP surgery is best left to the experts.

As a women's pelvic floor health advocate, every aspect of impact POP has to women is of top priority to me, every single layer - transvaginal mesh is just one of them. Pelvic organ prolapse is not an American women's health issue, it is a global women's health pandemic. There are 3 million women in this country alone with POP. It is imperative that the FDA is intricately involved in the global path to proper diagnostics and treatment for POP, along with coordination from NIH, WHO, & GHI; forward thinking will address the perception of POP as well as the reality of the status quo in all matters POP related including transvaginal mesh.

16

PREVENTION AND MAINTENANCE

POPS Patient Perspective: *My doctor told me I was the smartest patient he ever had; I would never have known what to ask if not for this group and Sherrie Palm!*
~PB, CO/USA

I t is extremely difficult to prevent POP. As an extremely pro-active woman who believes in preventative maintenance, I frequently wonder why there is no dialogue about POP during routine pelvic exams or childbirth classes. Considering that up to 50% of the female population may experience POP in their lifetime, and 2 of the most common life events women experience - childbirth and menopause - are the leading causal factors, it would be sensible to publicize POP awareness and incorporate POP screening into routine pelvic exams in an effort to diagnose the condition at an early stage. PC muscle strength and Kegel exercises typically become topics after the fact when women start experiencing urinary leakage or notice tissues bulging from their vagina.

> *I often get the question about a woman's prolapse: "Why didn't my doctor find this (prolapse) when he/she did my exam?" And my answer usually is "If you don't look for it, you won't find it!"*
> ~Sumana Koduri, MD

Many women are not aware that maintaining the strength of the PC muscle can have a positive value to address urinary incontinence as well as the amount of sexual sensation they can experience. By keeping this muscle toned and strong, it not only will help prevent urinary leakage, it will also magnify intimate sensation, potentially increasing orgasm frequency and intensity.

Since there are multiple risk factors and causes of POP, it will likely be impossible to totally prevent POP from occurring. However pelvic floor fitness activities may help contain the degree of prolapse and minimize the occurrence of urinary incontinence for many women. There is also the possibility that women who regularly perform Kegel exercises are more aware of sensations in the vaginal region, and would subsequently be more likely to notice changes occurring that may be indicators of POP. This could lead to diagnosis and treatment at an earlier stage of POP.

Weight management and exercise improve our health in every respect, including POP. Nearly all of us - me included - could use some improvement in our diets. I need to remind myself all the time to do the right stuff. Would I love to shove brownies in my face every day? You bet I would - I'm only human. But I resist the temptation as best I can and incorporate exercise into my daily ritual. Viewing our health from a maintenance lifestyle rather than flipping back and forth from healthy habits to unhealthy ones is much easier on our bodies. When I fall off the wagon and overdose on Dove dark chocolate (absolutely my Achilles heel), I recognize that the current day is a wash and get back on the wagon the next day with healthier choices.

Another area of focus that might help women prevent the start or progression of POP is paying attention to body stature. Good posture in general will optimize core strength, including the pelvic floor muscles. Monitoring our form and posture while lifting heavy objects, including our children, would truly help reduce downward pressure on the pelvic floor. Women usually forget to contract their PC muscle and hold their abdominal muscles in while lifting. It becomes reflex to lift without thinking about support to the pelvic floor, with the end result being pressure on internal organs and tissues. Every time I see a woman in public holding her child or grandchild on her hip, I wonder if she is contracting her core and pelvic floor, and I am quite sure the majority are not. We don't know what we don't know. Corporate America pays particular attention to protecting the back regarding employment that requires heavy lifting. Not a whisper is addressed regarding protecting the pelvic floor.

Vital to maintaining pelvic health are exercise regimens to strengthen the core and pelvic floor muscles. If you build strength and maintain tone in these areas, you are a step ahead of the curve in POP prevention and maintenance. These are pretty basic principles, but it is amazingly easy to forget about them. By bringing these few, simple practices to the awareness of women on a regular basis, it would be more likely that they would become second nature, and if women would try to incorporate them into their daily rituals, they would become more like habit.

> *The strength that comes from gaining voluntary control over your deepest core and pelvic stabilizing muscles is energizing and empowering. This is because, along with a healthy pelvic basket of muscles comes better posture, better control of your breathing, and a strong feeling of control of your own body!*
> ~Tasha Mulligan, PT

I question why PC muscle awareness is not introduced when young women have their first pelvic exam. If Kegel exercises were introduced at this point, and their significance explained from the intimacy, structural support, and potential to decrease damage during the childbirth perspectives (a healthy, strong PC muscle is more flexible during childbirth and heals more quickly after), women may embrace pelvic floor wellness as a part of daily fitness or feminine self-screening rituals. Women should be made aware of the value of contracting the PC routinely for pelvic floor strength as we do by brushing our teeth to maintain our oral health. If a woman was reminded about Kegels each time she went in for a routine pelvic exam just like she is asked if she has been doing self-breast exams looking for lumps, it could become second nature.

I am hopeful that as POP awareness advances, a shift in clinical screening and diagnostic protocol will emerge from treatment after the fact to establishing recognition prior to POP occurring. At the close of 2016, a standardized screening protocol for pelvic organ prolapse was not considered typical procedural policy during routine pelvic exams. Since childbirth and menopause are the two leading causes of POP, routine screening should certainly be implemented.

We need to shift forward with a more progressive attitude regarding women's pelvic floor health. It is vital that we recognize that women deserve health balance regarding *all* aspects of health. There is a fundamental need for all women to attain information and guidance regarding pelvic floor health concerns. By sharing knowledge of POP that we gain individually with all women, we shift women's pelvic floor health forward.

It is also vital that all players in the POP arena - patients, clinicians, researchers, academics, industry, and policy makers - collaborate to shift the POP dynamic forward, increasing awareness and treatment of pelvic organ prolapse. Together we can advance pelvic organ prolapse consciousness and redirect energy, generating dialogue toward advancing the least aggressive and most positive long term treatment outcomes possible.

~ 17 ~
MY POP EXPERIENCE

POPS Patient Perspective: *POP is not normal, nor should you be expected to live with it, it's an unacceptable way to live. POP can be very painful, debilitating and cause extreme emotional upset, despite what many health professionals say.*
~LM, UK

I have never had a "normal" female system: I spotted at the age of 15, had a light period at 17, and at 18 went on birth control pills to establish and regulate my monthly menstrual cycle. I went through fertility treatments in my early 30s, conceived at the age of 34, and had a hysterectomy on my 40th birthday to eliminate on-going reproductive organ issues; absolutely the best birthday gift I have ever given myself. The surgery disclosed a large cyst on one ovary, several large fibroids on my uterus, and aggressive adenomyosis - a benign inward growth of the uterine lining. I informed my gynecologist that I was tired of feeling miserable and pleaded for the procedure.

I asked my gynecologist "what happens to the organs inside my female area once my uterus is removed; what stops stuff from falling out?" The answer I was given was that the top of the vagina would be closed off, and it was not a concern. In retrospect, I often think back to that conversation and wonder why this did not initiate a discussion about the potential for pelvic organ prolapse. At that time, I'd never heard of pelvic organ prolapse and would not hear about it until I was diagnosed fourteen years later.

Prior to my hysterectomy, I experienced a symptom that should have generated discussion regarding POP, but it didn't occur to me to mention it to my gynecologist. I'd been having difficulty keeping a tampon in for some time. Once I had the hysterectomy, there was no further need to use tampons, so I didn't give it another thought. In fact, I didn't think about it again until I was diagnosed with POP, decided to write a book, started researching POP, and discovered in research articles I found that tampons pushing out is a symptom of POP.

The next symptom my body displayed about 13 years later was difficulty starting my urine stream; I had had this symptom for some time but didn't question it. I would wake up in the middle of the night to go to the bathroom and would become frustrated because I would be unable to urinate. I would spend 15 minutes trying several techniques, massaging my abdomen, listening to water run, closing my eyes and visualizing a man urinating off a waterfall (don't take offense guys, we ladies will do anything to start that stream), then would return to massaging my abdomen which would eventually work. I now know that my urethra was crimped from POP displacement of organs and tissues.

The symptom that really got my attention was the vaginal tissue bulge. After feeling a lump in my vagina for a few months, I finally became curious enough to get a

hand-held mirror and took a good look. I highly recommend women visually explore their vulva and vagina; if a look at what is occurring isn't enough to convince you to get to a doctor, I don't know what is. I was a bit shocked to see a walnut sized lump bulging out of my vaginal canal. I had no idea what it was, all I knew was that it wasn't normal and I wanted it fixed.

I went to see my physician, who is also a close friend, and she told me I had pelvic organ prolapse. I'd never heard of POP prior to my diagnosis. That was the beginning of a momentous shift in my life, both physically and professionally. My physician recommended that I try a pessary (another term I had never heard of, and I thought I'd been very pro-active with women's health screenings), and when I quickly became frustrated with the need to insert and remove a pessary daily, she referred me to the top urogynecologist that she knew - the third term I'd never heard of. The terms pelvic organ prolapse, pessary, and urogynecologist were clearly all cloaked in silence, and were about to radically change my world.

I'm not one to beat around the bush when it comes to self-educating regarding matters of my health. I went to see the urogynecologist armed with a sheet full of questions I wanted answers for. After she did a thorough pelvic and rectal exam, she patiently took her time addressing every question I had, and we then discussed the if-and-when of surgical repair. It was obvious that I had POP issues that needed repair (my prolapse was grade III; I needed rectocele and cystocele repairs and a large enterocele was discovered as well during surgery). I wanted the surgery immediately. We booked surgery a month out. I took advantage of that time to research POP in order to share this information with other women. I knew if I wasn't familiar with pelvic organ prolapse after being so pro-active with my health, other women likely weren't aware of it either.

> *Women aren't getting exams as frequently, doctor visits are short and there isn't a lot of time to ask questions, and women are often embarrassed to ask. Often someone might go for years without getting help. If you feel something is different – ask, and request an exam. Often women say they were told that everything is fine, but the prolapse goes away when they are in an exam position. If you have to stand to feel the changes, then make sure you recreate the symptoms during an exam, either straining or standing.*
> ~Katherine Stevenson, MD

I was exasperated that I needed surgery to fix something that was quite common but that I'd never heard of or read about. I questioned my surgeon how on earth that could be; she looked me right in the eye and stated matter-of-factly "Sherrie, women won't talk about POP". I was shocked and I was furious, I could not believe women would not talk about POP when they freely share the gory details of childbirth. My specialist told me a story about how she had tried to bring the subject up at a book club, a group full of educated women, and it still did not get discussed. She said it is something that women just don't feel comfortable talking about.

It did not take long for me to figure out that this is a subject that *all* women need to know about. We live in an enlightened society; the fact that we are repetitively subjected to every kind of physical, emotional, social, and sexual tidbit of health information on television and the radio as well as in books and magazines made me really question that so little information is readily known about this common condition. I started to discuss POP with other women, and found out that I was not the only person in the dark.

Once I made the decision to have surgery, it was full speed ahead as far as I was concerned. I've never been one to ignore a health concern, whether for a health issue that needed surgery or something that could make due with a bandage. I feel it is of great benefit for women who decide they want surgery to repair POP to go at it from the most positive angle - get checked, get fixed, get healed, get on with your life. Dwelling on the negative side of having POP or needing surgery to repair it serves no purpose.

Like most women with POP, I have multiple risk factors and will never know for certain what caused my POP issues, but I can make a pretty good guess. I have experienced one complication free vaginal birth at the age of 35, childbirth is the leading cause of POP. My mother had POP surgery for bladder leakage and rectocele issues, (I was not aware mom's surgery was POP surgery until I had my procedure, which initiated a dialogue), so there is a genetic factor. I was diagnosed with MS at the age of 30, and despite a very negative wheelchair bound prognosis when I was initially diagnosed, I have kept MS 'under control' over the years since my diagnosis. Women with neurological disorders may be predisposed to POP because of loss of muscle tissue integrity. I've been pro-active with my exercise routine for over 30 years as part of my self-help path to address MS. I've paid attention to core sensation over the years while I exercise, modifying my routine from time to time as need dictated to eliminate core or pelvic floor pressure. Although I've not regretted my hysterectomy for a moment, hysterectomy is a well-documented cause of POP. Years of chronic constipation from stress related IBS was another factor. I'm also sure a decrease in muscle tissue strength and integrity from menopausal estrogen loss added to my risk factor list. Additionally, I spent a few summers landscaping my yard that included moving large boulders and shoveling multiple yards of gravel, understandably detrimental to my pelvic floor health. Like most women with POP, I have had multiple risk factors and will never know for sure the exact cause, but that is not of great importance to me beyond adjusting causal behaviors.

One factor I do question is the possible connection of POP to my IBS (irritable bowel syndrome) or acid reflux issues. I am quite sure the IBS and reflux problems I've had over the years were related to being part owner of a stressful business that created a need for working an extreme number of hours at the same time as raising my son. Since two of the three POP repairs that needed to be addressed were a rectocele and an enterocele, repairs to the bowel and the intestines, I can't help but wonder about the POP intersect with my digestive issues. I questioned my urogynecologist prior to surgery about whether the POP issues could have caused or had an impact on degree of IBS or acid reflux; she said she did not think so. She also said she didn't think POP surgery would improve these conditions. Still, I went into surgery hoping that these other health concerns would improve. I did not have a recurrence of acid reflux until 7 years post-surgery, (I used to use a medication daily to control the acid), and it is currently sporadic, rather than a daily concern like it used to be. Unfortunately, POP surgery has not had an impact on my IBS. It did seem to get better for a short time post-surgery, but I'm guessing that was probably because I was just lying around in a relatively stress-free environment, not allowing myself to deal with anything demanding because I wanted to heal.

Additionally, over the year prior to my POP diagnosis I recognized a loss of PC muscle strength. I have always had good awareness of and strength in this muscle. The fact that I noticed I was having a harder time contracting this muscle, even though I really did not experience much of a problem with urine leakage unless I was jumping up and down and screaming while watching football, indicates that I had been cognizant of my body's red flags. I know that as I started my path into menopause, and my estrogen level dropped despite supplementing with bio-identical hormones, my PC contraction became weaker.

I highly recommend an exercise regimen for anyone who is attempting to recapture core or pelvic floor muscle strength, or to delay or prevent surgery, or for those who have had surgery and want to be proactive regarding long term maintenance. I've experimented over the past several years with multiple core and pelvic floor strengthening regimens and devices. I make it a point to continually review new programs and include a mixture of exercises from different programs within my regimen. It is crucial that women utilize a program that best fits their individual needs. We are all unique and what works for one may not necessarily be appropriate for another.

I'd like to pass along a few personal notes about my post-surgical period. I was very uncomfortable that first week after surgery, but I did go off narcotic pain medication on the third day post-surgery because I react negatively to nearly all pain meds which typically make me extremely wired up and miserable. By the second week I was up and moving around freely. I noticed the swelling and discomfort became more pronounced which of course was because I was upright and moving. By the end of the second week, I was walking relatively normally, by week three the bruising was gone. (There will be a lot of bruising, be prepared for a completely black and blue crotch.) At 3 weeks, I could also comfortably wear jeans. I was still using the beanbag heat pad for pain control at three weeks as well while I watched TV at night.

Several months after surgery, I noticed a pressure sensation when I was exercising. I went to see my surgeon and after a thorough checkup, she assured me everything was fine. Since I am fairly hands-on with weight training (free weights, ten-pound maximum), my surgeon recommended that when I lifted anything heavy over the next few months, I insert a tampon to contain downward pressure. I questioned whether I should use a pessary for this purpose, and she said that there should be no need to. Mesh was used to repair both my cystocele and rectocele; this was a protective measure to prevent POP reoccurrence because I am extremely active. I used the tampon support method while weight training for 1 month and after that, my tissues where strong enough to handle the load. I continue to evaluate whether items I must lift are too heavy however, to maintain my repair long term. Maintenance for life means assessing lifestyle behaviors and avoiding those that generate risk whether mesh is used for surgical POP repair or not.

On the sexual activity front, once I got past the initial post-surgical heal curve, I slowly resumed intimacy with no problems. As a woman who enjoys her sexuality, it was extremely important to me to be able to engage in an active sex life as well as truly enjoy it. I discovered that the core location of sexual sensation shifted, and the sensations seemed more intense. I'm not sure if this is because the pressure that the prolapsed organs put on the nerves in the area prevented sensation, or if there was no discomfort to distract from the pleasure sensations.

Every individual reacts differently to surgery. Since every woman's POP surgical experience will be unique, it's best to have some idea in mind of what is to come. The more questions you ask prior to a POP procedure, the less anxiety you will experience. There is zero doubt in my mind that POP surgery was a smart choice for me. February 2018 is my 9-year POP transvaginal mesh repair anniversary. At three months, I felt fairly healed up with minor pain at a couple of the laparoscopic incision sites. (I had 6 laparoscopic incisions plus vaginal incisions). It took six months to a year before I completely felt like I had prior to my POP procedure, but if I had to make the choice all over again whether to have the surgery to repair pelvic organ prolapse, I wouldn't hesitate for a moment to make the exact same surgical decision.

HEALTHCARE TUNNEL VISION

POPS Patient Perspective: The POPS forum has been priceless to me. Not only has it given me valuable information and support, it has also given me the courage and strength to break the silence and start a Danish group - the first one in my country.
~JM, Denmark

The problem with tunnel vision is we lose sight of valuable perceptions outside of the tunnel. Patient voice plays an integral role in the advancement of clinical practice. I engage in conversations every chance I get regarding pelvic organ prolapse; opportunities to discuss a health topic that has been shrouded in secrecy for thousands of years presents avenues to encourage healthcare evolution. As an advocate who guides women toward healthcare professionals for both surgical and nonsurgical treatment of POP, I encourage women to disclose symptoms and concerns that are often embarrassing to discuss. I feel strongly that we need to get past the discomfort zone and recognize that at its most basic level, pelvic organ prolapse is a health condition that is treatable, not a subject that needs to be hidden away behind closed doors.

POP is a common, cryptic health concern considered "not that big of a deal" by some members of the healthcare community, possibly because it is not life threatening as is cancer or heart disease. I'm here to tell you it is a big deal. This complex condition disables women from engaging in normal activities, reducing and often eliminating the capacity to engage, causes physical discomfort and emotional difficulties, impacts employment and fitness activities, engenders social isolation, causes sexual dysfunction and loss of self-esteem, and often result in multiple surgical procedures because of insufficient diagnostic clinician curriculum and inadequate screening and referral to women's pelvic health specialists. Every day I communicate with women in one of the various stages of this multi-faceted health concern. Every day I assure women that there are treatment options that can return their lives to balance. Every day I let women know they are not alone, that millions of other women are experiencing the same frustration the symptoms of POP generate. As a POP advocate, I'd like to encourage health care professionals who view POP as "not that big of a deal" to truly listen to their patients. And as a woman who has been surgically treated for POP and continues to do the right stuff to maintain pelvic floor integrity post-surgery, I am hopeful that in the near future we will be able to optimize pelvic floor health diagnosis and treatment. As of right now, we have a long journey ahead of us.

Clinicians obviously must base treatment on curriculum provided in medical school and residency, but too often insufficient emphasis is placed on listening to patient feedback. Women with pelvic organ prolapse simply want their clinicians to listen to them-to believe them-to treat them with the same respect we give our healthcare providers even if what we are disclosing to them flies in the face of what their schooling has taught them about pelvic organ prolapse. We need health care providers to see beyond it.

> *Listening and recognizing the challenges facing patients is critical to quality care. As a patient advocacy organization, we hear from women the frustration in their inability to communicate effectively with healthcare providers. We know that healthcare providers want the best for their patients, but as we better understand the patients emotional and physical challenges, then the better care we can provide.*
> ~Steven G. Gregg, PhD, National Association for Continence

The message is pretty simple - believe patients who express

they are experiencing pain or discomfort whether prior to treatment or after. Recognize that loss of intimacy is incredibly frustrating, and that POP invades the normalcy of patients' lives in a substantial way. The message to women is also pretty simple-hold your heads high, disclose your symptoms in entirety, and insist on your healthcare professional spending the time due you to discuss your treatment options. It is vital to remember that at their core, healthcare professionals are human, have good days and bad just like us, are incredibly busy treating a multitude of patients, and sometimes unintentionally get stuck in tunnel vision, treating all patients with pelvic organ prolapse the same when needs are incredibly unique from woman to woman.

Every generation of women since the dawn of the civilized world has engaged to some degree in forward momentum of women's awareness, health, and empowerment directives. In communications with women I've met along my journey to raise awareness of pelvic organ prolapse, I've heard countless stories regarding the physical, emotional, social, sexual, fitness, and employment POP quality of life impact to women's lives. Pelvic organ prolapse has been shrouded in silence for thousands of years; fortunately, the world at large is finally coming to terms with the reality of pelvic organ prolapse and as our voices become stronger and louder, women around the world will soon be familiar with POP.

The big picture regarding pelvic organ prolapse is as simple as it is for any other stigmatized health concern. There was a time no one could say the word breast out loud; we now freely and proudly shout our support of breast cancer, and encourage open dialogue regarding the impact to women's lives. The same holds true for erectile dysfunction (ED). Once stuffed in the closet, we now comfortably watch ED television commercials without flinching. The time has finally arrived to open the closet door and remove the stigma of the pelvic organ prolapse symptoms. POP is a health condition, nothing more, nothing less.

As we enlighten the world with POP information enabling women to comfortably share stories about their very personal experiences, and we become more educated about what is without a doubt one of the most common medical conditions women collectively experience, stigma will soften. Like most health concerns, awareness and open dialogue walk hand in hand to establish the new normal.

Studies frequently estimate that 50% of the female population will experience some form of pelvic organ prolapse. The dynamic varies a bit from country to country and from developed to developing regions of the world, but the bottom line is that POP is impacts the lives of countless millions of women globally. Since childbirth and menopause are the 2 leading causes of POP, women in every country in the world will continue to suffer silently with POP until we overcome symptom stigma.

It stands to reason that POP has been and will be around as long as women are. Regardless of location, socio-economic status, nationality, or religion, nearly all woman will have at least one risk factor for experiencing POP because most women who live long enough will experience menopause. It is unfortunate that many women currently choose to live out their lives in physical discomfort because they either don't understand what is occurring in their bodies or they are too embarrassed to discuss it with their physicians and the men in their lives. It is imperative that we change the status quo.

Above and beyond the quality of life impact of POP, is the basic need to feel healthy. When a woman must spend day after day with considerable POP impact to daily activities, it is difficult to functionally focus on anything else. As women, we are not trying to recapture the bodies we had at the age of 25. Superficial aspects of childbirth like stretch marks don't rattle our cages; that is a fair price to pay for the miracle of motherhood. We accept the shift in our shapes that comes after bearing children. All women with POP want at the end of the day is to simply feel normal again.

Ultimately, it is up to each woman as an individual to find the path that best suits her needs in the quest to address POP symptoms. For some it may be as simple as a pessary for support, for some it may be a combination of treatments, and for some it may be surgical repair. Every woman's needs are as unique as her body. Find a qualified clinician that fits your particular needs and move forward.

It is imperative that women with POP share what they learn along their journey and continue to push the POP dynamic forward so future generations of women can live in a world that recognizes, acknowledges, understands, and effectively addresses the extremely intricate and intimate impact of pelvic organ prolapse to our lives. Without a doubt, pelvic organ prolapse will generate the next significant shift in women's health.

APPENDIX A
TIPS AND TOOLS

TIPS

Bridging: Place the first two fingers against labia lips, apply gentle pressure to prevent a pessary from pushing out during defecation.

Splinting: Insert two fingers into the vagina and push against the vaginal wall to push a rectocele bulge back into alignment to enable defecation.

Heavy lifting: Avoid whenever possible. Contract your pelvic floor prior to lifting a child or other heavy weight. Hold a child or other heavy weight close to the body if you must lift.

Trust your judgement, avoid activities that generate pressure sensations to your pelvic floor.

Never strain during bowel movements despite constipation.

If possible, sit while coughing to reduce pressure on your pelvic floor.

Cross your legs and bend at the waist prior to sneezing to reduce downward pressure.

Request a standing pelvic exam if you have POP symptoms and a standard pelvic exam does not clarify POP incidence.

Be pro-active in addressing POP to optimize your quality of life.

Focus on what you can do, not on what you can't do, whether prior to surgery or post-surgery.

Say *no* to work, family, friends regarding activities POP inappropriate.

Whether or not you choose to have POP surgery, it is best to continue life-long POP maintenance for best quality of life.

Seek guidance from a women's health physical therapist/physiotherapist prior to choosing a fitness activity, particularly if you have a hypertonic (tight) pelvic floor.

Core, pelvic floor, posture, and hip stability all play a role in pelvic organ prolapse maintenance. Kegels must be performed correctly to be effective, contracting the pelvic floor muscles up and in. Posture is important to reduce pelvic pressure, pull your shoulders/chest up from your ribs with shoulders back. Contract your abdominal muscles, drawing your belly button up and in to support your core when possible.

APOPS recommendation for floor/core fitness training is the Hab-it DVD.

Eat a high fiber diet, preferably produce over grain based.

Increase water intake.

Raise knees with feet on a stool while sitting on the toilet to ease defecation.

POST-SURGICAL TOOLS
- Preemie baby diapers for ice bags.
- Hydrocortisone 1% cream.
- Colace Stool softener.
- KY Jelly.
- KY Ultra-Liquid or Liquid Silk.
- Foam or inflatable donut for sitting.
- Baby sippee cup or cup with attached straw.
- Sanitary napkins and panty-liners.

- Baby wipes.
- Loose clothing.
- Pain medication.
- Topical estrogen to aid healing of incisions if peri-menopausal or menopausal.
- Apples for fiber.

NON-SURGICAL TOOLS
- Pessary.
- Sea Sponge pessary.
- Impressa disposable pessary.
- Support garments.
- Heat.
- Rest.
- Rest with legs up a wall.
- Coconut oil for splinting, lubrication, and vaginal atrophy.
- ApexM medical device to strengthen pelvic floor.

CONSTIPATION TOOLS
- Magnesium.
- Miralax.
- Psyllium fiber (Metamucil)
- Flaxseed.
- Probiotics
- Increase water intake.
- Sodium docusate stool softener.
- Glycerin suppositories
- Squatty Potty or stool

FECAL INCONTINENCE AND FLATULENCE TOOLS
- Eclipse.

- Butterfly Pads.
- Imodium when traveling.
- Gas-X.

URINARY TRACT INFECTION TOOLS
- ❖ Cranberry supplement to help prevent a UTI.
- ❖ Drink ample water to flush system.
- ❖ AZO for burning.

APPENDIX B
RESOURCES

SUPPORT
Association for Pelvic Organ Prolapse Support (APOPS)
8225 State Rd 83
Mukwonago, WI 53149
http://www.pelvicorganprolapsesupport.org

HEALTHCARE PROFESSIONALS
Direct links can be found on the APOPS Practitioner Locator web
page at:
http://www.pelvicorganprolapsesupport.org/healthcareconnections/

Urogynecologists US/Canada: AUGS
http://www.voicesforpfd.org/p/cm/ld/fid=81

Urogynecologists Worldwide: IUGA
http://www.findurogynecologist.com/

Physical Therapists, Women's Health US: APTA
http://www.womenshealthapta.org/pt-locator/

Herman and Wallace Certified Pelvic Rehabilitation Practitioners
https://www.hermanwallace.com/list-of-certified-pelvic-
rehabilitation-practitioners

Women's Health Physiotherapists International, IOPTWH
http://www.wcpt.org/ioptwh

Myofascial Release Therapists
http://myofascialrelease.com/find-a-therapist/

Biofeedback Therapists, US: BCIA
http://certify.bcia.org/4dcgi/resctr/search.html

PHYSICIAN REVIEW SITES
http://www.ratemds.com

http://www.healthgrades.com

http://www.vitals.com

APPENDIX C
POP RISK FACTOR QUESTIONNAIRE (POP-RFQ)

The POP-RFQ can be downloaded from the APOPS website at: http://www.pelvicorganprolapsesupport.org/pop-risk-factor-questionnaire/.

If you are experiencing pelvic, vaginal, or rectal symptoms and suspect you have pelvic organ prolapse, this questionnaire provides preliminary information to initiate POP screening by a healthcare clinician. If you answer yes to POP risk factors detailed on this questionnaire, request POP screening by a primary care physician or gynecologist. Circle the applicable answer.

1. Have you had at least one vaginal birth?
   Yes   No   Number of births? _____
2. Did you experience a long labor, forceps, or suction delivery?
   Yes   No
3. Do you see of feel tissues bulging from your vagina?
   Yes   No
4. Are you in menopause?
   Yes   No
5. Do you leak urine when you sneeze, cough, or laugh?
   Yes   No
6. Do you have difficulty starting your urine stream?
   Yes   No
7. Have you experienced stool leakage?
   Yes   No
8. Have you had chronic constipation for over a year?
   Yes   No
9. Do you lift heavy weight at home or work (including children over 30#)?
   Yes   No
10. Do your tampons push out of place?

Yes   No

11. Have you had a hysterectomy?

Yes   No

12. Do you experience chronic coughing from allergies or emphysema?

Yes   No

13. Do you marathon run, jog, or engage in heavy lifting athletic activities?

Yes   No

14. Do you have back, pelvic, rectal, or vaginal pain?

Yes   No

15. Do you have vaginal or rectal pressure?

Yes   No

16. Do you have reduced sexual sensation?

Yes   No

17. Is intercourse painful?

Yes   No

18. Are you double-jointed?

Yes   No

This questionnaire is not meant to take the place of treatment from a health care practitioner. Always seek the advice of your physician on matters of personal health.

GLOSSARY

Adenomyosis: A benign inward growth of the uterine lining.

Biofeedback: A technique for making bodily processes perceptible to the senses so that they can be controlled or manipulated.

Bio-Identical Hormone Replacement: Natural hormones manufactured from soybeans or wild yams which duplicate and replace the hormones whose levels fall during peri-menopause and menopause.

Bladder: The sac in the pelvic region that retains urine until it is excreted from the body.

Bridging: Placement of the first two fingers against labia lips and applying gentle pressure to prevent a pessary from pushing out during defecation.

Catheter: A flexible tube inserted into the bladder to drain urine.

Coital Incontinence: Involuntary loss of urine in association with sexual intercourse.

Collagen: Fibrous protein in connective tissue.

Colpocleisis: A POP surgical procedure to close off the vaginal opening.

Cystocele: Prolapse in which the bladder shifts downward toward and into the vagina, pushing along with the front vaginal wall to the outside of the body.

Cystoscopy: A medical test for viewing the bladder and urethra.

Defecography (Proctography, dynamic rectal examination): A type of medical radiological imaging in which the mechanics of a patient's defecation are visualized in real time using a fluoroscope.

Elastin: A highly elastic protein in connective tissue which allows many tissues in the body to resume their shape after stretching or contracting.

Enterocele: Prolapse in which the small intestine shifts downward between the rectum and back wall of the vagina or between the uterus and front wall of the vagina.

Estrogen: A hormone in women that regulates sexual organs and their functions.

Female Pelvic Medicine Reconstructive Surgeon (FPMRS): A urogynecologist or urologist that specializes in clinical problems associated with dysfunction of the female pelvic floor, reproductive organs, bladder and bowels.

Fecal Incontinence: The inability to control bowel movements, causing stool (feces) to leak unexpectedly from the rectum.

Hormone Replacement Therapy (HRT): Synthetic or natural hormone replacement to supplement depleted levels.

Hysterectomy: Surgical removal of the uterus.

Incontinence: Inability to retain urine within the bladder or feces within the colon.

Irritable Bowel: A chronic disorder of the colon characterized by alternating diarrhea and constipation.

Kegel Exercises: Repetitive contractions of the pelvic floor pubococcygeus (PC muscle) used to control the flow of urine and to enhance sexual responsiveness.

Labia: The external areas of female genital lip tissue surrounding the vagina and clitoris.

Laparoscopic: Minimally invasive surgical procedure with small incisions.

Levator Ani: A broad, thin muscle situated on either side of the pelvis. It is formed from three muscle components: the puborectalis, the pubococcygeus muscle (which includes the puborectalis) and the iliococcygeus muscle, and is attached to the inner surface of each side of the lesser pelvis, forming the greater part of the pelvic floor.

Menopause: The natural regression of ovary function and cessation of menstruation.

Myofascial Release Therapy: A hands-on technique that involves applying gentle sustained pressure into the myofascial connective tissue restrictions to eliminate pain and restore motion.

Overactive Bladder (OAB): Urinary urgency, with or without urgency-associated urinary incontinence.

PAP Smear: A test for early detection of cancer of the cervix.

PC Muscle: The pubococcygeus muscle is a trampoline like muscle which sits at the base of the pelvic cavity, supporting the organs and tissues of the pelvic region. This muscle is also responsible for the ability to start and stop the flow of urine and impacts level of sexual sensation in the vaginal area. Also referred to as the pelvic floor muscle.

Pelvic Exam: A routine gynecological exam to check the internal and external tissues of the vagina, vulva, and labia.

Pelvic Floor Muscles: Refer to PC muscle.

Pelvic Organ Prolapse (POP): A condition in which an organ or organs and connecting tissues within the pelvic cavity shift in a downward direction out of their normal positions toward or into the vaginal canal, and/or to the outside of the body.

Peri-menopause: The period prior to menopause that is marked by fluctuating marked physical changes such as hot flashes or menstrual irregularity, due to a reduction of hormone levels.

Pessary: A synthetic device inserted into the vagina to support pelvic organs and tissues.

POP: Acronym for pelvic organ prolapse, a female health condition in which an organ or organs and connecting tissues within the pelvic cavity shift in a downward direction out of their normal positions toward or into the vaginal canal, and/or to the outside of the body.

Procidentia: The uterus pushes through the vaginal opening to rest completely outside of the body.

Pubococcygeus muscle (PC): A trampoline like muscle which sits at the base of the pelvic cavity, supporting organs and tissues above it, also referred to as the PC or pelvic floor muscle. This muscle is also responsible for the ability to start and stop the flow of urine and effects level of sexual sensation in the pubic/vaginal areas.

Rectocele: Prolapse in which the rectum bulges into the rear vaginal wall.

Speculum: Metal or plastic instrument used to hold the vagina open during a pelvic exam.

Splinting: Inserting two fingers into the vagina and pushing against the vaginal wall to push a rectocele bulge back into alignment to enable defecation.

Tibial Nerve Stimulation: Neuromodulation therapy used to treat overactive bladder (OAB) and the associated symptoms of urinary urgency, urinary frequency and urge incontinence.

Urethra: The tube that carries urine away from the bladder to the outside of the body.

Urethral Bulking Agents: A medical treatment used to treat urinary incontinence in women. Injectable materials are used to control stress incontinence.

Uterine Prolapse: Prolapse in which the uterus shifts down into the vagina and/or out of the body through the vaginal opening.

Urinary Incontinence: Inability to hold urine in the bladder due to loss of voluntary control over the urinary sphincters resulting in the involuntary passage of urine; stress urinary incontinence (SUI), urge urinary incontinence (UUI), and overactive bladder (OAB) are types of urinary incontinence.

Uterus: Hollow, pear-shaped organ that is located in a woman's lower abdomen, between the bladder and the rectum in which babies develop prior to birth.

Vagina: The muscular canal that extends between the uterus to the genital area outside of the body.

Vaginal Atrophy: An inflammation of the vagina (and the outer urinary tract) due to the thinning and shrinking of the tissues, as well as decreased lubrication.

Vaginal Vault Prolapse: The top of the vagina caves in on itself after the uterus is removed (hysterectomy).

BIBLIOGRAPHY

BOOKS
Culligan, Patrick J., ed, Roger P. Goldberg, ed. *Urogynecology in Primary Care.* London: Springer, 2007.

Goldberg, Roger P., *Ever Since I had My Baby.* New York: Three Rivers Press. 2003.

Reiss, Uzzi, and Mark Zucker. *Natural Hormone Balance for Women.* New York: Pocket Books, 2001.

Walters, Mark D and Mickey M. Karram. 2014. *Urogynecology and Reconstructive Surgery.* Philadelphia: Saunders.

PUBLICATIONS AND STUDIES
Abdel-fattah, M., Familusi, A., Felding, S., Ford, J., Bhattacharya, S. "Primary and repeat surgical treatment for female pelvic organ prolapse and incontinence in parous women in the UK: a register linkage study." *BMJ Journal* (2011) Accessed Dec 20, 2016. http://bmjopen.bmj.com/content/1/2/e000206.full

Alinsod, R. "Temperature Controlled Radiofrequency for Vulvovaginal Laxity" *prime-journal.com* July 23, 2015. Accessed Dec 20, 2016. https://www.prime-journal.com/temperature-controlled-radiofrequency-for-vulvovaginal-laxity/

Alinsod, R. "Transcutaneous temperature controlled radiofrequency for orgasmic dysfunction." *Lasers Surg Med.* 2016 Sep; 48(7): 641–645.

Published online 2016 May 19. doi: 10.1002/lsm.22537 PMCID: PMC5084776

Azubuike Uzoma, A., Farag, K.A. "Vaginal Vault Prolapse" *Obstet Gynecol Int.* 2009; 2009: 275621. (2009) Accessed Dec 20,

2016.
https://www.ncbi.nlm.nih.gov/pmc/articles/PMC2778877/#B3

Clark, A., Gregory, T., Smith, V., Edwards, R. "Epidemiologic Evaluation of Reoperation for Surgically Treated Pelvic Organ Prolapse and Urinary Incontinence." *Am J Obstet Gynecol.* 2003 Nov;189(5):1261-7. (2003) Accessed Dec 22, 2016.
https://www.ncbi.nlm.nih.gov/pubmed/14634551

Costa, Janitha, Towobola, Basirat, T, McDowel, C., Ashe, R. "Recurrent pelvic organ prolapse (POP) following traditional vaginal hysterectomy with or without colporrhaphy in an Irish population." *Ulster Med J.* 83(1): 16–21. (2014) Accessed Dec 22, 2016. https://www.ncbi.nlm.nih.gov/pmc/articles/PMC3992089/

Costantini, E., Porena, M., Giannitsas, K., Athanasopoulos, A., Balsamo, R., Masiello, G., Natale, F., Carbone, A., Mahfouz, W., Finazzi, Agrò E., Kocjancic, E., Illiano, E. "Coital Incontinence: Prevalence and Risk Factors in Incontinent Women."

ICS (2016) Accessed Dec 22, 2016.
https://www.ics.org/Abstracts/Publish/326/000299.pdf

DeLancey, J.O. "Anatomic aspects of vaginal eversion after hysterectomy." *American Journal of Obstetrics & Gynecology.* 1992;166(6, part 1):1717–1728. (1992) Accessed Dec 20, 2016. https://www.ncbi.nlm.nih.gov/pubmed/1615980

Downing, K.T. 2012. "Uterine Prolapse: From Antiquity to Today." *Obstetrics and Gynecology International,* Volume 2012, Article ID 649459, 9 pages. (2012) Accessed Dec 20, 2016. http://dx.doi.org/10.1155/2012/649459

Flynn, B.J., Webster G.D. "Surgical management of the apical vaginal defect." (2002) *Current Opinion in Urology.* 2002;12(4):353–358. Accessed Dec 22,

2016.https://www.ncbi.nlm.nih.gov/pubmed/12072658

Fowler, G.E. "Obstetric anal sphincter injury." ACPWH
CONFERENCE 2008.
*Journal of the Association of Chartered Physiotherapists in
Women's Health*, Spring 2009, 104, 12–19. (2009) Accessed Dec
22, 2016.
file:///C:/Users/sjpal/Downloads/fowler_hr.pdf

Handa, V.L., Garrett, E., Hendrix, S., Gold, E., Robbins, J.
"Progression and Remission of Pelvic Organ Prolapse: A
Longitudinal Study of Menopausal Women." *Am J Obstet
Gynecol.* 2004 Jan;190(1):27-32. Accessed on Dec 20, 2016.
https://www.ncbi.nlm.nih.gov/pubmed/14749630

Horst, Wagner. "Pelvic organ prolapse: prevalence and risk factors
in a Brazilian population." *Int Urogynecol J.* (2016) Accessed
January 7, 2017.
http://link.springer.com/article/10.1007/s00192-016-3238-7

Jackson S.L., Weber, Hull, A.M., Mitchinson, T.L., Walters, MD,
A.R.. "Fecal incontinence in women with urinary incontinence and
pelvic organ prolapse." *Obstet Gynecol.* 1997 Mar;89(3):423-7.
(1997) Accessed Dec 20, 2016.
https://www.ncbi.nlm.nih.gov/pubmed/9052598

Jelovsek, J. Erik, Brubaker, Linda, ed, Eckler, K, dep ed. "Pelvic
organ prolapse in women: Choosing a primary surgical procedure."
UpToDate. (2015) Accessed Dec 22, 2016.
http://www.uptodate.com/contents/pelvic-organ-prolapse-in-
women-choosing-a-primary-surgical-procedure

Kearney, R., Miller, J.M., Ashton-Miller, J.A., DeLancey, J.O.
"Obstetric factors associated with levator ani muscle injury after
vaginal birth." *Obstet Gynecol (2006)* 2006 Jan;107(1):144-9.

Accessed Dec 22, 2016.
https://www.ncbi.nlm.nih.gov/pubmed/16394052

Knowles, C.H., Horrocks, E.J., Bremner, S.A., Stevens, N., Norton, C. O'Connell, R., Eldridge, S. "Percutaneous tibial nerve stimulation versus sham electrical stimulation for the treatment of faecal incontinence in adults (CONFIDeNT): a double-blind, multicentre, pragmatic, parallel-group, randomised controlled trial." *The Lancet,* Volume 386, No. 10004, p1640–1648. (2015) Accessed Dec 22, 2016.
http://www.thelancet.com/journals/lancet/article/PIIS0140-6736(15)60314-2/fulltext?rss=yes

Larsen, W.I., Yavorek, T.A. "Pelvic organ prolapse and urinary incontinence in nulliparous women at the United States Military Academy." *Int Urogynecol J Pelvic Floor Dysfunct. (2006)* 2006 May;17(3):208-10. Epub 2005 Aug 3. Accessed Dec 22, 2016.
https://www.ncbi.nlm.nih.gov/pubmed/16077995

Lewicky-Gaupp, C., Margulies, R.U., Larson, L., Fenner, D.E., Morgan, D.M, DeLancey, J.O. "Self-perceived natural history of pelvic organ prolapse described by women presenting for treatment." Int Urogynecol J Pelvic Floor Dysfunct. 2009 Aug;20(8):927-31. doi: 10.1007/s00192-009-0890-1. Epub 2009 Apr 24. Accessed Dec 22, 2016.
https://www.ncbi.nlm.nih.gov/pubmed/19390760

Memon, H., Handa, V. "Vaginal childbirth and pelvic floor disorders." *Womens Health* (Lond Engl). May; 9(3): 10.2217/whe.13.17. (2013) Accessed Dec 22, 2016.
https://www.ncbi.nlm.nih.gov/pmc/articles/PMC3877300/ doi: 10.2217/whe.13.17

Parker, M. A., Millar, L. A., Dugan, S. A. "Diastasis Rectus Abdominis and Lumbo-Pelvic Pain and Dysfunction – Are They

Related?" *Journal of Women's Health Physical Therapy*: Summer
2009 - Volume 33 - Issue 2 - p 15–22. (2009) Accessed Dec 20,
2016.
http://journals.lww.com/jwhpt/Abstract/2009/33020/Diastasis_Rec
tus_Abdominis_and_Lumbo_Pelvic_Pain.3.aspx

Pitsouni, E., Grigoriadis, T., Tsiveleka, A., Zacharakis, D.,
Salvatore, S., Athanasiou, S.

"Microablative fractional CO2-laser therapy and the genitourinary
syndrome of menopause: An observational study." *Maturitas.* 2016
Dec; 94:131-136. doi: 10.1016/j.maturitas.2016.09.012. Epub 2016
Sep 16. Accessed January 15, 2017.
https://www.ncbi.nlm.nih.gov/pubmed/27823733

Serati, M., Salvatore, S., Uccella, S., Nappi, R.E., Bolis, P.
"Female urinary incontinence during intercourse: a review on an
understudied problem for women's sexuality." *J Sex Med.* 2009
Jan;6(1):40-8. doi: 10.1111/j.1743-6109.2008.01055.x. (2009)
Accessed Dec 22, 2016.
https://www.ncbi.nlm.nih.gov/pubmed/19170835

Slieker-ten Hove, Marijke C., corr author, Pool-Goudzwaard, A.
L., Eijkemans, M.J., Steegers-Theunissen, R.P., Curt W. Burger,
C.W., Vierhout, M.E. "The prevalence of pelvic organ prolapse
symptoms and signs and their relation with bladder and bowel
disorders in a general female population." *Int Urogynecol J* Pelvic
Floor Dysfunct. (2009) Sep; 20(9): 1037–1045. (2009) doi:
10.1007/s00192-009-0902-1. Accessed Dec 22. 2016.
https://www.ncbi.nlm.nih.gov/pmc/articles/PMC2721135/

Sokol, E.R. "Management of fecal incontinence – focus on a
vaginal insert for bowel control." *Med Devices (Auckl).* 2016; 9:
85–91. Published online 2016 May 10. doi:
10.2147/MDER.S86483 PMCID: PMC4869843

Staskin, D.R. corre author, Peters, K.M., Macdiarmid, S., Shore, N., Groat, W.C. "Percutaneous Tibial Nerve Stimulation: A Clinically and Cost Effective Addition to the Overactive Bladder Algorithm of Care." *NCBI*

Curr Urol Rep. 2012 Oct; 13(5): 327–334.
Published online 2012 Aug 15. doi: 10.1007/s11934-012-0274-9
PMCID: PMC3438389. (2012) Accessed Dec 22, 2016.
https://www.ncbi.nlm.nih.gov/pmc/articles/PMC3438389/

Subak, L.L., Waetien, E., Ven Den Eeden, S.K. "Cost of Pelvic Organ Prolapse Surgery in the United States." *Obstetrics and Gynecology* 98(4):646-651.
DOI: 10.1097/00006250-200110000-00021. (2001) Accessed Dec 22, 2016.
https://www.researchgate.net/publication/297610139_Cost_of_Pelvic_Organ_Prolapse_Surgery_in_the_United_States.

Weber. A.M. Richter, H.E. "Pelvic Organ Prolapse" *ACOG Clinical Expert Series* (2005) Accessed Dec 22, 2016.
http://www.themamasphysio.com/uploads/2/1/7/0/21707056/pelvic_organ_prolapse.pdf

Wu, J.M., Vaughan, C.P., Goode, P.S., Redden, D.T., Bugio, K.L., Richter, H.E., Markland, A.D. "Prevalence and trends of symptomatic pelvic floor disorders in U.S. women." *Obstet Gynecol.* 123(1):141-8. doi: 10.1097/AOG.0000000000000057. (2014) Accessed Dec 22, 2016.
https://www.ncbi.nlm.nih.gov/pmc/articles/PMC3970401/

Wu, J.M, Hundley, A.F., Fulton, R.G., Myers, E.R. "Forecasting the prevalence of pelvic floor disorders in U.S. Women: *2010 to 2050.*" *Obstet Gynecol.* 2009 Dec;114(6):1278-83. doi: 10.1097/AOG.0b013e3181c2ce96. (2009) Accessed Dec 20, 2016.
https://www.ncbi.nlm.nih.gov/pubmed/19935030

WEB ARTICLES
"Abdominal Separation (Diastasis Recti)." *WebMD* Accessed Dec 20, 2016.
http://www.webmd.com/baby/guide/abdominal-separation-diastasis-recti#1

Alinsod, R. "What are the Differences Between ThermiVa Radiofrequency and FemiLift/MonaLisa/IntimaLase lasers for use in Aesthetic Vulvovaginal Therapies?" *Linkedin*. (2015). Accessed December 22, 2016. https://www.linkedin.com/pulse/what-differences-between-thermiva-radiofrequency-use-alinsod-m-d-?trk=hp-feed-article-title-share

"Bladder Control Problems in Women (Urinary Incontinence)." *NIH* Accessed Dec 20, 2016. https://www.niddk.nih.gov/health-information/urologic-diseases/bladder-control-problems-women

"Bowel Control Problems (Fecal Incontinence)." *NIH* Accessed Dec 20, 2016. https://www.niddk.nih.gov/health-information/digestive-diseases/bowel-control-problems-fecal-incontinence

"Fecal Incontinence." *Voices for PFD* Accessed Dec 22, 2016 http://www.voicesforpfd.org/p/cm/ld/fid=141

"Hysterectomy" *National Women's Health Network* Accessed Dec 20, 2016. https://www.nwhn.org/hysterectomy/

Iglesia, C. "Transvaginal mesh for prolapse: Where are we in 2016?" *OBG Management.* Accessed Dec 20, 2016. http://www.mdedge.com/obgmanagement/article/107051/gynecology/transvaginal-mesh-prolapse-where-are-we-2016

Lee, Diane. "Diastasis Rectus Abdominis – Should we Open or Close the Gap?" Int Pelvic Pain Society. Accessed Dec 20, 2016.

http://pelvicpain.org/professional/blog/ipps-blog/november-2016/diastasis-rectus-abdominis-%E2%80%93-should-we-open-or-clo.aspx

Lukacz, E.S., Nager, C.W., Hsu, J.Y. "Kaiser Permanente Study Shows 1 in 3 Women has Pelvic Floor Disorder." (2008).

Eurakalert (2008) Accessed Dec 20, 2016.
https://www.eurekalert.org/pub_releases/2008-02/kpdo-kps022608.php

Rosenman, A. "Pelvic Organ Prolapse." *HealthyWomen.org*
Accessed Dec 20, 2016.
http://www.healthywomen.org/condition/pelvic-organ-prolapse

Siegel, A. "The Ins and Outs of the Vagina." *Our Greatest Wealth is Health*
Accessed Dec 20, 2016.
https://healthdoc13.wordpress.com/2016/11/19/the-ins-and-outs-of-the-vagina/

"Statistics and Research." *Running USA* Accessed Dec 20, 2016.
http://www.runningusa.org/statistics

"Uterine Prolapse" *Physiopedia* Accessed Dec 20, 2016.
http://www.physio-pedia.com/Uterine_Prolapse
Wakamatsu, M.M. "How much money do Americans spend coping with urinary incontinence?" *Sharecare* Accessed Dec 20, 2016.
https://www.sharecare.com/health/urinary-incontinence/how-money-spend-urinary-incontinence

INDEX

A

Abdominal pain 72
Adenomyosis 125, 146
Age related muscle loss 9
ApexM 53, 140

B

Biofeedback 143, 146
Bio-identical hormone
    replacement 9, 52, 146
Bladder 20, 27, 28-29
Bridging 138, 146

C

Catheter 9, 95, 146
Childbirth 3, 8, 15, 28, 123
Chronic coughing 114, 145
Coital incontinence 20, 26,
    31, 107, 148
Collagen 11, 55, 60, 145
Colpocleisis 82-84, 146
Constipation 8, 11-12, 26, 29
C-section 8-9
Cystocele 19-21
Cystoscopy 40, 44, 146

D

Defecography 40, 44, 147
Diagnostic tests 42
Diastasis rectus abdominus 8,
    114

E

Elastin 60, 63, 147
Electrical stimulation 46, 52-
    53
Enterocele 14, 22-23
Estrogen 9, 43, 51, 75, 113-
    114, 147
Exercise 16, 46, 57

F

Fecal incontinence 9, 26, 31,
    33
FPMRS (female pelvic
    medicine reconstructive
    surgeon) 36-37, 45

G

Genetics 8, 10, 115

H

Heavy lifting 4, 8, 12, 42,
    138
Hormone replacement
    therapy 9, 51-52, 147
Hysterectomy 8, 13-14, 22,
    27, 81

I

IBS 11-12, 29-30
Incontinence 49, 51, 58, 72,
    107

Irritable bowel 11, 129, 147

K
Kegel exercise 46-50, 121-123, 148
KY Jelly 99, 104, 139
KY Ultra Liquid 96, 98, 104

L
Labia 76, 98, 104, 138, 146
Laparoscopic 82, 94, 148
Levator ani 47, 148

M
Marfan syndrome 11, 115
Menopause 3, 9, 43-44, 61, 98, 148
Multiple schlerosis 15
Myofascial release therapy 42, 46, 54, 148

N
Non-surgical options 37, 45, 93

O
Obesity 8, 13, 115
Overactive bladder 60, 70, 148

P
Painful intercourse 26, 32-33
Pap 36, 61, 148
PC muscle 3, 39, 43, 47-50, 121, 148
Pelvic exam 3, 26, 39, 138, 149
Pelvic floor muscle 3, 8-11, 35, 47, 53, 57, 149
Peri-menopause 149
Pessary 50-51, 71-77
Pressure 11-13, 20, 22, 26, 30, 82, 122, 138
Procidentia 20, 149
Prolapse symptoms 40
Pubococcygeus muscle 43, 47, 149

R
Rectal pain 26, 30

S
Speculum 3, 40, 150
Splinting 20, 138, 150
Stool leakage 144
Support garments 42, 46, 59, 140

T
Tibial nerve stimulation 46, 53, 150
Treatment options 3, 37, 39, 134-135
Trimo-san 75

U
Urethra 2, 20, 29, 42, 44, 58, 150

Urethral bulking agents 46,
  58
Urinary incontinence 26, 28,
  42-43, 150
Urine retention 26, 29, 43, 59
Uterine prolapse 19, 21, 150
Uterus 13-14, 20-21, 81, 150

V
Vagina 22-23, 30-31, 35-36,
  41, 144, 151
Vaginal atrophy 32, 60
Vaginal vault prolapse 14,
  20, 22, 81-82, 151

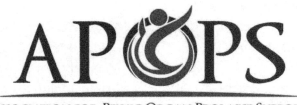

ABOUT APOPS

Association for Pelvic Organ Prolapse Support (APOPS) is a USA based 501(c)(3) nonprofit advocacy agency with global arms, founded by Sherrie Palm in September 2010 to generate awareness of pelvic organ prolapse (POP), to provide support and guidance to women navigating the physical, emotional, social, sexual, fitness, and employment impact of POP, and to bridge patients, healthcare, industry, research, academia, and policy-makers for the betterment of POP understanding and treatment evolution.

MISSION STATEMENT

APOPS mission is to advance global pelvic organ prolapse awareness, guidance, and support, and to innovate universal POP healthcare, education, and research.

VISION STATEMENT

APOPS vision is international evolution of pelvic organ prolapse awareness and understanding to optimize women's pelvic health empowerment.

> *Millions of women worldwide suffer in silence from the physical, emotional, social, and sexual ramifications of POP. Awareness of pelvic organ prolapse will not manifest until we freely share what we know with others. As we continue to nurture, guide, support, and network with women navigating pelvic organ prolapse, POP will become common knowledge.*
> ~Sherrie Palm

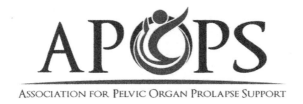

ASSOCIATION FOR PELVIC ORGAN PROLAPSE SUPPORT

September 8, 2010

From the beginning of this journey, I knew I wanted to connect with women on a deeper level about the impact POP has on our lives. Those of us who have already been diagnosed and treated for POP understand the distress women newly diagnosed are going through. It can be frustrating to dissect the information available; is the data we have access to accurate, which information applies to us personally, are treatments or surgery the best path. It takes a bit of time to figure out the right course to take.

My vision for APOPS is simple - women who are a bit further down the path of POP awareness connecting with women who are newly diagnosed. Together we will find the information that will assist our paths. Together we will guide, support, and nurture. Together we will shift the awareness curve by passing the information we gain on to the younger generation.

I have no doubt that with the strength and determination women bring to the table, we will change the mindset of the world at large regarding pelvic organ prolapse from a common female health concern that gets little acknowledgement to a widely-recognized condition that is addressed in terms of prevention, early recognition for less aggressive treatment, and maintenance for continuing quality of life. With your help, we can change the world.

My continuing gratitude to you all!

Sherrie Palm, Founder
Association for Pelvic Organ Prolapse Support

ABOUT THE AUTHOR

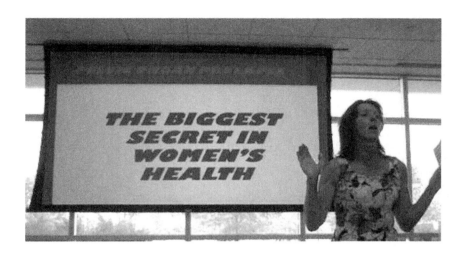

Sherrie Palm is the Founder/CEO/Executive Director of the Association for Pelvic Organ Prolapse Support (APOPS), a POP Key Opinion Leader, author of the award-winning book Pelvic Organ Prolapse: *The Silent Epidemic*, a speaker on multiple aspects of pelvic organ prolapse quality of life impact, and an internationally recognized women's pelvic health advocate. Sherrie's points of focus are generating global pelvic organ prolapse awareness, developing guidance and support structures for women navigating POP, and bridge building within POP healthcare, research, academia, industry and policy maker sectors toward the evolution of POP directives.

Submit queries about APOPS, pelvic organ prolapse, or Ms. Palm's speaking availability via:

APOPS landline: 262-642-4338
info.apops@gmail.com
http://www.pelvicorganprolapsesupport.org/contact

The Making of a 20th Century Woman

A Memoir

By Dorothy Marshall

Edited by David Edge Marshall

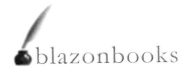blazonbooks

First published 2003
by Blazonbooks
239 Old Street
London
EC1V 9EY
www.blazonbooks.com

Copyright © The Estate of the late Dorothy Marshall
2003

Dorothy Marshall is hereby identified as the author of
this work in accordance with the Copyright, Designs
and Patents Act 1988.

David Edge Marshall is hereby identified as the
editor of this work in accordance with the Copyright,
Designs and Patents Act 1988.

ISBN 0 9545 7599 7

Dedicated to our father, killed in action on 10th May 1944, and our mother, who missed him so much.

David Edge Marshall
Nicholas William Marshall

3

Acknowledgements

Many people have worked hard to bring this memoir into being. Kate Perry, archivist at the library of Girton College, Cambridge, found most of the missing chapter on South Africa, and kindly provided access to many of the images throughout this book. Lancaster University kindly gave their consent to reproduce the transcripts in Appendix 3. The London School of Economics also kindly provided access to the images on page 206. Sarah Beauchamp Gregory contributed hours of her time transcribing the book to a publishable level. Chris Brennan provided valuable technical support and an introduction to Emma Cahill who delivered the book into the world. The support of many of Dorothy's friends, former colleagues and old students has been invaluable in keeping this project alive.

However, the greatest thanks must go to Brian Watkins, an old student and friend of Dorothy's, who has worked hard over many years to drive this project. Indeed, without his tireless and dedicated efforts, there would not be any chance of these memoirs seeing the light of day. For this, Dorothy would be immeasurably grateful.

David Edge Marshall
November 2003

CONTENTS

Publications by Dorothy Marshall   7
Editorial note   8

CHAPTER ONE: THE EARLY YEARS   11

CHAPTER TWO: CAMBRIDGE IN WARTIME.   41

CHPTER THREE: "THE HEROES" RETURN   69

CHAPTER FOUR: AUTUMN 1919   95

CHAPTER FIVE: THE SOCIAL WHIRL   123

CHAPTER SIX: GOING FOR GOLD   151

CHAPTER SEVEN: A CAMBRIDGE FIRST   183

CHAPTER EIGHT: THE LONDON SCHOOL OF   227
                      ECONOMICS (LASKI AND
                      FRIENDS)

CHAPTER NINE: THE VASSAR DIARY   247

CHAPTER TEN: VASSAR IN CONTEXT   273

CHAPTER ELEVEN: REFLECTIONS ON AMERICA
                      (AND THE WAY AHEAD)   301

CHAPTER TWELVE: WITWATERSRAND AND
                      SOUTH AFRICA   329

CHAPTER THIRTEEN: FAREWELL TO SOUTH
                      AFRICA   353

CHAPTER FOURTEEN: AN EPILOGUE   379

Appendices   389
Index   409

Publications by Dorothy Marshall.

1926   *English Poor in the 18th Century: a Study in Social and Administrative History* (PhD Thesis). Reprinted 1969 by Routledge; 1980: Kelley, USA.

1929   *The English Domestic Servant in History* A pamphlet published by the Economic History Association in 1949. First published as "The Domestic Servants of the 18th Century", Economica, Vol. IX, No. 25, 1929. Paperback edition 1968, The Historical Association.

1938   *The Rise of George Canning* London, Longman. Introduction by Harold Temperley.

1956   *English People in the 18th Century* London, Longman. Second edition 1980: Greenwood Press.

1962   *Eighteenth Century England* London, Longman. Reprinted in 1966, second edition in 1974, History of England in 10 volumes.

1966   *John Wesley* Oxford University Press

1968   *Dr. Johnson's London* John Wiley and Sons Inc..

1972   *The Life and Times of Victoria* London, Weidenfeld and Nicholson in their Kings and Queens series. Also in New York by Praeger in 1974. Paperback edition 1998, National Book Network.

1973   *Industrial England 1776-1851* London, Routledge. Paperback edition 1982.

1975   *Lord Melbourne* London, Weidenfeld and Nicolson.

1977   *Fanny Kemble* London: Weidenfeld and Nicholson.

EDITORIAL NOTE

As you will see from the first few words in Chapter 1, these memoirs were started in April 1987. My aunt, Dr Dorothy Marshall, died on the 13th February 1994.

In about 1988, she was asked to submit a sample of her manuscript. Her notes were always untidy and indeed her handwriting was extremely difficult to read, but for whatever reason, Chapter 12 got lost. Also, I think, she was very disappointed that her previous book 'Fanny Kemble', which was considered by many to have been her best work, was remaindered. These facts, plus her age (she was by then 88) caused her to lose heart, and she never pursued trying to get this published any further. She had appeared in a BBC television documentary and also in Angela Holdsworth's book of the same title 'Out of the Doll's House' that year, and had hoped to publish her autobiography to supplement this.

It was not until after she had died, and after all her papers were lodged in the archives at Girton College Cambridge, that the Archivist, Kate Perry, found the missing chapter. Even now, however, there are still some passages missing. This is sad because it is the culmination of her story, and sheds a lot of light on modern racial attitudes, how fascism spread in the thirties and the growth of apartheid in South Africa.

There are other quaint little incidents. For instance, how did anyone persuade her to get into a Gypsy Moth aircraft and allow herself to be flown in it? She was always afraid of flying, even in a modern Jumbo jet. I am afraid these little stories have now been lost forever. Also, because it was the lost chapter, it is not as polished as the rest of her writings. To me it seems jagged, like the rough diamonds found in that part of the world, being near Johannesburg.

In addition to these facts, she makes references to articles she had collected on her travels. Alas when her cottage in Old Hutton was cleared, some of these items went missing. Therefore, when reading these memoirs, these facts should be born in mind. I think however it would be wrong for me to alter what my aunt has written. To do so would be to change her autobiography, so I will therefore write an introduction to Chapter 12 and make notes where necessary.

Also, I will write an extra chapter, Chapter 14, which will in fact be an epilogue at the end of her first thirty years of the 20th century, and a summary of the rest of her life.

I find it odd that there were 13 chapters in, this book as my aunt was notorious for being superstitious. I remember on one occasion when we had attended an evening service, during which the vicar had preached a sermon on superstitions, my aunt insisted on bowing to the new moon seven times as we left the church. Poor vicar, he must have thought his sermon was preached in vain. There are many such amusing stories in these memoirs, which is the best reason I can think of for leaving the rest of the script as she wrote it.

David Edge Marshall.

CHAPTER ONE: THE EARLY YEARS.

I was born at Morecambe on Monday, 26th March 1900; I had my 87th birthday a month ago. The world I knew began to disappear with the First World War, which will always be to me 'The War'. I was born into one world; I shall die in another. I can just claim to be a Victorian.

The advantage of my long life is that I have memories of a world that most people today have never known. To the student of the eighties it must seem a quaint world, laughable or pathetic according to their point of view. My early world was bounded by my nursery. In the modern world only the well-heeled can afford a nursery and the equivalent of a nanny. 'Mother's help' is the term perhaps more accurately applied to the ruler of the non-aristocratic nursery, such as my own. After the age of seven 'governess' would have been the normal title. My father was a school master, not a salaried one but the headmaster of a school into which he had invested both his academic and his financial capital and there was always some one to look after me, my mother being much occupied with the domestic side of what was grandly known as Lancaster College. My nursery was a Peter Pan sort of a room. There was a high fender round the fireplace, a big rocking horse, an old fashioned rocking chair on runners, capable of being transformed by a child's imagination into a thing of magic. Behind a curtain was the toy cupboard. Teddy bears had not yet dominated the nursery world. My best beloved was a monkey called Beppo. He was made of natural skin and I can still recall the bare patch much loving had worn on his chest. I was never much of a 'little mother' type of child. Though I can vaguely remember an elegantly dressed doll that my parents had brought me from Paris I cannot remember having cared for any of my dolls. Indeed family tradition says that on one occasion, the window being conveniently open, I was heard to say, as I picked up one victim of my lack of maternal feeling and flung it out, 'There goes another heaven child.' At least my religious education must have started early!

My favourite toys were lead soldiers and a painted fortress. With these I could play endlessly. Perhaps this addiction was due to the fact that I was a war baby. When I was born the Boer War, like Queen Victoria, was nearing the end. The first song that I can recall was:

> 'Good-bye Dolly I must leave you,
>
> Though it breaks my heart to go,
>
> Something tells me I am wanted,
>
> To fight the foreign foe.
>
> I can hear the bugles calling,
>
> I can no longer stay.
>
> Good-bye Dolly I must leave you,
>
> Good-bye Dolly Grey.'

My first political memory also had war as its background. The war was the Russian Japanese war and the incident that impressed itself on my mind was the bizarre one when the Russians fired on the English North Sea fishing fleet under the delusion that it was a Japanese flotilla. Why this fragment of history should have been so remembered at so early an age I have no idea. I can only suppose that Morecambe, where so many men were fishermen, for some days must have talked of little else and some of that excitement must have penetrated into my nursery.

The first eight years of my childhood were closely linked with the sight and sound of the sea. My nursery window looked over the dramatic expanse of Morecambe Bay with its backcloth of the Lakeland hills. Even today when travelling North my heart takes a sudden lift as the train runs into Lancaster station. I am home again. I remember standing at my nursery window watching while a furious storm battered and broke the North End pier and seeing the shattered wooden pieces bobbing in the swirling water. Later my father took me out to look at the flooded houses in the vulnerable areas of the town. That was before the pier, and especially the pierrots, became a part of my daily life. By then my brother William had been born, an event that was etched on my memory. I was five years old. In those days babies were born at home and the household had clearly little time to give to me. It fell to my father to struggle to do up my little boots with a buttonhook before taking me to my grandmother who lived a few minutes walk away. I did not in the least realise the importance of the occasion.

What impressed itself on me was that it was my Father who was struggling with what was women's work. I can see those unevenly buttoned boots still. It was two years later that nineteen year old Minnie Abbot became our governess and that she and Morecambe Pier became an integral part of our lives.

It was on the pier that we took our daily exercise, a routine made more exciting by a pierrot troop who during the season gave performances on an outside stage. This was a far cry from the sophistication of today. They wore the regulation white suits and conical hats with black pompons on them. That their performance was given in the open air suited both us and our purse admirably. There was no entrance fee and such financial reward as they were able to secure was collected at frequent intervals in one of those conical hats. We had our own routine for dealing with the situation. The first time round Dabbott (William's infantile attempt to pronounce her name, which was to re-christen her for the rest of her life) put a penny in the proffered hat. Knowing the programme well from much familiarity when we judged that the time for another collection was approaching we would wander off, returning for another instalment when the financial danger was safely past. I do not remember the number of times this manoeuvre was repeated daily but I do know that I acquired a fine repertoire of popular songs, both sentimental and topical. Indeed decades later when lecturing on English History at Wellesley College in the USA, I illustrated a few outstanding landmarks in political or social history by singing, no doubt out of tune, such ditties as:

'In the year nineteen hundred and ten

We'll have Winston Prime Minister then,

But we'll muzzle him first, or with speeches he'll burst

In the year nineteen hundred and ten.'

The arrival of mechanical transport on our roads were selected by such songs as:

'Get out of the way, get out of the way,

Here comes the motor car

There's twenty bobbies after us,

And we don't know where we are.

14

We've killed a horse, and a donkey too

And a pig in passing by

Get out of the way, get out of our way,

Hi, Hi, Hi.'

The taxi cab we were told was:

'Better than taking a trip to Spain

Or having your honeymoon

Over again.'

While in more humble vein, Daisie was implored to sample married life on a bicycle made for two. Or more adventurously young ladies were invited to go, 'Up in the sky, ever so high, sailing in my balloon'.

With the sea almost literally on his doorstep and the fisher folk an important part of Morecambe life, my father too fell a victim to its lure. He bought a boat, a leaky small craft that to my delight he re-christened *The Dorothy*. From that day forward, until he was too old to handle one, messing about in boats became his interest and hobby. It was not an enthusiasm that my mother shared, nor looking back can I blame her, so I was usually my father's sole companion. I don't ever recall William and Dabbott joining us, and anyway, *The Dorothy* was not the safest of vessels for an active two year old. But to me to go fishing for dabs on a sunny afternoon was pure bliss, even though more than once my mother refused to allow us to eat the catch that we so proudly brought home, on the grounds that caught so near the shore, they were bound to be polluted. She was probably right. At that time there was a ship breaking yard for smaller vessels and I became something of an expert in identifying them as they sailed,

15

distinguishing a brig from a brigantine, a schooner from a yawl. Now even their names have half vanished from my memory and all my childish expertise is lost but the magic of an ocean voyage remains.

Though it was often to be renewed throughout my life this daily link with the sea came to an end when my father decided to move into quarters more suitable for a boarding school and rented Leighton Hall, near Carnforth, from the Gillows, although as my aunt lived at Blackpool I was never entirely cut off from it. Nor was my father. *The Dorothy*, who was old and leaky, he abandoned at Morecambe but he decided not only to acquire another boat but to have it built to his liking. It was the proximity of Arnside, with its small but prosperous boat building yard that made this a practical scheme. Saturday afternoons were the highlight of my week. Our link with the outside world was not, as it would have been today, the car but the horse and trap. My father rather fancied himself as a driver and often he would drive tandem. On hot summer days the hedges would be white with dust from the unmade road. Our routine was always the same. We would drive to the inn where we stabled the horses, my father always seeing that they had their oats and water before we left. Then we would walk to the shipyard where our boat was being built. At my request it was to be named *Maid Marion*: I was a devoted admirer of Robin Hood. Next came tea with boiled eggs before the horses were harnessed and another wonderful Saturday was over.

Later, *Maid Marion* having been duly launched, when the tide was in, we sailed her. Then it was not boiled eggs at the inn but sardines and tea in enamel mugs brewed from a kettle boiled on a primus stove, the milk being provided by Nestlé's condensed milk. My early familiarity with a primus stove was to prove useful later in my student days. In the years that followed I cannot claim to have been a genuine yachtswoman but teenage memories is the wonderful sensation of handling a boat and feeling it move beneath one.

My next encounter with the sea was to provide me with a romantic attachment to the Royal Navy and incidentally to the Royal Family in the person of the future George VI. I had been suffering from some childish ailment, mumps or whooping cough, it is immaterial which, and it was deemed advisable to speed my recovery by a change of air. Why Lamlash on the isle of Arran was chosen for this holiday I have no idea, but we could not have chosen a more dramatic place for my convalescence in the spring of 1913.

Lamlash Bay was a magnificent natural harbour and the Irish, under Sir Edward Carson, were threatening rebellion. So politically there was no more suitable a place for the first battle squadron from which to keep an eye on the restless men of Ulster. I was thirteen and Dabbott twenty five and we were both incurably romantic. We haunted the quay and watched the liberty boats chug to and fro. For me there was the additional thrill of one of them being commanded by a real live prince. Young Prince Albert was a midshipman. I worshipped from afar while Dabbott, preferring someone a trifle older, concentrated on a lanky sub-lieutenant, whose name we found out from the warrant officers always to be found on the quay, was Robert Bower. From the same source of information we also learnt that the Prince was known on board as the lobster, because he blushed so easily. My cup of delight was filled when it was he who was in charge of the launch that took visitors to the *Collingwood* when that ship was acting as hostess to the public on the Sunday afternoon.

When in August the first World War broke out the fleet was a reality to us. We had lived, however briefly, with famous ships such as the *Iron Duke*, almost on our doorstep. We were personally involved and Almighty Saviour Strong to Save became our favourite hymn and almost battle cry. The next time I was to see my prince in the flesh was when, as a student, I saw him from the gallery of the Cambridge Union.

If Morecambe was the first chapter in my life, then the move to Leighton Hall was the second. The mansion, for indeed it can be justly so described, the foundations of which went back to medieval times, stood in an extensive parkland. The grounds, excluding the park, made a wonderful background for a growing child. A large shrubbery provided trees to climb as well as a splendid setting for the exploits of Robin Hood and his merry men. There was a large walled kitchen garden and it was our joy, to the wrath of the crotchety old gardener, to climb onto its flat top and run round it. There was also a large artificial pond, known as the reservoir. What its original purpose was I never knew but it was a wonderful place for catching tadpoles in jam jars. Near at hand there was a large storeroom full of junk including several old fashioned hip baths, relics of the days before modern plumbing was installed. These made an excellent nursery for tadpoles and newts. These delights I shared with my father's pupils. My playmates were boys not girls and I did not find this strange.

The school itself mirrored the social pattern of Edwardian England. It offered a general education to boys whose ages ranged from nine to sixteen and over. Such schools filled an educational gap in that they provided for the sons of those people who did not wish to send their offspring to the Board Schools, but equally would never aspire to the public schools where 'the gentry' went. I still have an old prospectus that makes odd economic reading today. For boys below ten the basic fees were fourteen guineas a term, for those between ten and sixteen, eighteen guineas, and above that twenty. In addition there were extras such as drawing, music, and 3s.6d. for pew rent. The older boys could be described as young men and were mostly foreigners who had come to learn English. There were some Spaniards, one Erenisto came from Brazil, another Tewfik, who remained a life long family friend and in whose house in Istanbul I was later to stay more than once. Perhaps the most unexpected of the overseas pupils were three from Nigeria, Quar, Quamina and Isaac. How they came to board with us I do not know. Whether my father had no colour prejudice or whether he was tempted by their fees it would be interesting to know. My mother was plainly uneasy for her young daughter and I was watched carefully so that

I should not be left alone with them. There was no need for such caution. No one could have been more gentle or kind than my three black friends. I wonder sometimes if their presence so early in my life left any lasting impression on my mind, but I have never been conscious of racial prejudice. The only unpleasant experience I had during my five years as a member of a masculine community came from my own curiosity. I was perfectly familiar with the facts of life in so far as they appertained to rabbits and pet mice and cats. They carried their young inside them until, in due time, they produced their babies. I was however curious as to how these small creatures got inside their mothers and Edwardian parents did not think it suitable to inform their children on such matters. Accordingly, I looked for information elsewhere. Young Richards the gardener's son was our groom and seemed someone likely to know the answer. Probably I pestered him. Probably too, as a countryman he saw no great harm in satisfying my curiosity. He proceeded to unbutton his fly and bring out a repulsive looking object remarkably like a carrot. Some instinct made me turn and flee saying 'I don't want to see. I don't want to see.' This same instinct prevented me from ever telling anyone of this sudden revelation, but looking back, in all honesty I don't think it had the slightest influence on my later emotional development. I was too young and too innocent for it to register.

My own playmates were drawn from the younger boys with whom I shared my lessons in the classroom. One in particular was my boon companion. His name was Kenneth Crawshaw and his father was a Yorkshire woollen manufacturer. He must have been an amenable youngster; he was certainly my first boyfriend. We shared a special hiding place, which like mice, we had constructed under the roof of the Dutch barn where our hay was stored. We would sneak up the ladder when no one was about and wriggle through a disguised light barricade of hay into our hollowed out retreat. With what adventures we credited ourselves or played out in our hide-away I no longer remember, but for the ordinary sports in which school boys play I had very little desire or aptitude. True I did play a little desultory cricket with the younger boys, but a ball that landed on my nose and made it bleed put an end to my aspirations in that direction. My brother was made of sterner stuff. My mother was a keen amateur photographer and among our many family snaps there is a delightful one of him, aged about six, equipped with pads and holding his bat with a most professional stance.

Our equestrian achievements were equally different. William sat astride his pony with superb confidence. My experience was humiliating. He bolted with me and after that I refused to mount anything but our staid and docile donkey. As we had two very good tennis courts on which the staff and boys played, I ought at least to have become a reasonable player. It would have been a useful and lady-like social accomplishment but no ball ever seemed to come within reach of my racquet.

Our nursery was a large room with shuttered windows and deep window seats. Below one of these there was a long old fashioned couch where, when I was neither in the classroom or out of doors, I would curl up or stretch out, deep in a book. One of the uncoveted benefits of using autobiographical material is that through the spectacles of time one can see the seed bed from which my later major interests grew. These were books and the theatre, with its offspring the exciting new cinema. The source of both was James Barrie, the creator of Peter Pan, the boy who never grew up. I sometimes wonder if I too have ever quite left the Never Never Land behind, though it may be unfair to put the responsibility for this on Peter's shoulders.

When I went to Girton I believed myself to be a person who took a cynical view of the world. Now I know that I was an exceeding naïve romantic. I suspect that I still am in that I still read Georgette Heyer in preference to novelists like Margaret Drabble, even though, as a historian I am perfectly well aware that I have donned my rose coloured spectacles. When between the age of five or six I was taken to a matinée of *Peter Pan* at Manchester, I was totally bewitched by the magic of the theatre. My father had theories that children should not be given formal schooling before the age of seven and, according to family tradition, I taught myself to read so that I could recapture the magic of Barrie's hero, of Wendy and of Tinker Bell. The visit to Manchester became an annual event, the highlight of my year. When in due course my five year old brother and a young friend of his were to participate in this great occasion and, with masculine perversity, refused to save poor Tinker Bell's life by clapping to show their belief in fairies, I was outraged.

Many years later, with my Cambridge days long behind me, I made an unaccompanied nostalgic visit to a London performance. I wept because, unlike Peter, I had been trapped by the adult world. Even now, at the age of 87 I sometimes wonder if I am not still an escapist to the Never Never Land. *Jude the Obscure* is not for me, nor is the modern novel with its dissection of human motives and human pain. When I choose a novel I look first to see if it has a happy ending and rather shamefacedly retreat into the world which, as I know as a historian, never existed.

Stretched out on my sofa, as often as not sucking an orange through a lump of sugar, I read whatever came to hand. Fairy stories never appealed to me much; predictably I preferred Hans Andersen to Grimm. I took little delight in children being lost in unfriendly woods or being devoured by wolves, though I did have a soft spot for the ugly duckling. Apart from such books as *Little Women* or bound volumes of *The Girls' Realm*, which I had usually been given as presents, my reading must largely have been dictated by the fact that the books most easily available had been bought for the school library and were distinctly masculine in outlook. I followed the careers of Captain Marriatt's Four Midshipmen until in the final volume they had become Four Admirals. To the adventures of D'Artagnan, Porteus and I owed a colourful familiarity with French history. From Fennimore Cooper, who I must confess I found rather heavy going,

I gleaned much information about the Red Indian tribes. Winston Churchill (the American author not the British Prime Minister) in such books as *The Crossing* made the opening of the West a fascinating story and gave me an interest in American history. The list could easily be extended as memory delves into the many hours I spent sprawling on my sofa.

My early acquaintance with Scott I owed to my mother's great friend Elizabeth Preston, herself also a lover of the dramatic. When she came to stay with us in the school holidays she would read him aloud to us in her wonderful deep Irish voice, bringing each scene to life so that I thrilled to the doings of Ivanhoe and the clash of Norman and Saxon, of Saladin and the Crusaders, of Cavaliers and Roundheads. Looking back I am impressed by the wide background knowledge that I was acquiring of both European and American history. It would be churlish not to express my gratitude to Marjorie Bowen whose novels first aroused my interest in Dutch history. I could go on and on as long forgotten titles knock at memory's door among the *Westward Ho* and *The Cloister and the Hearth*.

By the time I was 14, unconsciously, history had become part of me, something that I took so automatically for granted that I never wondered why I studied it; or what use it was. Ask a mountaineer why he risks his life to climb to the summit and traditionally he is supposed to reply 'Because it is there'. That must be why I became a historian; like the mountaineer to discover what lay beyond the ranges had become to me as natural as breathing. A better metaphor might be to say that as a child I had prepared the ground and sown the seed; to harvest the crop when I became a woman was the natural consequence.

I was soon to be uprooted from my sofa and my masculine world. In my thirteenth year two events altered the pattern of my life completely. The first of these was when my grandfather, William Edge, the inventor and manufacturer of Edge's Dolly Blue, that then well known aid to a whiter wash before the days of the washing machine and the detergent, died leaving Thornlea, his country house to my mother. It was situated in what was then the rural village of Thornton-le-Fylde, midway between Blackpool, with its theatres and cinemas, and the fishing port of Fleetwood and was within two minutes walk of the tiny station where he could catch the train each morning for his works in Bolton. It was a pleasant family house, not large but comfortable but its glory was its garden which had been his joy and delight and which later was to be a millstone round our necks. The second event was the coincidence that the lease of Leighton Hall expired at the same time and the combination of the two led to my father selling the goodwill of the school, which moved to Kendal and we went to Thornton.

One of the first decisions that my parents had to make as a consequence of this move was what to do about my future education. Their views, for 1923, were enlightened. I was to go to a university and follow the family tradition: my paternal grandfather and my father had both been teachers. With this in view it had originally been decided to send me to one of the well established girls' boarding schools. Meanwhile for a year, as a stopgap, I went as a weekly boarder to a private school in Blackpool. I suppose it was well run and reasonably adequate, though I can remember nothing in its favour. I was utterly a fish out of water, or perhaps if I am to pursue the metaphor, a fish taken out of a swift flowing river of clear water into a small and rather stale tank. I had exchanged the company of boys who, except in holidays when occasionally female cousins came to stay, were my only playmates, and among whom I held a privileged position, for a gaggle of girls whose outlook and interests were as foreign to me as those of a foreign country. I had exchanged the freedom of woodland and park and farm for the dreary crocodile that took its exercise on hard pavements. How I disliked it and how I longed for the weekends that broke its monotony.

The sole piece of information which I acquired as a result of that wasted year I picked up in the dormitory when I learnt a surprising version of the White Slave Trade. This was that wicked men spirited girls away to South America where they were forced to have babies until they died. Few people today will remember the rumours that spread through middle class society when I was in my early teens. How great the real danger of innocent victims being so condemned to a life of shame I do not know, but perhaps it is worth remembering that even then, now considered something of a golden age when the streets were safe, parents were not without their alarms. Were the anxious warnings never to travel in an empty carriage, that was also before the introduction of the corridor train, never to speak to strangers or to go anywhere with them, part of social history and as such worth recording. Now it is small children who are at risk and old ladies who are mugged in the streets. The more things change? Throughout my teenage life these admonitions continued and even today, I feel a certain unease in lonely places, an unease reinforced by a year spent in Johannesburg in my late twenties, though it was the black man rather than the white slaver who was the local focus of fear. I am glad to report that neither my virtue nor my life has ever been threatened by either! Nevertheless those early fears provided one strand in my make-up; it is one which I should be happy to be without.

Had the plan to send me to one of the nationally recognized girls' boarding schools materialized I should have been as miserable as I had been at my Blackpool young ladies seminary, though the hockey stick rather than the crocodile would be my *bête noire*. From that fate the approach of the first world war saved me. In the uncertainties that loomed ahead it seemed wiser to explore the local possibilities than to send me away. To this search my father brought a persistence and acumen for which I cannot be too grateful. He made it his business to inspect at first hand all the possible options. His final decision was to send me to the Park School Preston, though this meant a train journey, followed by a long walk through Prestonville's drab streets to the park gates that gave the school its name. It was one of the new secondary schools and had only been opened in 1906 when Miss Alice Stoneman had been appointed its first Headmistress. It was a wonderful school and she a wonderful Headmistress. It was she, and the standards that she created that made my future career possible. Without her guidance and encouragement I should never have gone to Girton. No school could ever have given a better education; no school could ever have been more efficiently run. 'Stoney', as she was inevitably nicknamed was more respected and feared than loved by both pupils and staff.

The name suited her. I can see her still. Tall, gaunt with her hair strained from a face that might be described as having been roughly carved by a vigorous hand. With slightly hunched shoulders she strode through her domain. She never suffered fools gladly and her tongue was effective. She also possessed beautiful deep set eyes that glinted with amusement. Unlike my class mates, deeply as I respected and admired her I was never afraid of her. Perhaps this was because I was more at home with adults than with my own contemporaries; perhaps there was a rapport between us. But of one thing I am quite certain: no other pupil of hers at the Park School ever flung their arms round her and told her how much she liked (or was it loved) her. It was the done thing for pupils who were lucky enough to have a garden to present their favourite teacher with a bunch of flowers from it before morning school. Perhaps it was slightly unusual to signal Stoney for this honour, but apparently I had no qualms. She was a born teacher and in spite of her administrative responsibilities continued to play an active part in the classroom. Languages were not my strong point and even she could do little to rouse my enthusiasm for Latin grammar, in spite of the fact that she had read classics at the university. But in the classes that she took when the subject was English or Biblical studies, the effect was to create an interest that lasted. My horizons were permanently stretched. *Hamlet* under her guidance enthralled me. Of all Shakespeare's great tragedies it is the one that I know best. For many years when a new production appeared on the London stage I went to see it, collecting Hamlets as bird watchers observe their feathered friends. In contrast I found *A Midsummer's Night Dream* as taught by the English mistress, dull and boring which is some measure of Stoney's magic. She was equally responsible for introducing me to the fascination of Biblical criticism as an instrument in the understanding of the Scriptures. Before I was taught, like most children, they were a jumble of stories and moral behaviour that one took for granted.

By explaining the way in which the Gospels had been put together and by supplying the classical background to the Acts and Epistles here again she enlarged the boundaries of my mind. A deeply religious woman herself she was not afraid to apply scholarship to faith, to combine history and religion in a seamless robe. Inspired teacher though she was she can hardly have expected to be embraced by an over-appreciative 14-year-old which was the *lese majestie* that I committed when, overcome by my emotions, I presented my floral tribute. I don't know which of us was the more embarrassed!

In many ways during my early teens at the Park I continued to be a fish out of water though I benefited by now swimming in a larger tank. My class mates in the Upper Fourth, as I found out later, considered me an oddity. I was very well behaved and hard working, but I did not know how to make myself one of that lively form. In two respects I stood out. One was in English lessons when we were being introduced to *Palgrave's Golden Treasury* and by way of homework had to learn poems and recite them in class. Here my love of the theatre and my dramatic instincts overcame my diffidence and, whereas the rest of the form mumbled their way through the chosen piece, I, if called upon, recited my poem with all the intensity of an actress auditioning for a leading role. My other, and perhaps more useful quality was that as I found the members of the staff easier to converse with than my contemporaries, I could be relied upon, to our mutual contentment, to sit beside them at school dinners. If they felt I was 'teachers' pet' apparently they did not resent me. No one was unkind: I just did not belong.

By the time I reached the fifth form I had begun to make friends, two in particular, Mary Whitmore and Ethel Breakell, the latter tall and as bouncy as a young colt, with her mane of fair hair tied in a big bow behind. We became close friends and have remained so all our lives. It was she who later told me of the impact of my dramatic recitals had made on the form. The next milestone was when I was made a prefect; an honour that filled me with dismay and against which I protested vainly. Miss Stoneman told me blandly that she thought I would have a good influence over the younger girls. I hated responsibility; I always have. Stoney was shrewd enough to be well aware of this and may have been deliberately placing me in a situation in which I had to exercise it for my own good. Whatever her motives my reaction was to develop nervous dyspepsia. Instead of school dinners I was reduced to existing on a thermos of Benger's Food and cream crackers for my midday meal. To the dismay of my parents at this regime continuing for six weeks, my mother, in desperation at the doctor's failure to effect a cure, dosed me with a patent medicine, CICFA guaranteed to cure indigestion, constipation, flatulence and acidity. The effect on me was miraculous; I began once again to eat a normal diet. Alas CICFA has long departed from the market. Would I could still buy it for my digestion is still not what I could wish and I do like my food.

I should not grumble. This distressing episode brought with it a great compensation. I have always disliked games, having no physical aptitude for them whatsoever. Other girls could fly over the horse in the gym and climb a dangling rope. Invariably I stuck on the back of the first and failed to achieve more than the first knot of the second. So games on Wednesday afternoons were something to be avoided on any pretext. Though my periods caused me no inconvenience, because such matters were not talked about in those more physically modest days, I never could understand why they were considered a legitimate reason for being excused games. From the first to the last sign of this beneficent visitation I dodged the column. Basketball I could just tolerate but hockey I detested. My young brother jeered at my disconsolate recitals, commenting with exaggerated surprise when once I came home with a muddy stick. Now, due to my chronic digestive troubles I was excused games, an event over which I suspect the games mistress also shed no tears.

Release from the purgatory of the games field was a negative cause for rejoicing. I was soon to put my Wednesday afternoons to a more constructive use. History had always had a serious rival; my fascination for the theatre. Even before I could read I had been bewitched by the magic of Peter Pan and the fact that we always spent both Christmas and Easter with my Aunt Clara at Blackpool. This meant that from an early age, I was able to indulge this incipient addiction. Even before we had left Leighton Hall I was a hardened theatre goer and, as an extension of this activity, also a devotee of the new fangled cinematograph *The Picturegoer* was my favourite magazine. I cannot remember when I first read *The Stage* but even before we moved to Thornton I was beginning to bring an almost professional judgement to bear on the performances that I saw. Blackpool boasted two theatres, the Opera House and the Grand and each year at Christmas the D'Oyle Carte brought Gilbert and Sullivan to the Grand for a fortnight's season, while the Opera House was occupied by the Carl Rosa. I cannot remember at what age I demanded, as part of my Christmas presents, that I be taken to these performances, alternating between Gilbert and Sullivan one night and the Carl Rosa the next. Each night was an occasion for dressing up, not with the formality that the Royal Circle, where we always sat, would have demanded in London, but at least a pretty dress was *de rigour*. My favourite was a deep pink silky one, with a front panel edged with frills and decorated with small pearl buttons. These years were the hey day of the D'Oyle Carte with Henry Lytton and Barbara Lewis. *The Mikado, Iolanthe*, the *Gondoliers*, the *Yeoman* and *Patience* I knew almost by heart. *The Pirates* and *Pinafore* I liked less, while *Ruddigore* and *Princess Ida* were not performed at all. The Carl Rosa's repertoire was equally popular. *Faust* and *Carmen* were always given as were *Mignon* and such light operas, now consigned to the limbo of the forgotten, as *The Lily of Killarney* and *Mauritania*, in which I once heard Eva Turner sing the lead. Occasionally some Wagner might be included. This gave me the opportunity of hearing *Lohengran* and *Tanhauser.*

When we went to live at Thornlea, theatre going became a more regular pleasure. Fortunately for me my parents were fond of the theatre and, as this was the age of the touring companies, either before or after the London run, the great actors of the day all came to Blackpool, long forgotten Henry Ainley, Fred Terry and Julia Neilson in *The Scarlet Pimpernel* and a host of others including Mathesan Lang. It was the era not only of the straight play but of the musical comedy. My first introduction to this type of entertainment was *The Arcadians.* Though I have never been able to sing in tune and pitch (a mystery beyond my comprehension), I collected musical scores avidly picking out the tune with one finger. Now that I was freed from the tyranny of games I could indulge my passion for the theatre even more. Wednesday was matinee day and a seat in the Pit only cost a shilling. My parents were indulgent and I became a regular theatre goer. In addition I had long been a devotee of the silent screen; *The Picturegoer* was my favourite magazine. Today I might find little pleasure in seeing my old favourites now measured against the technical expertise of the modern screen, yet my memory insists that such films as *The Prisoner of Zenda* or *Far From the Madding Crowd,* despite the many versions of latter years, have never with more honesty or more magic been transferred from the printed page. To my enchantment with the Rudolf Rassendale of Henry Ainley and of Gerald Ames' Rupert of Henzau, I owe a further enrichment; an introduction to the novels of Anthony Hope. He is little read today, but the social historian of Edwardian England could do worse than study a novel like Second String when seeking illumination on the social nuances of the class structure of his England.

It had always been decided that after school I should go on to university and follow my father's profession and taken for granted that, as he had been a student at Owen's College (later to become the

University of Manchester) that it was there where I should go. It was Stoney who decided that I should go to Cambridge. Why I do not know. It can hardly have been due to my scholastic achievements up to date. My arithmetic was shaky, to say the least, my geometry pure guess work, plus theorems conned by memory. I never understood what it was all about. As for trigonometry after one week I was transferred to Botany, not that I shone in that either. My Latin and French were average, except that my pronunciation of the latter was so bad that when called to read in class even the upper Fourth laughed. Could anyone sink lower? Of my geography, after I had done better than my teacher had thought justified in an examination, her comment was 'The trouble with you Dorothy is that you are better on paper than in real life'. Looking back: I am inclined to agree; I still think most creatively on my typewriter. Even my English was marred by a chronic inability to spell. Today I should have been considered mildly dyslexic. Even history, my favourite subject, was not outstanding. Mary Whitemore and Ethel Breakell and I were equal contenders for the first place in tests and examinations. Whatever her reasons, I am eternally grateful to Stoney; it was she who made my future career possible.

If I were teacher's pet my friends did not resent it but were rather inclined to admire me for being able to sustain the role. This was demonstrated when, my brother having contracted some infectious disease that might have ended in my being in quarantine on the eve of my French paper for my School Certificate, Stoney decreed that I had better stay with her during those vital nights. The prospects left me unperturbed, justifiably so as Stoney was the least frightening of hostesses and I thoroughly enjoyed her company in the evening. But when I returned to school next morning after the first day of incarceration I was greeted as Daniel might have been when he emerged from the lion's den.

If I were to be entered for Girton there were some practical difficulties to be sorted out. It was the era before university grants were available and I certainly was not of scholarship standard and by 1917 the Marshall financial future in the face of war time conditions seemed uncertain. The Little Go, as the entrance for admission to Cambridge University examination was traditionally called, was better fitted to the curriculum of a public school than that of a Girls' Secondary. Latin and Greek were essential and Miss Stoneman, who had read classics, was the only member of staff qualified to teach it. In itself the standard of Greek required was not exacting. All that was required was a translating knowledge which, with the help of an interlinear crib, was not too difficult to acquire. But knowledge so obtained was not so foolproof. Examiners had a nasty trick of omitting an occasional sentence or two out of the set passage and to translate what was not there was hardly likely to impress the examiners with my mastery of Greek.

So Miss Stoneman devoted a couple of hours a week to coaching me in Greek and the set books, the *Fifth of Zanophen* and *The Gospel according to St. Luke*. Though today I doubt if I could stumble through the Greek alphabet, I am still grateful to have been forced to read Gospels in the original tongue. With equal nobility, indeed with possibly more, as I realised when for two years I became a school mistress, Miss Woodham Smith sacrificed some of her precious lunch break to giving me dictation. Here I fear she had little success; my spelling is still, to say the least, uncertain. The second subject not taught in the Park School, nor I imagine in any other, was Paley's Evidence of Christianity. This I was left to wrestle with alone.

Thus armed and prepared I faced the ordeal of Little Go and to my joyful surprise not only passed but even got a respectable second even in maths and French. Though Woody's efforts made no lasting impression on my spelling the advice that she gave me when I left Preston proved invaluable. 'Always wear good corsets and remember that she who would have friends must show herself friendly.' The first admonition I tended to disregard but the second was to be a lifebelt in my first term at Girton, almost swamped as I was when the safe haven of my tank had been exchanged for uncharted seas.

When I went up to Girton in 1918 I was no longer living at Thornton. In 1917 the family had moved to a small village, Old Hutton, about five miles from Kendal in what was then the country of Westmoreland. This year was also another landmark. I was developing literary ambitions and had started to keep a diary. For the benefit of posterity I started with a description of my family and explained why the move had become necessary:

> 'We should not be the family that we are if it wasn't
> for money troubles. We ought to have plenty. Mother
> and Daddy have about £1000 a year between them,
> only it never seems to join. Ever since I can remember
> overdrafts have been burning topics of conversation
> and it was Daddy's plus Mother's plus the War that
> finally buried us in the country.'

That we came to Old Hutton was one of those haphazard chances that change a life. Thornlea was too expensive to run; the garden was a constant drain. I was to go to Girton and William was now old enough to become a boarder. The war showed no signs of ending and our expenses must inevitably grow. But deciding that Thornlea must be sold was one thing; deciding where to go was more debatable. Until that could be decided Mother determined to rent a country cottage where we could store our furniture rather than entrust it to a Repository in which she had little faith. So we found a small house with a small garden and moved some of the furniture there, just enough for us to camp out during a summer holiday. As a family we have lived there, though not in the same house, ever since.

My father did not accompany us. This was not as heartless as it sounds. He was too old for the army and as a trained chemist was working at what was then the United Alki Works at Fleetwood. He went to live with his sister, my aunt Clara, who was still living at

Blackpool and came to us only for holidays. It was my first introduction to village life and there I put down permanent roots. Villages in the twenties were still communities. Kendal, our nearest market town, was five miles away; five hilly miles and the only means of transport the horse and cart or carriage as the case might be. We had our bicycles if we wanted to make the journey. For the necessities of life that was seldom. We had an excellent village shop and tradesmen's vans or carts called once or twice a week, the butcher and the fishmonger, whose wares in the heat of summer suffered somewhat from this leisurely transport, the grocer and the greengrocer and the chandler, who supplied the paraffin for our lamps.

There was no electricity and, though we had running water and the luxury of a bathroom and WC the water came from a spring further up the hill and arrived by gravity. Where it went to I don't know, but probably into the beck that ran at the bottom of our garden. We were as self-contained for our entertainments as for our necessities. A village concert was a rare event to which everybody went and where there were no class distinctions, either in the performance or the audience. In the village class distinctions were so taken for granted that they had no inhibiting effect on personal relationships. In the absence of other diversions we walked or cycled and when the weather was especially inclement we read or, in the evening Dabbott and I sang at the piano or, converted into one of those new fangled pianolas, my mother played her favourite pieces. The sound of the Hungarian Rhapsody or the Moonlight Sonata still brings back nostalgic memories of that lamp-lit room. There are still a few people to whom I am Miss Dorothy. At last I had somewhere I belonged; somewhere to which I could always return, some fixed and stable place I could find peace. 'Once the northern hills pull you' I wrote in my diary 'nothing has ever quite the same eerie quality of fascination. Its lonely roads, looping over hill and valley, seem to lead into the heart of romance.'

Though Thornton, with its proximity to Blackpool, had fed my love for the theatre and Old Hutton had deepened my love for the hills and moors of the North, they had done little to prepare me for the unfamiliar world of Cambridge and Girton. I had led a curiously secluded life that had afforded me little opportunity to acquire a veneer of social expertise. This was something that the Park School did not supply; politeness and good manners, yes, but how to behave at a party or when meeting strangers, no. In normal times this would have been supplied by my family's social commitments but as a child I had been limited to the company of boys or visiting relations during the holidays and by the time we had moved to Thornlea, where my social horizon should have expanded, the War had put a stop to many social activities.

The fact that I had no friends of my own age who lived locally contributed to my social isolation; there were no birthday parties to which I should automatically have been invited. Nor were there the informal incursion of friends and neighbours, not even a local tea room where the local ladies could congregate and gossip. Even if there had been my mother would not have been one of their number. My description of my family is illuminating on this point.

> 'There never was any social life and what there was we dodged', I wrote, 'there were four exits from our living room, so escape was easy. Occasionally my mother would put on her best things and pay a long overdue call. When she returned she always said that she had had a rotten time and had to be revived with tea, her panacea for most of the ills of life. Daddy had a boat on the river Wye and was only happy when he was sailing and with his sailing cronies.'

My parents were people who should never have married. But in those days well brought up Methodists did not even exchange kisses until they had become engaged and to break an engagement was considered flighty on the part of the woman and a thing no gentleman would do. Today there would have been an amicable divorce but in the twenties, when adultery was the main escape hatch, for my parents this would have been unthinkable. They put a brave face to the world but their lack of common interests and common friends was an obstacle to social activities.

At Old Hutton the scene changed once more. When we first went there my father was engaged on war work. Transport was difficult and his appearance at Old Hutton was confined to holidays. My mother's close personal friends came to stay and later I brought my Girton friends. The lack of transport combined with a social hierarchy which did not include entertaining one's inferiors to dinner, though tea was extended to borderline cases, meant that our circle was confined to Mrs Brown, who lived at the so-called manor, the vicar and his wife and Dr McCallum who lived in Kendal and who was an old friend of Elizabeth Preston.

Apart from the Doctor it was an odd assortment of folk. Mrs Brown was county but had married her groom and been ostracised by her family, or so gossip said. The vicar, Mr Grier, was Irish, charming and eccentric and a disaster in the pulpit, or even when he dropped in, because whether preaching or conversing, like Tennyson's brook, he went on forever. His wife was Italian, completely charming but she was a cat lover whose standards of hygiene were not high and the vicarage stank of her pets. So our social life was hardly exciting nor a useful preparation for Girton.

Mrs Brown did however bring one new experience into my life that gave me a foretaste of the pleasure and thrill that could be derived from the company of young men as opposed to mere boys. She introduced us to THE NEW ZEALANDERS. I write their joint names in capitals to emphasize their importance. Whether as an act of patriotism or for financial gain I am not clear, but Mrs Brown had three young New Zealanders to stay and recuperate after a spell at the front. There was nothing for them to do in Old Hutton and hopefully she brought them over to us. For men starved of female company, we must have seemed a gift from the gods, and certainly an improvement on the company of Mrs B and her very ordinary and dull spouse. My mother could not have been much above 40. She was a beautiful as well as a charming woman, warm and welcoming in her own house. Dabbott was what might be described as 'a comely wench' by a historical novelist. She had long flaxen hair, a disposition as romantic as my own and was only 29. For the next week they practically lived with us. They played on our pianola from morn to night, sang songs round the piano, which Dabbott played, walked with us, talked with us and filled our days with excitement. My mother, who was used to masculine admiration, took our new friends in her stride, but Dabbott and I were soon wallowing in a treacly sea of sentiment.

The three musketeers in the curtain raiser to the brave new world of maids and men of which I was to become a part next year were Olive Begg, Will Spratt and Bill Hutton. Will Spratt who was the oldest and, looking back I should judge to have been the most amorously inclined, concentrated his attentions on Dabbott. It was to Bill Hutton that I lost my heart. Lovingly I described him as:

> 'A huge six footer. A sleepy individual with great
> shoulders, a bull neck and a mop of flaxen hair
> brushed back a la knut. He had a round, rosy, placid
> face with sleepy blue eyes. When he smiled his face
> suddenly lit up and became charmingly boyish and
> confiding. His manner stamped him as belonging to
> the early twenties, self confident and of the opinion
> that his was the last word on any subject. He drawled.
> To him everything was 'delightful' and every statement
> was met with a 'Is that so?' He reminded me of a
> sleepy ox and I could not decide whether I liked him
> or disliked him.'

We got into a fierce argument over a long forgotten novel *Sonia*, I admiring the hero whom he dismissed with crushing contempt, loftily dismissing my opinion as 'A woman's view', so that I wrote 'I could have murdered him'. Later that evening I capitulated, writing:

> 'He had a beautiful voice when he wasn't too lazy to drag himself out of his chair, melting my heart by his rendering of such sentimental numbers as 'Less than the Dust' and 'If only I could come to you with all my love confessed.'

Next morning we took our visitors to see the local waterfall, Dabbott walking ahead with Mr Begg and Mr Spratt, so that I had Bill Hutton to myself. That evening I confided to my diary:

> 'I enjoyed this walk. I felt quite grown up walking beside him and looking up at him. Disgraceful admission for one who pretends to be as superior as I do. When he called me 'chield' in that drawling voice, I protested that I was not so much younger than he and older than I looked. His reply was 'You carry your age all over you'. Oh it was a far reaching conversation. Among other things we discussed the English habit of kissing and the fact that women matured more quickly than men.'

I thoroughly enjoyed every minute of it. I think I was getting to like Bill Hutton very well.

The idyll was soon over. Their leave ended and they went. The last evening was bitter sweet. I comforted myself that:

> 'As Mr Hutton sat lounging in his chair I thought his eyes looked sorry and next morning he held my hand and said "Goodbye Bambino".'

The rest of the entry was so pathetically naïve that even now, after all these years, I hesitated as to whether to include it, yet not to do so would leave incomplete the key to understanding the mixture of immaturity and romantic idealism with which I was equipped to face the unknown world of college and university.

> 'Their going brought a gap of desolation into our lives.
> They had so entwined themselves with our intimate
> things, even our songs sang of them. Yet I am glad,
> very glad that we met them. They have revolutionised
> my whole outlook on life. I know now that men can be
> brave and straight, clean, true and God fearing with the
> gaiety of schoolboys and the depth of men. I know
> now that a man can be his own master and I know
> now that nothing is greater than moral cleanliness and
> that there are worse things than death. I want to put
> this down now so if ever in future I doubt and hesitate
> I may remember that I have met such men, that please
> God they are no dream. I want to resolve now never
> never to give myself to any man who is not one of
> these, I will never scoff inwardly at good men and
> marriage again because I have met these three.'

By the end of August I was slowly recovering, writing:

> 'I am beginning to forget the NZ a little but sometimes
> a wave of longing for their return comes over me.
> I won't pray for it because I don't think it wise but,
> though I try not to think of them but it is hard not to
> long.'

Not until September, when Mr Spratt wrote to say a last farewell, as they were due to sail to New Zealand next day, did I give up a lingering hope that they might return. Now I realized that:

> 'So I can give up my restless expectation and dismiss
> them from my mind. It is just as well. I wonder if I

would have fallen in love with Mr H if I had had the chance. However I can't see anyone falling in love with me. Nearly every girl I know takes the wind out of my sails. I was alone here. That is why I had such a good time. They were perfectly mad evenings but I must never behave like that again.'

Mad evening! Even by the standards of 1918 I must have been the greenest girl ever to enter the door of Girton College.

CHAPTER TWO: CAMBRIDGE IN WARTIME.

Regrettably my first impressions of Girton are sketchy and full of gaps. For there are two reasons, the more fundamental one being that I have been cursed with an almost non-existent power of recall, both visual and factual. Had I been forced to rely on my memory alone these reminiscences of Cambridge and Girton could never have been written. The second reason hinges on the first; for some unknown cause, there are no entries in any diary I can find between 19th September and 11th November 1918. The only reference to the fact that I was to go to Girton in the October is the bald statement on 3rd September that I had been vaccinated and that it had not hurt much. One of the college regulations was that students should have been vaccinated which I had never been, my father having objections to the practice of infant vaccination.

Apparently I had only started to keep a diary in the August of that year and it had been intended to provide the basis for a novel but it is almost incredible that my memory should have retained practically no recollection of all the preliminaries that must have taken place earlier in the year. I do not remember even whether I went to Cambridge to sit my Little Go examination or whether I was allowed to do it under supervision at Preston. I have only the vaguest impression of having been interviewed by Kitts, as I was later, like everyone else, to call Miss Jess Blake, the Mistress. If I did, and I must have had some interviews as well as an entrance examination to have been admitted, then I think it improbable that I made the journey to Cambridge alone. Most likely my mother came with me and we stayed in a hotel and that when I left Old Hutton in October I was facing the world on my own for the first time.

The first lion in my path was the change at Bletchley. The conditions of travel were very different than those of young people today. They travel nonchalantly staggering under huge backpacks containing their possessions. I travelled nervously, my possessions being incarcerated in a piece of luggage called a cabin trunk which it would have been impossible for me to hand handle. They were apparently designed to fit under the berths of ocean going passengers, being oblong in shape, often covered in a sort of canvas and bound by wooden hoops and were the then modern substitute for the old dress trunks which they had superseded. To handle them, porters were needed and porters could be elusive and needed tips. So much heavy luggage needed not only porters but special luggage vans and the prudent traveller, before settling in the carriage, saw the trunk safely bestowed into the van. Then, on arriving where a change took place, the first thing to be done was to dash to the precise van wherein the precious trunk nestled and wait anxiously until a porter removed it, put it on a trolley and moved off to the correct connection. On this, my first journey alone, at least the change at Bletchley caused no problem. Suddenly the platform seemed to be swarming with young ladies all with cabin trunks and all bound for Cambridge, a chattering foretaste of the days to come.

My next hazard was getting myself and my luggage from Cambridge station to the college which was on the other side of the town about two and a half miles along the Huntingdon Road. If I recollect aright there was a cart or van on which the porters placed our trunks to convey them to Girton but personal transport we had to provide for ourselves. This meant taxis. No student ever indulged in one for herself; as many as could be crammed in shared both the discomfort and the fare. It was a free for all as we claimed our trunks, left them to fate, and seized one of the waiting taxis. I no longer remember how I fared in the scrummage; possibly I was merely swept along with the throng.

The rooms assigned to me were in Bear Pits; how they got that name I do not know. As they were near the main entrance it may have been that they were noisy. They were also central and convenient. The building, of red brick, was dominated by the Tower through which was the main entrance to the college. On one side was the portress' lodge and the lobby that contained our pigeon holes where we looked for letters or notices. The door on the other side led to the corridors along which our rooms stretched.

The quarters assigned to me were next but one to the entrance through the archway. In those spacious days, with the exception of a few larger rooms, students had a bedroom and study each. The two were divided by a wooden partition and were basic in their equipment. In the sitting room there was a kneehole desk, a bookcase, a small table, a chair or two and an unpromising looking small arm chair. That disposed of the furniture in the study. The bedroom, a mere slip of a place, was equally spartan consisting of a narrow bed, an old fashioned washstand and basin, a chest of drawers and a small wardrobe. Lighting and heating conformed to the same comfortless standards. There was an oil lamp in my sitting room and a candle had to suffice for my bedroom. The lamps were supposed to be filled and trimmed every day but they did not encourage the burning of midnight oil. By then they had probably spluttered and gone out and there was nothing that even the most prudent virgins could do to husband their stock. As I rarely worked late at night I was less affected than some, but one of my closest friends has reminded me how she used to have to take refuge in the corridor outside her room which boasted of a gas lamp under which she used to stand and industriously read with her book held close to it, keeping her studious vigil far into the night.

Heating arrangements were equally limited. Each study had a fireplace and was supposed to be given a scuttle of coal each day. Scuttle itself is a vague term; not all are equally full. Even at best a warm fire and comfortable room needed careful planning and in my time our precious fuel was cut off by rail strikes and miners' strike and keeping warm became a major problem. I can still remember searching through Woodlands, that part of the College grounds that stretched from Girton corner fringing on the Huntington Road as far as the main gates, searching diligently for even a fir cone or small branch with which to augment my stock. In the struggle to keep warm I was better equipped than any of my friends. Owing to the many days spent with my father in Maid Marion, I was used to both the advantages and the vagaries of the Primus Stove. I wonder are they still in use today or have they been utterly replaced by bottled gas.

It was a dangerous form of heating. First it had to be filled with paraffin, then pumped up until the flame turned blue and burnt steadily. But the stove could flare up and fill the room with smoke. On one occasion, according to my diary, the methylated spirit, with which the flame had to be started must have spread over the kettle which blazed up. 'I flung it into the hearth where it blazed merrily' much to the dismay and fright of Soulie who refused to allow me a second attempt. So we had to go to bed on half cold cocoa. Had the college authorities ever known of my solution to the heating problem they would have been horrified and justifiably so. I could easily have set either myself or my room alight.

Lamps I was used to, coal fires I was used to: both were normal for lighting, heating and cooking in villages such as Old Hutton. The sanitary arrangements of the college could best be described as modified eighteenth century. In country cottages and farms the 'privy' at the end of the garden, often known as the 'Necessary House' or 'Nessy' was the normal convenience. But I had never lived in a house without a water closet. So it was a shock to discover that these adjuncts to civilized living had not yet reached Girton. True the privy was no longer to be found at the bottom of the garden or housed in some external building. On each floor except the ground floor there was a room divided into discrete cubicles fitted with the usual seating arrangements except for the lack of water. A lever released a flow of either sand or sawdust, I cannot remember which. Every afternoon at tea time, when the young ladies were in Hall, munching, if I recollect correctly, bread and margarine, or some equally unattractive substance, a party of men used to come up in the service lift and empty the stinking buckets. It was all very discrete, within its limits efficient, but I never found it pleasant. When eventually Girton moved into the twentieth century and installed water closets I was delighted.

The provisions made for personal hygiene were better, and indeed may have been superior to some, if not most of the men's colleges. What their 'bogs' were like I have no means of knowing. In the twenties this was not a subject for social conversation. But the bathing facilities for Trinity men were plain to any Girton student who had a nine o'clock lecture. Often have I been amused by the spectacle of young men clad in dressing gowns, sponge bag in hand, making their way to the bath house. To the older generation of dons this institution was an unnecessary pandering to modern fads. According to one oft told Cambridge legend one elderly don is reported to have asked peevishly, 'why do the men want bath houses? They are only up for eight weeks.'

Later I learnt the reason for Girton not having succumbed earlier. It had been a question of money. To move from Hitchen, the site of the first woman's college, had been financially a daring experiment. To build the new college and to finance it had strained every financial resource to breaking point and it was not until 1913 that the college could afford the luxury of modern sanitation and electric light. Plans were well in hand when the imminence of war made it impossible to put them into practice. With the coming of peace the project was revived. What surprised me when I exhumed my diaries after 70 years was that nowhere could I find any comment on either their existence or their disappearance. Owing to the fact that I was not keeping a diary when I first took up residence explains the first omission, but I should have expected the removal of these links with the past to have been greeted by me with expressions of joy and not with a blank silence.

If I found Girton weak on 'mod cons' I found it vigilant in creating and upholding the dignity of the college in the matter of traditions and formalities. However scattered our activities throughout the day our evening meal, Hall, was a corporate ritual. One 'changed' from one's day time attire, as in the twenties any young lady living at home would be expected to do, and suitably dressed we stood silently behind our chairs. It was the only meal of the day at which we were waited on by the gyps as we, in accordance with Cambridge custom, called our domestic servants. Wearing spotless black dresses with white caps and aprons, all 32 were drawn up in a line in front of the hot plates or serving hatches. Silence prevailed as the Mistress followed by the dons made her stately progress to the High Table. Then came the familiar grace, and we sat down. Immediately the silence was broken by the clatter made by the gyps' boots as they hurried to place the soup before us and by the sound of our voices raised in conversation. When the noise became too overwhelming Kitts would ring a small bell and request us to talk more quietly. When our exuberance overcame our manners as a last resort in her most acid voice she would command total silence until further notice. Attendance at Hall was obligatory; we had to sign in before the meal and if for any reason a student or group of students had been given permission to leave early before the departure of the Mistress and her dons, the etiquette was to turn and bow to the High Table. From the tales that we heard of the behaviour of the men, one gathered that their behaviour was somewhat less decorous.

Between the end of Hall until nine o'clock was a period devoted in theory and generally in practice, to study. These were Silence Hours, another Girton institution intended to preserve academic calm and prevent the lazy or the idle from chattering in the corridor. When this occurred the victim, whose concentration had been shattered, opened the door and called out 'Silence Hours please'. This was known as jumping, or being jumped. It was a democratic privilege enjoyed by all. Even a humble fresher could jump a third year who then had to make a formal apology. A casual apology of 'sorry' shouted back was not acceptable. At nine o'clock Silence Hours ended and social life began. Like much of Girton ritual it was based on an earlier tradition when the college had provided students with a small jug of milk each to be used in making a comforting cup of cocoa before retiring for the night. Hence the name JUG. This could be informal or solitary. For the fresher who came up as I did without friends it was the time when one became most conscious of how lonely one was. This was accentuated by the ease with which the product of boarding schools, used to mingling with their kind and often with a school mate to keep them company, could form little groups. The coal shortage encouraged this gregariousness; automatically the group drifted into whoever had a fire in their room. There they congregated in cheerful groups, gossiping or setting the world to rights, both popular activities.

Formal jugs were a different matter and had their own ritual. They were the means of introducing the freshers into the social life of the college. This task was undertaken by the second years as a social obligation. They, usually acting in pairs, sent out a formal invitation hoping that Miss so and so and Miss so and so could come to jug on such and such an evening. These were placed in the letter racks under one's initials in the Portress' Lodge. They were my social life line. I don't know how often I looked hopefully to see if there might be one for me. How effective they were I am uncertain. One arrived at nine, made polite conversation and met other freshers, possibly as shy as oneself. One was not encouraged to outstay one's welcome and our departure was governed by what was elegantly known as 'the chuck'. This was an indigenous device by which after an hour to an hour and a half the member of the group of guests whose name came first in the alphabet, had to rise, explain that she had an essay that she must complete for tomorrow or some such conventional excuse, and with thanks for a pleasant evening withdraw with her companions. As M. was safely in the middle of the alphabet chucking did not often fall to me. Poor Miss Alcock got plenty of practice. It was a civilized custom which, when I in turn became a don, I could have wished had been adopted by the students whom I was entertaining, when even my desperate allusions to last buses failed to dislodge them.

Shy and diffident as I was I might have fared badly had I not been lucky in my neighbours in Bear Pits. On one side Jessie Belfield, a second year, was kind to me and with her great friend, Helen Harvey I struck up a friendship that was to last for many years. Helen had her own coterie of friends, but they were of an essentially serious turn of mind, more interested in ideas than in men and the more frivolous side of life. Had I only belonged to their group I should have missed much that Cambridge had to offer and from this I was saved by my neighbour on the other side.

Ruth had not particularly wanted to come to college; she had a good brain but was in no sense an academic. She intended to enjoy Cambridge, she was out-going and good at making contacts and soon collected a group around her. To this I found myself belonging, partly through proximity but partly because, though I had very little faith in my ability to be cultivated for myself I had one trump in my pack. Rationing, plus a belief that academic women had a soul above food, had done nothing to cultivate our gourmet instincts. College food was at best dull, reminiscent of Virginia Woolf's strictures in *A Room of One's Own*. I do not however recollect her having to eat lukewarm curried tripe or go hungry. That was the fate of students who, because they had 12 o'clock lectures, got back to lunch late and had to be content with other people's leavings. Even Girton only sank so low once a week but I have no compensating memories to balance against cold curried tripe. Writing home I reported:

> 'I spend shillings a week on food. Cambridge just seems laid out with food suitable for study consumption, tins of cafe au lait, cocoa and milk and a delicious confection known as Honey Sugar. Have I told you the story of the Newnham porter? When he was asked what the students did he replied 'Well, ma'am, the young ladies eats and eats and meanwhile they has meals.' It is horribly true. What it was like before the war I don't know. Officially we were really well fed apart from study feasts but I shall be horribly fat by the time I get home.'

Honey sugar, which we could usually get at the little grocers at the top of Castle Hill, certainly had never known a bee and there was a current belief that it emanated in some way from a by-product of brewing. It was certainly fattening but we were thankful for small mercies, and when I could get hold of a jar of jam very nobly I saved it for my brother believing that at school his need was greater than mine. Perhaps many of my fellow students were more hardened to war time catering having spent the last few years in a boarding school, or in an urban setting where they had less access to a modest black market than I. Rationing in a country village was a less restricting business. Though groceries and such foods were on ration even when purchased at the village shop, we had friends among the farming community. Butter, though not plentiful, was at least obtainable; so were eggs and the occasional chicken. Rabbits too, which were not on the official meat ration were plentiful.

Even butchers' meat, particularly when the son of a local farmer, when most slaughtered their own beasts had a weekly butcher's round, was more generous than the official ration. We had three different butcher's vans that called each week and if the weather should chance to be hot it was plain wastefulness to allow the meat to go to waste so it was made available to regular customers. Certainly no one at Old Hutton seemed to be short of food. As a result of the general laxity of the countryside my mother was able to send me an occasional food parcel. The arrival of a chicken was a matter for celebration; butter was easier to get and arrived more frequently. With this I could bait my trap. When I asked my friends to Jug I could regale them with hot buttered toast as an accompaniment to the inevitable cocoa. This stratagem proved successful. I had a point of contact, something to offer which gave me self confidence. I became a member of a group.

Another Girton institution that provided some access to social success was 'The Prop'. Having left school days behind us as young ladies we conformed to the conventions current in society. To address a mere acquaintance by their Christian names was unthinkable; that was a privilege confined to family and friends. Yet in the close knit community of the college, to remain Miss Marshall within the orbit of my new friendships soon came to feel over formal. The Prop was the social mechanism to make an easy translation. The phrase 'To Prop' was itself a shortened version for the even more formal politeness of Edwardian England. It was shorthand for the considerable mouthful 'May I propose to call you by your Christian Name?' This, even in 1918 would have seemed stilted. Freshmen could not however prop indiscriminately; seniority had to be observed and to take the initiative was confined to one's equals. A fresher could only prop a member of her own year. I could prop Ruth or Elspeth but not Helen or Jessie, who were in their second year. One must wait for the honour of being propped by a second year or, more lofty still by a third year. I discovered that one slipped easily into the use of Christian names among one's first year friends, but to be propped by a senior was rather like collecting stamps or scalps. It was therefore always reassuring to one's self-esteem to be propped by a senior. It meant that in some way you had stood out from the freshman hordes, but to be propped by an outstanding second year was like acquiring a rare stamp, something about which, with a casual air, one gently boasted to one's friends.

The treasure of my collection was Theodora Llewellan Davies, the senior student of the second year and the niece of Emily Davies, one of the founding females of Girton. I thought how like Mr Hutton she looked, writing:

> 'Indeed there was a real resemblance. She was a tall squarely built girl with a face like a placid cow. Her fair hair was dragged back and usually straggled a little. Her eyes were blue and far seeing, so that she usually ignored you if you met her in the corridor. But when she did see you her smile was sweet. She had a peculiar drawl in her voice and used to say "plaise" instead of "please".'

Altogether she was a remarkable looking girl, not a beauty but at times beautiful. Personality poured out of her. I have seen her sway a General Meeting, so that it ended by doing just exactly what it had originally proposed because of her skill in handling it. It was my fate to worship from afar. Apart from a few kind words and having propped me in my first term, apart from the privilege of calling her Theo if she ever happened to remember my existence, I gained nothing except perhaps a little kudos. She read law and promised to put her talent to good use in that she was one of the first women to be called to the bar. But, though I often wondered what had finally happened to her, half expecting to find her like Barbara Wootton, a member of the Lords, only recently did I discover that she had opted for the role of wife and mother.

If there was still a touch of the school girl in my feeling for Theo there was equally a boarding school flavour lingering in some of our other corporate activities. This I feel was particularly displayed in our tribal ritual of 'College Songs'. This happened once or twice a term and entailed all the students, though the freshmen may have sung them with the greatest enthusiasm, joining together in an expression of college solidity. Today I doubt if even the memory of that past tradition remains among the sophisticated students of today. It is hard to imagine them as, joining enthusiastically in such gems as:

> *'Play up all the college cried,*
>
> *Pass it to the wings girls,*
>
> *That's the sort of thing girls*
>
> *Lord, I thought I should have died,*
>
> *Knocked it through the Newnham goal.'*

sung to the tune of *'Knocked them in the Old Kent Road.'* Another favourite, reminding us all of the ordeal that lay ahead was:

> *'Fare thee well, for I must leave thee, Do not let the parting grieve thee,*
>
> *But remember that the best of friends must part must part.*
>
> *I have a Tripos to get through, to get through.*
>
> *I can no longer stay with you, stay with you.*
>
> *I spend my days in the Baptist school room now,*
>
> *And may I never get a....'*

at which point a bellow of protest drowned the fatal word *plough*. The Baptist schoolroom was the venue for the Tripos examinations and the word plough signified a failure. Even before I went down the

52

enthusiasm for college songs was waning.

In the early days of the college Girtonians had been very conscious of standing alone, of having to balance the traditions of the men's colleges by traditions of their own. They were traditions that had within them no place for the physical appearance of men. One of these I always described as 'the dancing'. My memory of this is now extremely vague in so far as I cannot now recall whether it was a weekly or fortnightly or only an occasional event, but it certainly smacked of the boarding school in that the dancing was ballroom dancing, or party dancing if thought of in connection with something less formal than a ball. It took place after Hall and we danced together with our friends.

To some extent it was a useful social mixture in that it widened acquaintanceship between the years as well as between the members of one's own. I was not a natural dancer and, owing to my rather unconventional teenage days, I don't think it ever included dancing lessons, though I certainly had them in elocution So I viewed attendance at 'the dancing' with mixed feelings. Perhaps I should not have had the courage to go at all had it not been for Jessie Belfield who in my early days marched me off firmly and danced with me kindly. This unisex dancing and revelry was extended to more important social events in that each year acted as hostess and gave an annual dance. Here is my account of the dance given by the third year when I was in my second.

> 'I went to the third year partly meaning to stay only
> a little time and then slip away. I enjoyed it and
> stayed on. I liked Dorothy Tait immensely and also
> Churchman. Ruth dances awfully well now, she says
> mine has improved.'

Then came an episode even more reminiscent of the schoolroom:

> 'We came away and I put my kettle on. Soulie (who

was the college organ scholar and boasted a piano in
her room) started playing, and a group of us, I in my
pyjamas, danced for half an hour in the passage. It was
great fun and better than the real dance.'

Looking back; 'good, clean fun' might have been a more
sophisticated comment. In addition to such activities the college
had its own Dramatic Society, whose standard did not impress my
critical mind, and its own debating society, though this, when the post
war thaw took place, was sometimes intruded by invitation into the
masculine world of the Cambridge colleges.

More practical and regarded as a praiseworthy activity was the Fire
Brigade. In a letter home, written in the early November of 1918, I
described how:

'Of course I joined the Fire Brigade but fortunately it
is going to be reformed, only 36 instead of all the year.
The bad ones are going to be thrown out at half term,
so I am distinctly hopeful. At present we poor recruits
have to be up at 7.30 three times a week to practice
roping and hosing. My knots are weird and wonderful
but not I fear really effective.'

I was duly thrown out. So uninterested was I, in spite of the sporting
ardour of our college songs, in any kind of game, that I almost
forgot to mention that naturally Girton had its hockey team, and
for all I can remember, also one for basket ball but the only allusion
that I can find in all my diaries is to record that once out of a sense
of loyalty I did watch half a match with Newnham before slipping
away with enthusiasm to watch the Lent Bump races. Nor did I try
to avail myself of the tennis courts which were much in evidence in
the summer.

One last college institution which played its own decorous part in Girton life was the fact that we had our own chapel, a fact that in Cambridge would have been so taken for granted that, unless for its architectural eminence would hardly have merited a mention, had it not been that our rival Newnham, by its charter had been prohibited from any official place of worship. Attendance was not obligatory and my attendance probably somewhat spasmodic, nevertheless it was part of my college life with which I should have been sorry not to have had.

Though it can hardly be described as an institution no account of Girton life would be complete that omitted part of our grounds known as Woodlands. Though memory portrays it as more extensive than it was, or perhaps it has shrunk since I was a student and grown shabbier, for me it was a place of retreat and solitude, a place where one could be alone or where in the cool of a summer evening one wandered with a friend, or picnicked with one's group. In my diary it figured more prominently than did the chapel. Here are two word pictures, one of winter and one of spring that I hope convey the feeling of Girton as I knew it.

'I wandered round Woodlands alone. There was not much daylight left and the sun had gone... The night was cold. Each tree and twig and leaf was crusted with white, like a soft Shetland scarf thrown over their nakedness. The path was broth with fallen leaves but the undergrowth being mostly evergreens, still retained its colour though coated with frost... Above the sky was blue, so cold and far away the white trees seemed to merge into it except where the sun's rays had left a belt of pink, almost as cold and aloof as the blue. The moon was a pale yellow. Not a thing stirred; it was utterly and completely silent, so that all the past was present. So still that the future seemed here. The coldness of the world seemed to end just beyond the bend of the path. I began to sing, waiting for something indefinite to come, for some spirit to enter me. I sang of the dead brown leaves and the cloudy white trees, of those that would follow and of those who were gone. Then I sang of us, how, like leaves, we blossomed and fell and hoped that like leaves, we too might mean a richer life for those who came after.'

Later I was to rejoice in the sudden glory of the spring when Woodlands burst into life again when one morning, very early, I realized that winter was past and life was beckoning me forward; that the present was all sufficient. I wonder do the students of today still find, as I did, a place for dreams and visions?

In 1918 the position of women students perhaps could be described as being, 'neither fish, flesh nor good red herring'. We were allowed to sit the same Tripos examinations as the men and to receive a certificate stating that we had done so and the class that we had attained and we were allowed to attend the same lectures as the men but we were not members of the university. A student from Newnham or Girton might get the most brilliant of Firsts but she could not assume the title of BA. In applying afterwards for a post or in facing the world all that she could quote by way of qualifications was limited to that certificate. The 'don' of the women's colleges had no say in the setting of the Tripos or the contents of the courses that were required to sit it. It was a man's world and the women were there almost on sufferance. Yet though the war had not persuaded the university to grant women degrees, it had done much to improve their standing. Most of the men of military age were at the Front. Only the conscientious objector, the physically unfit, the foreigner and the wounded provided the skeleton numbers in the men's colleges, while many of their dons, too old to fight had gone to swell the wartime ministries. The women predominated at lectures and were even being asked to take on the role of lecturer. Eileen Power, the Director of Historical Studies, had been so distinguished and lectured to first year students on English economic and social history.

Eileen Edna Power, EEP in the College shorthand, was one of the most outstanding academic women of the immediate post war period and I consider it to have been my incredible good fortune that for my first two years she was both my tutor in college and also through her lectures laid the solid foundations of social and economic history which later was to be my own special field. I owe her more than I can say in more ways than one. When I came to Girton I was an intellectual snob. I thought of academic women as being a superior class apart. Dress, appearance, female charm were all beneath me and I must have been a sore irritation to my poor mother when I was so patiently indifferent to the wardrobe which she was providing me. As a protest I even tried to read a book when it was being tried on. Eileen Power changed all that. She was a charming. beautiful creature, open and friendly in her manner, well groomed, well dressed and so attractive. She built no barriers between herself and her students. A tutorial in her delightful room in the Tower was never a stilted occasion. Often a chocolate box was at hand, the substitute of the male don's offering of sherry to his college students, and always a friendly smile.

She was the cause of one of my most gauche remarks to another member of the staff. This was later, when the men had just begun to return after the war and whom, duly chaperoned, we were allowed to ask to tea in our rooms. Miss Dean was one of the kindest and most good hearted of women but hardly a dame fatale and she was therefore much in demand in this role of which she must have grown heartily sick. Once, when I was planning a tea party together with one of my cronies and asked her to officiate, she asked me, 'Why don't you ask Miss Power?' to which I made the truthful but devastating reply, 'Oh, she is much too attractive'. If our prospective guests were likely to fall a victim to EEP's charm rather than to ours at tea parties, there were some functions for which she was much in demand. At college balls or society dances she could be relied upon to concentrate on her own partner, only collecting her brood in time to get them back to college before the witching hour of midnight.

If only the debt that I owed to her had been that academic brilliance and feminine charm were not mutually exclusive that debt would still have been considerable as far as my personal life was concerned. Even more important than this lesson, which given time I might have learnt for myself, was that she taught me the tools of my craft. Any success that I had in my professional life in later years I owed to her example and influence over me in my first two years at Girton. Because she used her tutorials to bridge the gap between don and student, because she seemed friend as well as tutor, when I found myself in her position instinctively I adopted her attitude. I tried to produce the carrot before the criticism, to give the student something on which to build. Unless I thought that a student was trying to take a rise out of me and was doing it deliberately, which few of them ever did, I would do my best to treat their views with respect while still arguing for my own.

EEP was not only a good tutor: she was a brilliant lecturer. How brilliant I only recognised when I had to follow in her footsteps. What she had to say seemed so simple, so interesting, so uncluttered that taking notes was no problem. Then, at the end of the lecture she would suggest further books to be consulted. Having spent hours doing so it was only to discover that everything vital to the understanding of that particular subject was in essence in EEP's so simple sounding lecture. Only later, when I was no longer a student did I discover that she was giving the course for the first time, keeping ahead of her class by a couple of lectures. When, in my turn, I had to be responsible for structuring a course from her example I distilled two principles. The first is to capture the interest of your audience, so that they want to listen, that done the next vital step is to give them the essentials on which they can build and finally, never, never leave them in a muddle. One lecture should be content to lay the foundations of the building. What appears above ground should be the work of the individual student.

The First Year course for part I of the History Tripos consisted of four papers, Medieval European History, English Constitutional History from the Tudors upwards, Political Theory Part I and the aforementioned English Economic and Social History. Each entailed two lectures a week, the writing of essays, Time Papers and the subsequent tutorials. Dr G Coulton, a distinguished if unorthodox scholar, lectured on Medieval European and as this was totally unknown to me, I foundered badly, knowing nothing of the Fall of the Roman Empire or the wanderings of such people as the Vandals and Visigoths. He was not a good lecturer and I found the subject confused and not particularly interesting. Yet somehow by the end of the year his enthusiasm had brushed off on me and I had a feeling for the Middle Ages. Though I have long forgotten the substance of his course I think, if confronted by a fragment of some interpretation of Medieval I should still know instinctively if it felt right.

I am also grateful to Dr Coulton for a less flattering reason. If EEPs' lectures were a demonstration of her brilliant presentation, then his lectures were an example of how not to lecture. I can see him now, striding up and down, pouring forth a torrent of words, with little attention to the structure of his thought, a defect made worse by the fact that as he marched away from where I was sitting I often missed the vital clue to his rambling sentences. In other ways too he typified the helpless intellectual male. Once when a group of us were discussing him one member of it declared 'I always know when his wife is away because he comes to lectures in cracked boots'. Barbara Bliss then electrified us by stating 'One day he came in in a pink collar and nothing else'. As I wrote in my diary 'Doubtless this enormity of Dr Coulton's was a trifle exaggerated.' Yet in spite of all his deficiencies by the end of the year somehow I acquired an understanding of the medieval roots of western civilization, whereas in my third year Reddaways' lectures on modern Europe were hours of boredom.

Dr Tanner, who lectured on Modern English Constitutional History, was in every way a complete contrast. Constitutional History is not a subject that necessarily lends itself to anecdotal treatment. I never remember Lapsley of Trinity, who in our Second year pontificated on the stronger meat of the medieval period, which was considered too difficult for us First Years, hence the cart before the horse approach, so enlivening it. Dr Tanner spiced his investigation into the growth of the Constitution with the more amusing details of its makers. This made it difficult for him to cover the course within his allotted span of lectures and as its end drew near, if my recollection is correct, he was prone to leave out the more prosaic details of statute and law in favour of a more personal touch. From the point of view of students facing an examination this might have been something of a disadvantage had he not most obligingly edited that most useful compilation of Constitutional Documents on which his lectures were so obviously based. So we could relax in his lectures and he, though I did not think of so sordid a point at that time, could enjoy our appreciation and his royalties.

Somewhere on my bookshelves there must still lurk my Tanner on which I too came to rely when it was my turn to introduce a new generation of students to the glories of the English Constitution. That, and Maitland's *Constitutional History* were both for examinations and the writing of lectures a very present help in time of trouble. So I remember you very kindly dear Dr Tanner with your walrus moustache and the impression that you gave us of imparting to us the things that you found entertaining.

In Part I of the Tripos Ancient History of Political Science were alternative papers and for the latter it was required to have a working knowledge of the history of classical Greece and as I wanted to take Political Science, somehow I managed to persuade whoever sanctioned my courses that my knowledge of the ancient world was sufficient for me to take that subject as read. It was in fact extremely limited, consisting mainly of the doings of their gods and goddesses supplemented by one text book carefully mugged up. It was a most interesting course being largely a study of comparative constitutions from those of Athens to those of the United States and modern Europe. Jordan, who gave the course was both stimulating and entertaining. I still remember one of his quips, or quotations, when explaining the functions of the Vice President of the United States, namely 'That a woman had two sons, one of whom was lost at sea and the other became Vice President of the United States and neither was ever heard of again'.

Though I calculate that I could not have been up more than a month to five weeks I had already settled down to a regular routine and had begun to make friends. The day's programme was dictated by the time of lectures which took place in Cambridge and were usually given in the morning, whereas tutorials and study tended to be concentrated on the college. Between the two stretched a mile and a half of the Huntington Road, not then as now lined with houses and the overspill of Cambridge once Castle Hill had been left behind. For those who had no other means of transport, which in practice meant those who could not or would not cycle, the college provided a bus which left the college in time to get students to nine o'clock lectures and brought them back after the last ones of the morning had ended around one. This meant that the 'Busites' were condemned to lunch on whatever had been left by the more fortunate students who were not so regimented. Even this bus was something of an innovation. Originally the young ladies from Girton had been conveyed to and fro in a fleet of taxis, a practice still exhumed by male members of the university as affording material for jokes on the subject of Girton students.

It is not surprising that those who could elected to cycle, but this too had its disadvantages. On cold mornings hands became almost too frozen to grip the handlebars or manipulate the brake going down Castle Hill. On windy ones the problem was to prevent our hats being blown away, for to go to a lecture without a hat would have been unthinkable. Windy nights in winter were even more of a problem because our bicycle lamps, smelly difficult things filled with oil, had a trying habit of blowing out and the police did not always accept in friendly fashion the explanation that the wind had blown it out. Nor had it always; wicks spluttered and failed or oil ran out and no one wanted to walk back pushing a bike. If the expedition involved party dresses unfitted for the ubiquitous bike then we would club together and crowd into a taxi so that the fare came to a shilling a head.

Even for those of us who were independent of the Girton bus it was often necessary to spend an hour or two in Cambridge between lectures and to meet this need the college provided a waiting room off King's Parade where, in theory, one could work. It was even possible to have lunch there if one had to remain in Cambridge for the afternoon. Its culinary standards were not high. Having eaten there one morning on pressed beef, rice pudding and fruit, I expressed my opinion with one word 'Ugh!!!' It was a place to be avoided and generally I did.

For students wanting to work between lectures the much pleasanter alternative was the Seely Library. This was open to both men and women, though the etiquette of the lecture room, with its segregation of the sexes ruled here too. In both the men and the women sat apart and never exchanged a word. Young ladies did not speak to men to whom they had not been properly introduced. Had they done so I wonder sometimes if my own life would have been different.

During my first year I became increasingly conscious of a certain young man who shall remain nameless. Perhaps I noticed him because until after the Armistice the women much outnumbered the men in lectures. As he walked with two sticks he was obviously a war victim and I managed to acquaint myself with his name as at lectures lists were still passed round to be signed by those present and a little calculation, based on the seating pattern, enabled me to attach the correct label to the object of my interest. I had a feeling too that he was not unconscious of my presence. But, though we attended some of the same lectures for three years, we only spoke to each other once. That was in the Seely Library. One day the men had manoeuvred so that we should be forced to sit among them and I sat next to him. My pencil broke and none of my friends had a penknife, so he lent me his. That night I recorded in my diary 'That was enough thrill to last for some time'. It had to suffice. It was not until four years later, when I was working at the London School of Economics under the direction of Dr Lillian Knowles that I came up against K.B. again, then a junior lecturer there. This time the initiative was his. 'I believe we used to go to the same lectures at Cambridge' he asked. My instinct had been correct; he had been as aware of my presence as I had been of his. We became very good friends but it was too late for romance. As the Granta once observed 'Marriages are made in heaven but one should not entirely disregard the Seely Library', did not apply to my secret romance. Now there are men students at Girton. Probing is a forgotten tradition and Christian names are derigour from the first encounter. The adage that 'The more things alter the more they remain the same', as far as the conversations are concerned, does not apply to the students of the Twenties and those of today.

The beginnings of change came, though very gradually, with the Armistice, which in 1919 was to fill the men's colleges to overflowing with young men who, having escaped death, meant to enjoy themselves. The War, with a capital W had dragged on so long that peace seemed to take me by surprise. By November I had settled into the routine of Girton life, lectures, essay writing and the beginning of tentative personal relations. We cycled in on Saturday mornings not to work but to indulge in a cup of coffee and an iced cake, currently known as 'deadlies' at Mathews, a cafe much frequented by students. I might then do a little modest shopping or buy a plant at the colourful market, generally an inexpensive and long lasting cineraria, a plant that still brings those Saturday memories back.

Early in November my mother had planned to come to Cambridge for a short visit. This no doubt was partly to see how I was faring but also for the more practical purpose of making my spartan study somehow more comfortable. On the morning of the 11th November we set out to buy a more comfortable armchair, some cushions and a few pictures to break the monotony of my walls. One, *moonlight over a placid sea*, still hangs in my bedroom. I have always loved the moonlight on water. We also bought a tea set for when I entertained and an inexpensive pewter teapot, sugar and cream jug. So equipped I was ready to play the hostess when the occasion arose. My mother, with some justification doubted my judgement in such matters and the family budget could not stand the risk of mistakes.

Budgeting my personal expenses was necessarily my own responsibility. I had ten shillings a week, plus £5 a term for books. Such prices in view of the enormous change in the value of money since 1918 can mean nothing to most readers today. So to give the cost of my college fees and board and lodging may be helpful by way of comparison. In 1918 these were £105 a year which was even then reflecting pre-war prices and by increments these had to be increased until by 1920 they had reached £150 per annum.

We were busy choosing materials for curtains and to make a loose cover for my armchair when there was a sudden wild clanging of every bell in Cambridge. That night I wrote in my diary, so long neglected,

> 'Today the Armistice was signed and Cambridge went
> mad. Students and cadets climbed roofs, careered
> round on buses, including the Girton one, flew flags
> and blew whistles. These diversions they varied by
> breaking the windows of Cambridge shops and
> lighting a bonfire in the market square at night. The
> whole town was filled with excitement. Men, women
> and children marched madly round the town, shouting,
> cheering and blowing trumpets. When we left we
> found some people on Castle Hill silently worshipping

at the shrine of two unshaded street lamps. The blackout was over.'

That was not the end of that historic day. My diary continued:

'At 1 am that night I woke to the sound of fire rattles and shouts as I thought of alarms. Up I jumped, flung on some clothing and groped my way down the passage, trying in vain to find an unlocked door to the engine house. Then I came back to my room intending to get out of my window. But luckily I went upstairs to be informed that it was an undergraduate rag. Furious I retired to bed. The sanctity of Girton had been invaded.'

Next morning the exuberance was over. The town was quiet as Cambridge people remembered its dead, the young men who would never know its colleges and courts, or, who having known them briefly would never return. The Thanksgiving service at Great St Mary's, the university church, was packed and many more were turned away. To be there was an unforgettable experience, not a joyful celebration of victory but a memorial to the price of young lives with which it had been bought. To me the hymn *'For All The Saints Who From Their Labours Rest'* still brings back that poignant memory. It was their ghosts that were with us in St Mary's that day. To them we paid the tribute of our thanks. I was very near to tears and the service over I took refuge in King's, not in the chapel but in the utter peace of the river. Inadequately that evening I wrote 'I felt queer all afternoon'.

That evening the living took control again. Half way through Hall the Fire alarm disturbed its chatter and the student members of our fire fighting squad rushed out to take their places. The fire, whose flickering flames we had seen, came from a bonfire in the court. All was excitement and half the freshers followed. I nearly did but, as I afterwards boasted in my diary 'I am glad to say I didn't'. Kitts, who had departed to deal with the disturbance, came back and made a speech asking us not to disgrace the dignity of Girton. We all cheered her and then rose to our feet, then got through Hall somehow. The men then found ladders and broke into the college. We retired to our rooms, drew up the shutters and drank cocoa, experiencing all the virtue of a beleaguered garrison, as they stamped down the corridor. Kitts again turned them out and again we cheered her. Some of the second and third years tried to persuade Kitts to let them join the roistering males but she refused. Then the bulldogs came up and these brave housebreakers slunk away except for one youth who was lame. For the sake of the uninitiated I should explain that the bulldogs were not four legged creatures but the stalwart men empowered to enforce the discipline of the university on recalcitrant members. So ended the invasion of Girton and we, as victors, let off steam by holding an impromptu dance.

For the remainder of the term Girton and Cambridge returned to the normal routine of lectures, essays and tutorials, interspersed with jugs, 'the dancing' and elevens at Mathews on Saturday mornings. The loneliness, and feeling of defencelessness in an alien world was being replaced by the tentative growth of new personal relationships, so that I began to develop a sense of belonging, of being one of a group, of having friends. Ruth my neighbour in Bear Pits was a gregarious creature and through her I found myself being merged into a loose coterie that included Elspeth Giles whose friendship became very precious to me.

If Ruth fostered my social life within college it was to Elspeth that I owed an entry into the newly awakened life of Cambridge when in the May term the men came back. Her father, Dr Peter Giles, was the Master of Emmanuel College and there, as our friendship grew I was to become a welcome guest. Through my work I also acquired another, and in many ways, very different friend in Winnie Lamb. She too was reading History. We went to the same lectures, sitting side by side, and in College spent time discussing our work. So from the end of my first term within College I belonged to two worlds, that of serious, conscientious non frivolous Winnie and her friends with whom I discussed History and religion and that of Ruth and Elspeth who took life and learning more lightly. From both I gained much. I was beginning to slot in.

CHAPTER THREE: "THE HEROES" RETURN

In the spring of 1919 Cambridge was reborn. THE MEN WERE BACK. No theatrical impresario could have contrived so magical a transformation scene. Nor a cast so varied to complete an academic career that had been interrupted, others to one planned but never started. Now they looked forward to three years of Cambridge life. There was no need yet even to think about the Tripos, let alone to worry about it. These men had learnt to take short views of life. Each day was a day to be enjoyed. If this was true of undergraduates who expected to stay up three years, it was manifestly more so for men who were only up for a short period. Such were the members of the naval attachment who had a special glamour in my eyes. But most prominent of all, at least to my socially minded friends, were the Americans.

When I returned for the May term Elspeth informed me that there would be many Americans about. They were officers in the American army, university men, who were sent to get a taste of English life. She told me that it was really part of the friendship stunt propaganda. John Harvard had been an Emmanuel man before he had sailed to America and founded Harvard. So all the Harvard men in Cambridge made Emmanuel their headquarters even if they were attached to other colleges. That meant that the Giles' had to do a great deal of entertaining. Elspeth told much about one set of men they had had into tea during the Easter vacation.

The house was full of visitors and the duty of showing them round the college had devolved on her. There was a Mr Blake, Mr Sherry, who was very good looking, English and charming. I fancy she had concentrated most of her attention on him. Anyhow she told me how nice he was. There was also a tall, solid red faced young man who had attached himself to the party but hardly opened his mouth during the whole afternoon. His name I did not catch, though later he was to be, like Sherry, of some importance. Elspeth was wearing her soft liberty greyish voile dress with the fissure. She told me that she was in fine form that afternoon so I can guess how animated and sweet she looked.

The British men who had returned might have returned also to the pre-war attitude of the university to the women students and have taken little notice of them. That was not the American way. They were out-going, informal, friendly and, to quote a later musical, thought that there was nothing like a dame. It was they who gave their own particular brand of excitement and colour to the Cambridge scene when I returned to Girton in the April of that year though for the first part of the term I was an onlooker of the social activities of Ruth and Elspeth rather than an active participant.

Under the pressure of this invasion even Girton began to move out of its female isolation. Under carefully controlled conditions we were allowed to entertain male visitors. Not of course when we were supposed to be working, but as a special concession on Sundays and I think also maybe on Saturday afternoons. For this privilege the permission of the Mistress had first to be obtained and this was something of an ordeal. Kitts was a formidable person, partly because I think she was a shy one and partly because her position set her apart. This was emphasised by the size of her room and the position of her desk behind which she sat to receive you. Having knocked and having been told to come in the first problem was when to say-'Good morning Miss Jess Blake.' To do so as soon as one entered meant having to advance silently over what felt like a vast intervening stretch of carpet. This silent approach made one feel very conscious, wondering what to say next. On the other hand to approach without this formality, reserving the greeting until reaching the desk somehow seemed lacking in politeness. The request made, Kitts was apt to ask 'Do your parents know these young men'. In most cases the answer must be 'No' but fortunately this was not a barrier to permission being given but rather an opening gambit. Kitts was taking no risk with the proprieties even in allowing this limited freedom; in a man's world, with the hope that discrete conduct would lead the sooner to the granting of degrees, she had to watch her step.

So the next step was to secure a chaperon. I can no longer remember whether the name of this victim to convention had to be produced when asking permission to hold a tea party or whether it was enough to give the names of the other Girton members, for tea parties were always joint affairs. Generally some kind hearted don was pressed into service and to the more approachable this must have been a considerable nuisance. Perhaps they exerted some pressure on Kitts behind the scenes for though a chaperon was still required for a tea party held in a student's room, with proper permission picnic tea parties given by two or more students came to be held without a chaperon.

The first barricades had been stormed and later even the presence of that guardian of our conduct was waived so long as the hostesses were two or more in number. To this glamorous world of tea parties I should never have been able to enter on my own initiative. I was far too shy, far too inexperienced. Ruth had no intention of this fate becoming hers. Even when the men had broken into Girton on the night of the bonfire in the court, in spite of Kitts' disapproval she had been one of those who had dashed out to see the fun. She was a natural 'dame'; Elspeth's situation was different. Because her father was Master of Emmanuel it was inevitable that she would be involved in the returning hoards of masculinity. As Master he and Mrs Giles had to entertain their young men, and the pressure to do so was increased by the fact that Harvard had been an Emmanuel man, their daughter was more than welcome to bring her Girton friends with her to those traditional Sunday afternoon tea parties at the Master's Lodge. So between Ruth, who sometimes needed me to complete one of her tea parties, and Elspeth, I began to find my feet in this new exciting world of men.

Sunday tea parties can hardly have taxed even my courage over much but this was soon to be put to a more alarming test. On Elspeth's birthday Dr and Mrs Giles decided to celebrate it with a small dance to which I was invited. By then Elspeth had already collected a swarm of admirers, most of them American, so there was no danger of my lacking partners. Had she not asked me I should have been desperately hurt as I had never been to a dance before, but the prospect was terrifying. I was not a natural dancer, having very little sense of rhythm, and such practise as I had had I owed to 'the dancing' with my fellow students at Girton. Even then my proficiency was of a low order and faced with strange men I feared the worst.

It was with trepidation that I put on my first evening dress; white georgette with big pearl trimmings and a lace scarf to drape round my shoulders. Elspeth and Ruth were very reassuring, telling me that I looked very nice, a judgement with which I privately agreed. Even small dances in the twenties were conducted with almost the same formality as had prevailed when Fanny Burney's *Evelina* took the floor at her first dance. Describing the evening I wrote:

> 'It was awful. The Girton contingent followed Elspeth
> in shyly and stood in a solid block near the door while
> the men lined up on the other side of the room. At
> first I thought they were never going to ask us to dance
> but eventually they broke ranks and advanced towards

us. There were an even number of men and women so you stood by the door until a man came up to you and asked 'Have you a partner for this dance?' You said 'No' and he asked 'May I?' and away you went. Dancing was not nearly as difficult as I had feared. The men get hold of you and sort of glide and you do your best to let your feet glide too. At the corners one turned a bit and sometimes swayed about.'

My first dance was memorable for another reason. It was the first time I had met an American in the flesh, though having been an ardent picturegoer, I was familiar with their screen image. My impression of them as partners was distinctly favourable. I described one of them as:

'A very tall American who was rather funny. He was very, very American with an accent you could cut with a knife. He danced beautifully though, sort of glided along, so that it seemed quite easy. When we went into the garden it was getting dark and somehow he conveyed the idea that he found me brilliant and charming. Inexperienced as I am in these matters it was my private opinion that he was flirting with me. I would like to know if I was flirting with him. It is a thing I know nothing about of course, so it is difficult to tell.'

I was then nineteen, even by contemporary standards very green: by those of today's, incredibly so.

My favourite partner that evening was another American, a Mr Martin, whom I described as:

'Short, with a tiny French moustache and a little of a French manner. He hustled round the room and then had to mark time at the corners. He was always bumping into people but we got on very well together. At first he tried to stuff me about America and Indians running amok in New York and Harvard, but when I mentioned that I had always understood that Indians lived in reservations he stopped. Then I got my first lesson in American politics from an American, such previous knowledge as I had, had been confined to D W Griffith's great screen drama *The Birth of a Nation* and to Jordon's lectures on Poly Si. Now I learnt that Democrats are usually Southerners and believe in State Rights, while Republicans are Northerners and believe in high tariffs. Wilson is a Democrat. Apparently the Klu Klux Klan still exists as Night Riders and in practice negroes don't vote in Southern States.'

I returned to college in a happy mood feeling that I had broken the ice though in honesty I had to add 'that the aftermath was even more pleasant than the actual dance'.

It is difficult to generalise; one's own experiences loom too large and that experience is limited. Looking back I can see that my delayed, adolescent excitement as I took my first exciting steps towards womanhood were not typical of the majority of Girton students who were either more socially adept or less interested in men. Throughout my first three years at Girton I had friends in both groups. My diary, by concentrating on my own emotional development, the experimental, the new, the exciting, distorted the balance of my day to day life. This was dominated by lectures, by concentrated reading and by essays and time papers.

For this side of my life my friends were different. Chief among them was Winnie Lumb. We worked together as a pair, absorbed in the purpose for which we had both come to Cambridge, the study of History. I cannot imagine her going to dances or having her heart fluttered by an American. I never remember men figuring in her conversation. That was also true of Helen Harvey, a second year History student with whom, because her great friend Jessie had the study next door to mine, I became a close friend. Between them Helen and Winnie steered me away from the tepid Methodism, in which I had been brought up, towards the Church of England. It was due to them, together with the influence of the Cambridge colleges and traditions, that later I was confirmed.

These were the friends who stimulated my intellectual interests and broadened them. It was with them that I discussed not only religion but the problems of the day. I have no statistics, no firm evidence, only impressions but these are that the majority of my fellow students were in essence what one would call career women, who went serenely on with their way of life, taking advantage of their intellectual opportunities, such societies as were open to them, but essentially rooted in a female world. They were the head-mistresses, the teachers of the future; that I too expected to be my own future. I might be full of romantic ideas which I expressed in verse, I hesitate to call it poetry, but I don't remember ever looking forward to marriage, while sex, as an emotion, was still a closed book to me. Perhaps that is why, if I thought about marriage at all, I fancied the idea of a sailor husband on the grounds that I thought I could be an awfully nice wife for a short period but that once he sailed away, I could devote myself to my own concerns. I am not sure that I was not showing a greater self knowledge than I realised when I harboured such thoughts. In spite of the wonderful burgeoning of early summer all around me, in spite of the thrill of my first dance, what loomed most largely on my horizon was not men but the imminence of Mays.

In non-academic terms perhaps Mays may best be described as a trial run over the Tripos course. They were University examinations, they were important in that they indicated the probable form of the future runners, but they carried no penalties for a poor performance, To prepare for this ordeal we had Time Papers modelled on the actual type of question that we would have to answer, so that we could accustom ourselves to regurgitate the information that we had acquired in all our First Year courses within the prescribed three hours. In addition there was an essay Paper, designed to test not our knowledge and understanding but our ability to tackle a general topic for which we had not been prepared.

I wasn't unduly worried at the prospect of sitting Mays. I had done rather well in my Time Paper on Economic History, getting what EEP described as a shaky First, really a border line paper between a First and a II.1, and my Medieval European and Political Science papers had been respectable. My own forecast would have been that I was likely to come third in the college list after C F and W T, the acknowledged stars of our History Year. The night before Mays I felt less calm, cool and collected, suffering from pre-examination blues. On Sunday I wrote:

> 'The day before Mays ... Until this evening I felt
> awfully bad, as if nothing would ever come out of
> my head again. However having been assured by
> Winnie that I should get a First, which of course is a
> lie, and had a bath, I felt better; ready to conquer or
> die in fact. When the exam was over I felt that I had
> done neither, being neither pleased nor displeased
> with my performance. I believed that I had made a
> mess of the last question on my Economic paper, on
> which I had hoped to do well and that the topic I had
> chosen on the Essay paper had been the wrong choice.
> Compromise would have been a more interesting
> topic than Divine Right. So that though I might have
> secretly hoped for a II.1, now expected a II.2 and put
> the results out of my mind. When the results came out
> I was still in residence as I had night to keep.'

This obscure phrase referred to the university regulations that decreed that to qualify for the Tripos, students sitting it had to put in a minimum number of nights in college. Because of its financially precarious position Girton students normally only came into residence for this minimum period and if for any reason a student failed to do this the missing nights had to be made up at the end of term. In my case I had come back late after a bout of flu. So I was still in college when C P Jones appeared in my room saying 'Congratulations.' Looking up from my book I asked without much interest 'Why?'. 'Don't you know? You are top of the Mays History List.' Jumping to my feet I exclaimed 'I'm not, I'm not' in tones of unbelief. I rushed up to Miss Dean's room and was assured that this miracle was true. In spite of my own assessment, which was also true. So far we did not seem a distinguished year; I had my expected II.2 but I did head the list. I had expected to come third but never first and I felt that something very strange had happened to those lists. To be truthful so did everyone else and many and varied were the theories to explain away my success. I tidied and dressed hoping for a visit from EEP but Phil Taylor carried me off to jug so I missed her. I was in a state of such wild enthusiasm that I felt no joy could equal this.

After Mays there had seemed no point in doing more work. I had felt free to indulge in the idleness and pleasure that was the hallmark of 'May Week' with its bump races and its balls. I had no likelihood or even desire to attend the latter but the Races were a spectacle enjoyed by gown, town and women students on equal terms. It was on the tow-path that I first felt that sense of belonging, of belonging to Cambridge and that Cambridge belonged to me. This reaction was unexpected. The first day I had not gone; it was raining and I was not interested. Boats chasing one another down the narrow Cam did not sound exciting. Elspeth however was quite firm, insisting that the May Week races were important and that I ought to come when she went next day.

So I went and within the first half hour had become enthusiastically addicted to the magic of the tow-path. It was not a mere flash in the pan: for the next three years I was keenly interested not only in the more glamorous May Races but almost as much in the often cold and rainy Lent Races. I followed the fortunes of my favourite colleges with the keen interest of any race goer and my later diaries often contain the names of an entire crew. As my social life developed in my second year I even had a more personal interest; a member of the eight was also one of my dancing partners. In my diary I was obviously at some pains to try to capture something of the excitement that my first introduction to this university tradition that I could fully share. 'It is difficult', I wrote, 'to get into words that May Day scene. The river was so broad and smiling'. Here I can only have been contrasting it with its breadth as seen from the Backs, the only part I had hitherto known. To describe it as 'broad' was certainly a euphemism. More justified was my next. observation,

> 'So peaceful in contrast to the swirling mass on the tow-path. It seemed to throw into relief the bright blazers, the light dresses of the women. There was the brilliant scarlet of Lady Margaret men (the St John's crew) while the blue and cherry of Emmanuel contrasted with the sober green of Queen's. Then the serenity of the river was broken as one by one the Eights came up to their stations, proudly, gracefully, as if to show their watchers their worth. I watched the graceful boats, admiring the rhythmic swing of the oars and the gaily coated coxes with mounting excitement. The magic of the May Races was beginning to work. By the time we had reached Ditton Meadow it seemed as if all Cambridge had poured onto the tow-path. There the bank was lined with small boats and still more people. The Meadows afforded the best, or at least the most popular place from which to watch. So as neither I nor Elspeth had any small change, as to enter them a charge was made in order to limit the crowds that, without this discouragement, would have swarmed over them, it was lucky that our

escorts were prepared to do the gentlemanly thing and pay for us.

Dramatically the babble of voices hushed, then came a prolonged murmur 'the first gun'. The babble was renewed but now there was a strain in it. Everyone was waiting. Again, like corn in the wind, came that mutual murmur 'the second gun'. Then silence. Then from a distance a faint; noise. It grew louder as the full throated hurrahs grew nearer. Then it seemed as if the tow-path heaved, like a huge serpent as the cheering men, encouraging their college crew, forced their way through the standing spectators. At that moment a boat's prow appeared round Ditton Corner, close behind it came a second, struggling to make a bump. Because the Cam was too narrow for the Eights to race side by side, rather like a game of croquet, each strove to eliminate its rival by catching, up and bumping prow to stern. Then the boat that had been 'bumped' and its successful rival drew into the bank. In the races next day the victor and the vanquished changed place, the final prize being to become head of the River by the last day. When, as we watched, there was a gap in the procession we knew that there must have been a bump in the early reaches and as Emma 2, (which being translated meant the second Emmanuel boat) must from its delay in appearing have made a 'bump' Elspeth was jubilant. When the races for the Division were over a stately procession of victor and vanquished, of the bumpers and the bumped, marshalled in their correct order, re-rowed the course, the former with flags flying vigorously cheered by their supporters on the banks, the defeated trying to look unselfconscious. That evening victory was celebrated by a Bump Supper in a way which I suppose men do celebrate when there are no females present to restrain them.

The Second Division races were in a sense an appetizer for the thrills of the First Division, contenders for the proud title of Head of the River, Lady Margaret in their distinctive scarlet, Pemmer (Pembroke) in their light and dark blue, and then, third in the line up Trinity followed by Jesus, their black and white oars flashing in the sun. When the last boats had taken up their stations, once again there came that strained no man's land of sound, broken by the sudden murmur as the marrons were fired, then the faint cheers growing nearer, accompanied by the clamour of fire rattles and the clang of bells. Once again the crowd on the tow-path heaved and parted as round Ditton Corner came the noise of a boat its oars splashing in haste. All heads were craned to see 'Who was it?' Again the sun caught the red on black oars. It was Jesus leading still but hard pressed by Trinity Third. Then came Pemmer with Lady Margaret close behind. In two minutes it was all over, the long graceful strokes of the First Division already only a memory.'

I was hooked and each afternoon until the races ended found me on the towpath. I had the fever and was determined not to miss a single day.

There was another feature of May Week that I sampled for not only my first time but for the returning men, though it appealed to a more selective group. Cambridge had a long dramatic tradition both serious and frivolous undergraduates. This was its first post war show. I cannot remember the title of the show but the plot of their current musical was a tangle of skit and comment on the new post war Cambridge, on the world in which they found themselves.

It purported to deal with the establishment of a new college devoted to the study of self advertisement, the crest of which was to be the Archangel blowing his trumpet. The tangle of inconsequential happenings do not matter, though the climax was interesting. The students contrived to steal the degrees, only to discover that the dons had gone one better and stolen the Blues. This was too much to bear. By general consent the old order was restored on the grounds that 'One has one's whole life to attain a degree but only four years in which a man could get a degree'.

One member of the cast I thought quite outstanding. He was a N C Hulbert who played a Yankee so convincingly that I thought he must be an American, his accent was so perfect. It was only later that I discovered him to be Claude Hulbert, the brother of the then distinguished musical star of the musical comedy stage Jack Hulbert. He later followed the same profession. Though Footlights did provide an opportunity for budding actors to show their talent this privilege was limited to members of the university. As in Shakespeare's day it was an all male cast and so conditioned were we that I did not even comment on our exclusion. We were still living in a man's world. Not all the members of Footlights aspired to a theatrical career. An eminent social historian once told me that he had played the leading young female part in the Footlights' performance of his day, dancing and singing no doubt with his usual zest and determination which has marked him throughout his life. I withhold his name to spare his blushes!

Nevertheless Girton and Newnham were beginning to make ascent in this exclusively male world. Whether the social barriers, the outward barricades as it were, would have crumbled so rapidly or so easily without the impact of the Americans, I have often wondered. They were unencumbered either by the necessity of taking their academic obligations seriously or by the conventions of English society and the female company on which they normally relied was on the other side of the Atlantic. As a wise old father of a friend of mine used to observe 'Great is the God of Love but greater is proximity'. We were there. We too represented a new generation of students for whom life was no longer quite so real and so earnest as it had been for the pioneers of university education for women. 'The way of a man with a maid' was taking over and for those of us who had the inclination and the opportunity of meeting them, the Americans certainly speeded up the process.

Left to myself I should have had neither. Whether on the tow-path or at Footlights I should have enjoyed them exclusively in the company of my female friends. Ruth and Elspeth were both madly social but apart from her birthday dance until almost the end of the term my male contacts were very few and those I owed to my friends. It was Elspeth who had taken me first to the Bump Races and it was she who had provided our gentlemanly escorts who had paid our entrance to Ditton Meadows. The next day I went with Ruth and the pattern was repeated.

This time we paid for our own entrance to the Meadows, to Ruth's annoyance. She preferred the more gregarious tow-path crowd so it was not until we were returning along the towpath that she ran into two Americans that she knew. She introduced me but I was tongue tied and while she chatted away I walked in stony uncomfortable silence until we got to the Pike and Eel, where we had left our bicycles. Next day I went to both the Footlights and the Races afterwards with Helen. So far my encounters with the Americans had not been encouraging. It was only after the end of my Mays that I even took part in a mixed tea party and that was to help Elspeth, who was the hostess but who still had a last paper to sit that afternoon. I cut what I described as 'the most beautiful cucumber sandwiches' and we had bought 'deadlies' from Mathews. Another friend of Elspeth, Susie had also been invited to help hold the fort until Elspeth arrived. So far my social debut had been hardly distinguished.

I was soon to be faced with a more formidable hurdle. It was decided by the powers that be that Girton too would give a May Week dance. Who the instigator was I never knew but certainly without Kitts' approval this break with the past could never have happened. She was a wise and understanding person, as I came to realise when I had more personal contact with her in my senior years, and must have been as aware that Girton stood on the edge of a new era. If her students were to play a part in the social life of the university there were advantages in their doing so under the auspices of the college and not in clandestine meetings. Moreover to join in the celebrations that graced May Week was to claim a stake in what before had been the domain of the men's colleges.

Because numbers had to be limited only to the second and third years to grace this festivity which was to take place after the first year had departed. But because I had night to make up after having missed the first few days of term I was still in residence. So was Ruth and because Elspeth lived in Cambridge she too would be able to come. Apart from any fears that I might have I had also to solve a more immediate problem. Ruth and Elspeth had swarms of young men, so that the need to invite a partner caused them no difficulty, unless it were which of their attendant males to so honour. I alas had no prospective partner. Resourceful as ever my friends decided that the Mr Martin, with whom I had danced several times at Elspeth's birthday dance and whom I had liked would be my most suitable guest. Accordingly they helped me to concoct an invitation. I was half horrified at my audacity and half relieved when he accepted. But at least I had a partner.

The dance was less of an ordeal than I had expected. I put on my white georgette dress trimmed with pearls and hoped for the best. My reliance was mostly on my appearance, which my friends assured me was 'very nice' for my dancing was atrocious. I could not have had a more understanding partner than Mr Martin. He introduced me to all his friends and so practically filled up my programme. Later, when I recorded the events of the evening I observed, somewhat condescendingly:

> 'He was one of the best type of Americans, a
> gentleman, which I imagine is rather rare over there. I
> suspect he had rather a boring time but he thanked me
> very nicely at the end.'

Having met so few Americans I was hardly in a position to judge or to know how characteristic of his countrymen in his kindness and courtesy my Mr Martin was. My Mr Martin; how formal we were in those days; I never even knew his Christian name and would certainly not have used it if I had.

Since this is not an autobiography I shall not dwell on the individual partners that Fate or Mr Martin provided. One partner however, speaking of his war experiences presented me with a fragment of history too fascinating to omit. In addition to the Americans there was also a naval contingent up on a short course, some of whom I had met at Elspeth's birthday dance. Tonight, being for once without a partner the long suffering and good hearted Miss Dean introduced me to a naval lieutenant. I think his name was Story. I described him as 'The best dancer I had that evening; he even made me feel that I too could dance.'

Perhaps long periods afloat had made him determined to gather rosebuds while he could. I don't know if he regarded me as a rosebud but he nearly squeezed the breath out of me. Though I have been in some tight corners before I have never been held so closely by a man. I had no option but to follow where he led. The dance over, we wandered into the sweet. smelling dusk of the grounds where we found two chairs. Here I became expansive, telling him how romantically I had been attached to the Navy ever since, as a fourteen year old recovering from mumps at Lamlash on the Isle of Arran, I had been fascinated by the spectacle of the First Battle Squadron anchored in that magnificent bay. In the spring of 1914, Northern

Ireland was thought to be on the verge of armed resistance to the latest attempt to introduce yet another bill to settle the Irish question and the navy was waiting in the wings. Dabbott and I spent hours on the quay watching the liberty launches go to and from the great ships and talking to such of the warrant officers who would answer our eager questions.

Perhaps the greatest thrill of all was to learn that Prince Albert (later George VI) was a midshipman on the *Collingwood*. Here before my eyes was a genuine prince and I feasted them on the slim fair youth whenever he was in charge of the liberty boat and collected every scrap of information that I could about him, including the fact that on board he was known as 'the Lobster' because he blushed so easily. As I was never likely to meet a prince I settled very happily that evening for my naval lieutenant and, wishing to impress him began to parade my knowledge of the ships of the fleet, I even boasted that I knew how many funnels each class possessed. He challenged me, asking in a teasing voice, 'How many funnels had the *Queen Mary*?' 'Three, then I hesitated, 'No, Two. She was a battle cruiser'. Then with a sudden inspiration I asked 'Was she your ship?'

'Yes, I was on her when she was sunk; I was one of the fifteen survivors out of 1500. It was soon after I had joined her.' He continued in answer to my plea that he would tell me the full story. 'We were suddenly ordered south and everyone was frightfully keen. But nothing happened so the men were piped down to breakfast in the middle of which the enemy were first sighted. Everyone rushed to action stations. I was in one of the gun turrets and for half an hour we peppered one another. Then one of our guns was put out of action and soon after that the other was blown straight through the ship and the cordite caught fire. I thought it was about time to be getting out when I discovered that the ship was split in two. I flung my coat and waistcoat off and one shoe. I was stopping to untie the other when the ship was blown up and me with it. I went down with her, sucked down by the suction. I thought I was done for alright.

There was just time to breathe a prayer or two before it was all over. To hasten matters I tried to swallow as much water as possible but it tasted so beastly I determined to have another fight for it. Up I came to the surface gasping for breath and swallowed a mouthful of oil . . . ! Well I kept up for about half an hour, then a destroyer came hovering round. I tried to signal but after a bit she picked up some men and then went off because an aeroplane was dropping bombs above. However she came back and I was picked up. Once aboard I was violently sick but the First Lieutenant made me swallow some Bovril and brandy.'

I exclaimed at such a strange mixture and was told that it was excellent in a case like that. After a hot bath and a sleep he insisted that except for a splitting headache he felt alright and was able to take part in a night attack. When he returned to base he was given a month's leave. When I asked what affect this terrible experience had had on him, all the answer that I got was 'That no man need ever go to pieces unless he wanted to. Another fellow who was picked up with me had to have six months sick leave; went all to pieces but it was his own fault.' Was this bravado on his part and was it true I had no means of knowing and I was too thrilled by the recital to spoil the memory by enacting the role of a doubting Thomas. By the time we had gone inside the dance was nearly over. How many partners I had cut I did not know and regrettably did not care. Tired but happy I went to bed. It had been a wonderful night and my self confidence was growing.

With the Girton dance the excitement of May Week came to its end. But for me, one last experience that was to complete my picture of Cambridge still lay ahead. First however there was a more domestic interlude between me and my last thrill. I still had nights to keep and my Father took the opportunity to come to stay when I had no work to claim any of my time. I showed him all over college and took him to pay his respects to Kitts. This was at his insistence and hers. I suffered from the inherent fears of the young that in some way their parents will say or do the wrong thing. For instance he might show off an unjustified pride in my ability, a sentiment that she might not share. It was only while he was with me and after the interview that I heard the glorious news that I had topped the Mays History list. My fears of course were groundless. We went round the colleges and spent much time in Mathews and other places of refreshment but it was very hot and after the excitement of Mays Week, now that the colleges were emptying that the Cambridge scene had suddenly gone flat. I wished he had been able to share in the cheerful hullaballoo of the tow-path, he would have enjoyed that, just as he would have enjoyed Footlights. I wished he could have seen the Cambridge that I loved and not the half dead town that remained when the university had gone down. I might even have taken him to a baseball match. Ruth and I had gone together to that and my diary contains a long description of what I supposed to be the rules of the game. Personally I had not been over impressed, writing that

> 'Baseball seems to me to be a kind of glorified
> rounders. There is nothing graceful about it to watch.
> The players wear dirty grey flannel shirts, baggy
> bloomers and jockey caps.'

Not prepossessing was my verdict. My father would have agreed. Boats and driving tandems were his hobbies, though after we had left Leighton Hall, dog carts and horses were things of the past.

My nights having been duly kept and my Father having departed, I was no longer a student in residence bound by college and university regulations. Instead I was to stay with Elspeth for a week and then she was to come back with me to be introduced to the Lakes, where she had never been. While I had been concentrating on my Father she had been concentrating on the Americans and when we met for elevens at Mathews, after I had seen Daddy off at the station, she told me that she had found a man she liked better than Mr Sherry, a Mr Lathrop. She went on 'You may meet him tonight. We heard that the

Americans were leaving Cambridge tomorrow, so Mother has asked all the Harvard men in for coffee. Emmanuel being John Harvard's college they always feel there is a link between us and them. It's going to be rather fun and at the end we are all to have a cider cup in the Long Gallery. All the Harvard men are going to drink healths out of the cup that Harvard presented to the College. Later we heard that they were not going for a couple of days or so. By the way Sherry and Lathrop are going to take us on the river tomorrow. We went out, quite a lot of us, to Granchester on Monday. Mr Lathrop and I went exploring in the churchyard and all round the old vicarage. Well they wanted to fix up another day. I said I had a friend staying with me so they said bring her too. I think it will be rather nice. I hope you will like them.'

Had Elspeth's parents been ordinary parents, though I might have felt some nervousness at staying for a week with people I hardly knew, I should not have got into my taxi, when it arrived at 4 o'clock in an agony of trepidation. But Dr and Mrs Giles were not ordinary parents and to stay at the Master's lodge was not like being a guest in an ordinary family. Dr Giles was an important person, very active in university politics and a well known figure. It was rather like, if not quite God, at least being the guest of one of the archangels and spending a week in one of the heavenly annexes. The Lodge was not, of course, completely unknown territory. Elspeth had taken me to the Giles' Sunday afternoon tea parties more than once in addition to my debut at her birthday dance. But on those occasions I had been in a group of young men, some of whom may have felt as awed as I did. Now I had to face the family alone. The Giles had two other daughters, Margaret the eldest and Taffy – why that nickname I did not know – the youngest. Elspeth took me straight up to the drawing room where Margaret and Mrs Giles did their best to make me feel at home calling me Dorothy. All the same I should have been glad to have Mother to hide behind. However, she was safely tucked away at Old Hutton. I did my best to act the polite lady and hoped I appeared more self possessed than I felt. It seemed strange to have Elspeth also playing a new role, that of daughter of the house. Dinner was even more of an ordeal graced as it was by Dr Giles.

After dinner came the American deluge; there seemed to be hundreds of khaki figures; I believe there were about twenty. Elspeth introduced me to Mr Heard, the Senior Tutor. He was one of those dark, ugly attractive clergymen. I liked him and felt safe with him. Hugh Walpole had apparently parodied him in 'Prelude to Adventure' which had made Elspeth very indignant, the more so as certain of his mannerisms had given grounds for attack. Alas as a refuge he proved a broken reed instead of affording me sanctuary as any good cleric should surely do. In other words saying 'I must not let an old fogy like me monopolize you. You must talk to some of the younger men.' He then handed me over to an extremely dull specimen of that species whom luckily I managed to discard when we moved from the drawing room where we had been drinking coffee, to the garden. Elspeth was wandering round with a man I presumed to be Sherry, in tow. She was very much the grown up daughter that night as she handed round cigarettes. Her face was animated and, with her short hair fluttering, she reminded me of a flower head on its slender stalk. Then we went up to the Long Gallery.

The lights were lit and the panelled walls looked mellow. In the confined space the hum of voices and the clink of glasses was intensified. I felt a queer exhilaration in the air, a sense of brotherhood and excitement. It was almost as if I saw a great thing taking place under my eyes. We sang Auld Lang Syne and then the party began to break up. Elspeth introduced Mr Sherry and somewhat hastily I decided that I did not like him. He was medium sized with a limp hand shake with the air of being just about to drop off to sleep. His complexion was pale and he had a tiny blonde moustache. I was not prepossessed. When I asked about Lathrop I was told he had not come. After the departure of the crowd we sat around for a little time and then departed to bed, tired but happy, feeling that this was life indeed.

Next day I tasted for the first time what even after all these years, still distils for me the magic of Cam, a river picnic. Though during the glory of early summer I had soaked myself in the beauty of the Banks, standing on Clare bridge or sauntering past the weeping willows that fringed the river at St John's and which always made me think of mermaid hair with their long green tresses. But I had never been on the river itself, nor had I ever cherished the expectation of ever occupying one of those punts poled lazily by young men in immaculate white flannels. Now at the eleventh hour this delight was to be mine. To my surprise I found that we were not to be a foursome in a punt but to take to the water in canoes, a craft firmly forbidden by Girton rules. But, for this one week these did not apply. Elspeth, who had got everything planned out, informed me that I was to go with Mr Lathrop but that on the return we would change partners, which I thought was rather significant of her feelings. After lunch we dressed. I wore a flowered voile dress, light and pretty looking with a big tilting hat, pink underneath and biscuit on top with swaths of pink ribbon. If excitement could make me pretty then I was pretty that day for my cheeks were flushed and my eyes glowing. Elspeth was wearing her green dress with white collars and cuffs that made her look more like a mischievous boy than ever with her short, dark, curly hair. Mr Sherry called for us at the Lodge and at the boathouse a tall figure was waiting. My first impression of Julian Lathrop was of long white flannel legs and a blue blazer, very naval looking. He had dark curly hair, hazelly grey eyes, very straight and kind and the general look of the strong, silent type. He had a firm handclasp too: instinctively I felt he was a man one could trust. At first we drifted past the banks, almost in silence until Elspeth and Sherry tried to emulate the races and bump us with the nose of their canoe. Then we fell apart again. By now I was beginning to feel that in my condemnation of Sherry the previous evening I had been over hasty. His hazel eyes were nice and twinkly and he had a whimsical mouth when he smiled, though he still put the paddle in the water as if it was almost too much trouble. To be with a man I hardly knew had left me tongue tied, then Lathrop broke the silence as we passed Trinity by asking me what

90

the library reminded me of. As Mr Sherry had told me that Lathrop was interested in architecture, I tried to think of some intelligent comment to make but no inspiration came. He then informed me that to him it resembled a railway station. I would never have thought of so mundane a comparison but found I agreed. Near Bates Bite we beached our canoes and prepared our picnic, sandwiches, deadlies, strawberries and cream with tea brewed on a methylated stove. It was a lazy, leisurely happy meal and disgracefully late before we started to paddle home. It was getting dark by the time that we reached the lock. Everything was grey and rather chilly: from the other side of the river there came the sound of gramophone. When we reached the backs it was almost dark, mysterious and grey where John's rose from the water and the Bridge of Sighs spanned the water and so at last we came to the boat house. The men suggested hopefully, that as they were sure that dinner at the lodge would be over by now, would we come back and have something to eat at Sherry's house. Elspeth very firmly said NO and equally, firmly dismissed them when they walked with us back to the Lodge. She realised what her mother's reactions would be at our returning so late without the respectability of a chaperon. Because I was a visitor under her roof Mrs Giles tempered her stricture in the interest of politeness while making it clear that to return at 10.50 pm was not to happen again. It had been a wonderful, wonderful day. The men suggested that we repeat it on Saturday; devoutly I hoped that they would.

The invitation was repeated though Mrs Giles' response could hardly have been described as enthusiastic. Nor was the weather co-operative. The morning had been dull and rain threatened. As we sat in the drawing room armed with umbrellas and macs waiting the arrival of Mr Sherry, we must have looked quite a quaint, very British, specimen of a prospective river picnic. Mrs Giles suggested tea in the Long Gallery but we persisted that the sun would come out and our optimism was justified. It did. After our previous expedition I regarded Sherry and Lathrop as old friends. My feelings about the former had changed completely. This was partly because as we paddled back in the evening I found his conversation interesting and well informed and perhaps I was influenced even more by the fact that Elspeth had told me that he had found me 'absolutely charming'. How could I fail to like him after that! It was a marvellous picnic in which we behaved more like school children than ladies and gentlemen. We went as before in canoes, and as before it was Julian who brought Elspeth back but the picnic itself was almost a riotous affair. The men had a race to see which of them could eat a doughnut the faster, nearly choking in their eagerness to win. Then in trying to light the methylated stove to boil our kettle Lathrop singed Elspeth's hair and set the bag with the strawberries and chocolates on fire. That tragedy I averted smothering the blaze with one of the cushions from the canoe. I also received an example of the fact that the same words in American and British language did not necessarily convey the same meaning, when Sherry, leaning over me and picking something from my head remarked conversationally, 'Excuse me but you have a bug in your hair'.

This was the end of our Midsummer madness. Though on the Sunday the Giles' gave a last tea party to some of the departing Americans, it was a formal, frustrating affair in which there was no chance of even a private word of farewell. Moralizing as usual in my diary I wrote

'To be attractive to men should not be an aim in life
but only an incidental. It usually leads to trouble and a
funny feeling inside. It is better to confine oneself to
one's own sex and one's work if you want peace and
quiet. In future I will be an iceberg.'

So my first year at Girton came to an end with this wonderful script of happiness behind me, I was making new friends, I was gaining social self-confidence and all this had been a bonus. My work had not suffered, I was learning the skills of my craft and in a surprising academic spurt, had even headed the History Mays list. In that field at least my ambitions had been aroused. When I came back in the October of 1919 as a second year, I was ready to enter more fully into what not only the female world of Girton could offer but the wider one of the university. My initiation was over.

CHAPTER FOUR: AUTUMN 1919

When I returned to Cambridge in the autumn of 1919 that first fine careless rapture was a thing of the past. It vanished with those innovating birds of passage, the Americans. The university had returned to its self-contained existence. Whatever their private memories, their hopes and fears the soldiers of yesterday had become the students of today. Even so they brought to the university a maturity that, looking back, I can see gave a depth to all its activities from the union debates to the performances of the ADC. This was the world that for the next three years was to shape and mould me, the world in which I began to find and develop my own maturity, the world that was to dictate my future, so that when the fighting men returned from the Second World War the roles were reversed. A lecturer myself, used to students straight from school, I had the satisfaction of dealing with men of experience leavening the lump of callow youth. Was Cambridge, I wonder, ever again to have the flavour of those magic years when I was at Girton and permitted, albeit on the fringe, to feel myself part of it.

We were the fortunate few. For many ex-soldiers returning to civvy street the prospect was less entrancing. In the first heady euphoric months of victory they had looked forward to the rewards of the victors, 'a land fit for heroes to live in'. The reality was to prove far otherwise and by that autumn disillusionment was beginning to express itself in industrial unrest and strikes. From time to time this world impinged on our cloistered existence and when this happened I fear that EPP's lectures on economic and social history had done little to arouse my sympathy for the English working class, particularly when their actions threatened my convenience or comfort. Indeed though she dwelt with some emphasis on the shackling of Irish economy by the British Parliament, leaving a lasting impression on my mind, I remember very little time being spent on the social exploitation of the Industrial Revolution. As a consequence I was much put out when in late September the Railways went on strike. It was a double blow as the strike caught us away from home, and threatened my return to Girton. Today, with so many alternative means of transport being available and so many families possessing cars, rail strikes can be more easily circumvented. In 1919 that was not the case and as a social historian, writing for posterity I hope I shall be forgiven if I include a few extracts from my diary to illustrate my own reactions.

Though there had been rumours of the possibility of a rail strike we had not taken the threat seriously and, as we had already planned to stay with relations in Bolton before I returned to Girton, we went. It proved an unfortunate decision. When the railways did go on strike we were stranded. Today the situation would not have seemed so difficult. In 1919 towns were not linked by regular coach services and the number of private cars was limited. We were lucky in that one of our relations' husbands actually was the proud possessor of a Crosley. So cherished was it however, that to persuade him to allow us to be driven home in it required a mixture of skill and perseverance that would have done credit to a diplomat. Eventually we set out. Here is my description of our journey home.

> 'I sat in the front and talked to the driver. He had
> been in the army since 1914. In France, Belgium,

Holland, Italy, Spain and Germany and he liked the
latter the best. He was pretty disgusted with the strike
and declared his willingness to take a rifle any time
– seemed to think it would come to bloodshed – a
pretty prospect. The roads were teeming with traffic.
Great charabancs.

(I wonder were they horse-driven, like the ones which tourists
explored the Lake District, or early motorised vehicles? I wish I could
remember? However they were propelled I seem to have taken them
for granted, continuing)

There were motors piled with luggage and we even saw
some people travelling in a hearse. Once we saw a train
and I cheered.'

Home once more I felt impelled to record this historic journey in
verse that, had he ever heard it, must have convinced McGonigall that
he had a serious rival. I refrain from recording this masterpiece in its
entirety but here, to show that my boast; was no idle one, here are the
first two and the last verses,

'Oh what a happy land is ours,

Where nought but strikes abound.

What formerly cost us ten bob

Now costs us over a pound.

On Saturday the railway struck

It gave us quite a shock

When we found that British labour

Had run so much amok.'

After no less than thirteen verses composed in a similar style. I concluded

'And when, a white haired lady,

They ask with awe and fear

What did you do in the great strike?

I'll say 'travelled from Bolton here.'

We returned on the 30th September and, though we were back at Old Hutton the shadow of the strike continued to dominate my thoughts as I was due back at Girton on the 10th October and this time there would be no Crosley to come to the rescue. It was difficult to get firm news. I wonder do people realise today how much they rely on the BBC? Owing to the strike we even had no post. My diary is full of suppositions as I struggled to make sense of this upset in the nation's life.

> 'The public are pretty mad. The Government says
> the food is alright, so if the miners and transport.
> workers don't come out it may win. Still in a few days
> more most of the mills and mines must cease, (I wrote
> pessimistically) for lack of transport and it remains to
> be seen if this will incline the people working in them
> towards the Government or the strikers. Mr Thomas
> seems perfectly mithered. I should like to think
> hotheads behind are pushing him on against his better
> judgement and because of their presence and probable
> mistrust he has to show an uncompromising front.'

At the 2nd October I was still moaning, that 'the strike still goes on' though I did find one item of news that amused me. Apparently when Sir Edward Carson was stranded at Penrith the only remark made by that distinguished politician, which I recorded for posterity was 'what the dickens am I to do about my breakfast?' Then on the 6th, via the postman, we heard that the strike was over.

Returning as a second year was very different from that apprehensive journey of a year ago. I belonged and rather naïvely observed that 'It was rather nice to feel yourself one of a great body like a university.' This time changing at Bletchley and arriving to face all the bustling confusion of students at Cambridge station held no terrors. A friend brought my case up while economically I cycled to avoid the expense of having to share a taxi. This was not altogether a successful scheme. In transit my rear lamp had fallen off, so that I had to buy a new one and, because I had trusted to Providence and Cox's cart to bring my trunk up with the other Girton luggage instead of seeing to it myself, it was left behind and I did not get it until after the week-end and I was 'pretty mad'.

It was easy to slip into the old routine since though the subjects of my courses were new the pattern was the familiar one of lectures, essay-writing and tutorials – a pattern shared basically between the members of the university and the students of Girton and Newnham, I imagine. I imagine however, that we wore our rue with a difference though this is only supposition on my part. We did not talk to the men who shared our lectures and the men whom we met socially never talked 'shop'. I never remember meeting socially a man whom I recognised as a budding historian. I doubt however if male noses were quite so close to the grindstone as ours. Girton students read Honours only; not for them the less time consuming Pass degree. Nor could they compensate for a poor third by the proud attainment of a Blue. Not in my wildest dreams did I ever believe that I should see a member of a women's college coxing the Cambridge crew on Boat Race Day. Though there were a few good time girls among us, who took the chaperon rules as lightly as they dared, on the whole we were a hard working lot disciplined by the need to attend lectures. Cutting was not encouraged and boring though at least one course that I attended in my Third Year was, only very occasionally did I fail to turn up. Our work load, like Gaul, was divided into three parts: lectures, essays time papers and tutorials, and private reading.

Though lectures were the least mentally exhausting segment in this three part division of labour they were the fixed stars in our universe round which the rest of our academic activities revolved. Like fixed stars they varied in luminosity. Our first year courses had been what were considered the easier options; the infant food for budding historians and as such easily digested. In the second year we moved on to more solid food though the bill of fare consisted of two rather than three courses. These were a second paper on Political Science and Medieval English Constitutional History. The former traced the development of theories of Government from Plato and Aristotle, through the Middle Ages to modern times. Predisposed to be interested by the study of constitutions the previous year, and fortunate in Dr Jordon, who was an excellent lecturer, clear and stimulating, I found the subject fascinating. A by-product of which I was certainly sufficiently interested to accept Helen's suggestion that we cycled into Cambridge to listen to the modern philosopher McTaggert who was lecturing at 5.30 in Trinity.

> 'The room was crowded, men sitting on the window seats, on the mantelpiece, on the floor, while standing round the walls were more men notebook in hand.'

Surprised by so dedicated an audience I added:

> 'This caused me to observe that the mere male delights in nothing but pleasure is an idea that is forsaking me, seeing the lectures are entirely voluntary. All types and colours flock here, honestly and seeking knowledge.'

For outstanding lecturers there was always an audience. For the series that Sheppard of Kings gave on Homer, anyone who wanted a seat in his auditorium had to be there half an hour before he began. He was himself almost a Cambridge institution. I described him as

> 'A dear little man, with thick wavy hair, now almost
> grey, and a comical, creased face, quite plump.'

Another new enchantment was EEP's Sunday readings. These were open to all third year students who wanted to come and to second years reading History and they, like Sheppard's lectures were something not to be missed. On this first evening her chosen poet was Browning and I was literally as charmed as a snake by the skilful playing of the charmer, confessing

> 'I didn't understand half of it. Oh but her voice is like
> running water, I could just listen and listen while she
> read on. She reads so well, every inflection marked, a
> slow clear rise and fall and pause, then on again. I can
> see that they will be a very great joy to me. I was not
> to be disappointed though the diet she provided was
> not always to reach the soaring heights. On another
> evening she read first Squire and then what I described
> as 'some killing parodies'. We screamed with laughter.
> EEP is a joy forever especially when she refers to
> revolting people who steal her books and then hopes it
> is no one present. She gurgles with laughter.'

Whether it was under her inspiration or not I do not know but the next few pages of my faithful diary is full of my own poetic efforts of a sentimental character. I wonder do the young today still find the need to express their emotions in verse? Reading them now, and the prose pictures in which I also indulged, it is a shock to realise how young and vulnerable I was. These were secret things. I did not share them with my friends. Now I wonder how many of my fellow students indulged in such outpourings. Was I typical or a sport? I shall never know how reliable my memories are or to what extent I shall mislead that hypothetical student struggling with a Ph D on women students in the twenties.

My other new course, medieval constitutional history failed to capture my imagination and remained an unloved subject. There were several reasons for this. Perhaps the fundamental one was my lack of political background. Tudors and Stuarts seemed to occur again and again in my school curriculum but my knowledge of medieval history might, though it had not been published then, have been gained from '1066 and all that'. Quite mistakenly the academic powers that were assumed that if we had not been specifically taught Medieval English History we would acquire it independently; a task surely not beyond students who were aspiring to Honours in History in the Tripos! Alas there never seemed time to do so and I floundered through Stubbs Charters with very little grasp of what it was all about, though the darkness was pierced in places by Maitland's enlightened prose. Even before my first lecture, while I was still struggling to complete a paper for Miss Firth who was to be my tutor, I confided dolely that I did not know

> 'What I have written is to the point as I don't know
> what the point is, my only hope is that the Firth won't
> either.'

It was not an auspicious start and alas Lapsley, brilliant medieval scholar, had an appalling delivery. He spluttered and coughed and was almost inaudible. Moreover the situation was not improved by the fact that he resented having to condescend to having women there at all. We were the swine before whom he was forced to cast his pearls and he made the distribution as impersonal as possible by seating us in the body of Trinity Great Hall while the men sat round him on the dais. Not surprisingly I came back moaning that

> 'The Lapsley was awful. Hardly heard a word he said

– beastly man – most depressed. I made myself some coffee when I got back without asking anyone to have any and took an aspirin.'

As we got more accustomed to his voice we did contrive to take reasonable notes but his lectures were never enjoyed by me because fundamentally I never understood their deeper significance.

Apart from attendance at lectures and tutorials we were free to organise our work as we pleased. It was largely a matter of temperament. Some tackled it with enormous bursts of intermittent energy, others by a more methodical planning of their days. I belonged to the latter and tried to do a consistent seven to eight hours a day which included lectures in the morning in Cambridge. In connection with our lectures we were expected to get through a mass of private reading. Unless one had a magnificent memory which I most certainly had not, this meant the taking of innumerable notes for future reference and I frequently suffered from mental indigestion. The following extract is typical of many scattered through my diaries, writing at the end of a boring day

> 'I think six hours a day solid reading is beastly. I have only had one lecture and no papers to do and solid reading is an awful strain. I have been counting up: I did 300 pages of varied stuff yesterday, either Poly Si or Stubbs medieval charters etc. and heavy going and it's all concentrated stuff, not like economic or medieval European.'

Another typical grouse was 'Potted Pollock and Maitland until my hand refused to write.' The monotony of solitary reading was punctuated by crises of hectic activity, when a batch of essay subjects appeared on the History notice board. These were on specific topics and had to be handed in by a certain date, later to be followed by the appropriate tutorial. Generally they were focused on current lectures and were intended to make sure that we students were keeping up to date with their reading and had understood it.

Life was not however all work. There were social duties as a second year and social pleasures. The social duties were concerned with being pleasant to the influx of freshers who had to be entertained at jug and generally initiated into the traditions of the college. My first impressions were not over favourable, writing

> 'the freshers are a most unpromising lot – mostly specs
> – all brains and no beauty. However I like them slightly,
> some are quite pretty. Elspeth and I are giving a jug to
> Miss Wetton, Foxwell and Le Maitre.'

Miss Wetton, Soulie, was a new neighbour in Bear Pits where, because I liked my rooms, I remained through my time at Girton. She was our new organ scholar, very pretty, very charming and she soon became one of our group, which shows the fallibility of sweeping generalisations.

One of the bonuses of a second year is that one has accumulated a more or less permanent group of friends, consisting of a small inner ring who did things together, either because of proximity or congeniality, so that we habitually dropped into each other's rooms, or frequently had an informal jug together. To some extent this sociability was due to circumstances rather than inclination. Whether it was due to rail strikes or coal strikes or both I do not now remember, but for much of the time I was cold. Among my first entries for the autumn term was the lugubrious entry

> 'It is the first time I have been warm today. Until I
> went to have jug with E and R. I sat wrapped in my
> great coat reading STUBBS; such is life."

Sharing fires however could be a mixed blessing. Two days later I was complaining,

104

'I am sitting nursing my fire, mercifully alone. I am a wee bit sick, R is always here and well I know coal is difficult but!'

My closer friends by now had tended to split into two separate groups. It was not so much a division based on academic ability as on their other interests. Friends like Elspeth and Ruth enjoyed young men and dances and tea parties. Winnie Lumb and Helen Harvey were more serious minded. They were more inclined to discuss ideas than 'to gather rosebuds while they may'. I owed my introduction to Rabinth Tagore to Helen who was forever quoting 'None lives for ever and nothing lasts for long. All is done and finished in the eternal heavens, keep that in mind and rejoice.'

It was under Elspeth's wing that I first ventured out into the social life of Cambridge. To both I owed much. Winnie was my working partner: we went to the same lectures, read the same books and talked 'shop'. My pleasure loving group were inclined to damn them with the adjective 'worthy' and when I had Winnie to jug I did not ask Ruth. Joan Bedale, with whom my friendship deepened in my second year was a link between the two. She was a member of a dance Club, of which more anon, but as a clergyman's daughter, like Winnie and Helen she was a convinced Anglican. The Methodism of my childhood had grown dim and when I went to chapel it would be the college chapel. All around me was the beauty of Cambridge and the jewel of that beauty was King's College Chapel. I won't say that I was an easy convert for I gave the matter much thought but whether I should have taken the final step of being confirmed without my friends taking the practical steps that were necessary I much doubt. Towards the end of the Michaelmas Term, Helen having prepared the ground, I found myself being interviewed by the vicar of Holy Trinity as a candidate for confirmation. Then came the Christmas vacation and I missed an important part of that instruction. However when the vicar's brother, who was Bishop of Peterborough came to Cambridge in the February of 1920, it was decided that in spite of gaps in my preparation, I should be confirmed. In this the Fates were kind. I do not wish to sound irreverent, but swallowing theology has never been my strong point and looking back I think the less theology I knew the more the faith in which I believed. Having borrowed her white confirmation dress from Joan I cycled down and went straight to Holy Trinity feeling, I wrote,

> 'Cool and yet dazed and the whole thing left very
> little feeling. I remember the shock of seeing Theo in
> her white veil. Her face was nearly as white. Then we
> prayed, or dazedly tried to pray, until the Bishop came.
> That is my second picture, the Bishop in his white and
> red sitting there in the chair, and Theo and I sitting
> all in white, one on each side of the chancel with our
> friends beside us, just that and the half dazed feeling
> with which I knelt before the Bishop and felt his hands
> press heavily on my head.'

Next morning I cycled down to take early communion at King's College Chapel. Could anyone have a more beautiful setting, for their first communion service? Again, writing my diary that night I confessed to the same dazed feeling but

> 'I think that when I know the service I shall find peace
> and strength in it but that is not yet. My senses are
> too numb to take in the words and their significance.
> Even now it seems miles away; the grey stone with the
> early light just filtering through the coloured windows,
> the slender candles burning, the priests in their white
> surplices round the altar. The grey stones and the
> surpliced figure just as it had been for hundreds of
> years, though men have come and gone and those who
> prayed there are dust.'

I have indeed found that peace and strength in the communion service for which I hoped but it was not the doctrine of the Anglican Church that converted me from my luke warm Methodism, but my Girton friends and above all Cambridge itself. Had it been otherwise to have included something so personal in what never set out to be an autobiography would have been unjustified. But it was an integral part of what Cambridge meant to me, that and my Girton friends who together have made me, in so many ways, the person I am.

Though we were not members of the university it was still true 'that a cat may look at a king' and Cambridge had much to offer which at least we were allowed to observe men doing though we could not participate. It would have been unthinkable for women to become members of the Union or even as guests to play an active role in its debates. Indeed as far as my own knowledge and memory goes among the invitations to the public figures of the day there was no distinguished woman so honoured. Lady Bonham Carter was invited to the University Liberal Society, not to the Union though she would surely have been worth hearing. It is illuminating that I never remember that this exclusion of my sex caused me any resentment. It is even more illuminating that I should have felt women taking part in the debates was almost sacrilegious. To my shame I have to confess that some lingering feeling that it is very odd to have a woman as President is still my gut reaction, just as I dislike the idea of men undergraduates at Girton. In 1920 it was still a masculine preserve, a training ground for British legislators of the future: there was no place for females in its deliberations. We were however, like women in a harem, permitted to look down from the gallery above. Even this eerie access was carefully guarded. Admission was only to be allowed by courtesy of a member of the Union, who alone could provide the necessary ticket. Even then, to insure that we should behave with all decorum some godly, or at least obliging, matron acted as a chaperon for women students. That I was able to attend my first debate on 18th November 1919 was due to Ruth having got tickets for us both from one of her numerous swains. In the future I found her a useful supplier of these necessary documents.

The motion before the House was 'This House disapproves of any decrease in our armaments in the near future.' The proposer was a Mr Reaid from Emmanuel, the possessor of a cherubic countenance and a tiny moustache, a smiling, practical type who made little impression on me. The second speaker I described in some detail

> 'The opposer was Mr Abrahams (Peterhouse). He was
> tall, very white skin, good speaker, a little languid and
> sardonic.'

He was a regular speaker and I rarely failed to make some comment on him; he intrigued me and I wish I had also recorded his initial. Could he have been the Abrahams who later was to attain fame as a runner? But the man to whom I lost my heart that evening and about whose possible identity and future there was to be no doubt was Sub-Lieutenant L Mountbatten. His speech was well – nautical! He started by converting the Gardaiene swine into submariners, told funny stories and mixed things up with surprising statements and changes of front. 'Amusing, vigorous, nautical' was my verdict. The other speakers, as far as I know, were to be of less interest to posterity but two members on the floor of the house also belong to History. The Princes were there, Albert and his younger brother Henry. It was the first time I had seen Prince Albert since my hero worshipping days at Lamlash. Alas the Union in general and Mountbatten in particular had altered the focus of my interest. My earlier feelings were not however totally eclipsed. I thought him

> 'better looking than Henry. He clapped a bit, chiefly
> Mountbatten. He looked thinner and sharper featured
> than before.'

That night I was in the grip of a new interest, one that was to continue to hold me for my next two years at Cambridge. My final verdict was

> 'It was glorious. The sea of faces, the lights, the
> padded chairs, above all the speaking and the good

humoured give and take. It intoxicated me like wine (this was poetic licence as I was still a teetotaller) or an opera, or anything that makes your pulses throb and the blood rush round your body. I am quite ready to fall in love with any young man at the shortest notice if he will get me tickets for the Union.'

This was no mere flash in the pan; the union debates continued to have a strong fascination for me and during my second and third years I managed to get tickets for several debates a term. I am not sure of what this fascination consisted. To some extent the debates had the appeal of a soap opera. Though the episodes, in the shape of motion, varied the setting was the same and so were the actors. I became very familiar with the style and personalities of the officers and also of the regular speakers from the floor and I criticised their performance in much the same way that I did that of the actors when I went to the theatre. In addition the setting appealed to my sense of the traditional and to my feeling that I was sharing in something that was essentially Cambridge. I did not feel excluded, I felt a part of it. The debates also gave me the sensation of being in touch with the wider world of politics. There were many problems about which to argue in the difficult years after the end of the war. At first there had been euphoria with the British expecting the fruits of victory to fall into their laps and to be able to subsist on them without further effort. But by the twenties it was growing ever clearer that there were old problems to tackle, as we still thought of Britain as an imperial power.

The next debate that I attended highlighted the bitter political tension of the immediate post wars. Lloyd George, who had ousted Mr Asquith the leader of the Liberal party became Prime Minister in 1916. In order to concentrate the country in its struggle first for survival and then victory he had formed a Coalition Government with the Conservative party, and fought the election of 1918 in alliance with them, a policy of which Asquith disapproved. That split the Liberal party, the majority following Lloyd George and Asquith going into the political wilderness. Lord Haldane, who had been minister of war in 1914, and who had been blamed for having made too many concessions to Germany over their naval policies, had been invited to speak on the motion 'That the pre-war Liberal policy was both deceptive and dangerous.' Because Lord Haldane was so controversial a figure, tickets had been hard to get and the House was packed to overflowing. Members had even swarmed over the barriers intended to control them. It was an excellent debate with the big guns speaking third and fourth; the well known barrister, Sir Earnest Wild proposing the motion and Lord Haldane opposing it. I described the latter as

> 'A funny man. He stands on his feet very stumpily,
> almost as if they were two blocks of wood. Also his
> little fingers are very small indeed and his face looks
> as if someone had taken a piece of plasticine and
> had made it into a face. He is nearly bald, with just a
> few hairs combed over and he speaks in a light half
> squeaky voice.'

In spite of this unflattering portrait Lord Haldane still managed to give an impression of authority and I found him more convincing than the polished Sir Earnest Wild KC. One of the more exciting aspects of the Union debates was their custom of inviting public figures to debate contemporary problems. In the two years that followed I was to see in the flesh men who otherwise would have been mere names to me.

The Haldane debate, though it arose out of the bitter divisions in the post war Liberals roots, lay in the past. The majority of debates that I heard were concerned with the problems of the present, but as in the Irish question with its unhappy legacy of bitterness and revolt the present was the product of the past. In 1914 it had been the Ulster Protestants under Carson who had been on the edge of open defiance. After the war it had been Sinn Fein that was demanding the removal of the British. Even during the war it staged a brief rebellion in Dublin in 1916. Though the rising had been easily repressed Sinn Fein continued to grow in strength and, in an effort to satisfy it, Lloyd George made tentative attempts to introduce a home rule bill for Ireland. This again gave rise to bitter controversy and ended in the South proclaiming an independent republic in 1919. The Government then sent in the Army. The notorious Black and Tans put down the resistance but their success left increasing hatred of the English. This was the background of the debate to which I went in the October of 1920 when the motion before the House condemned the reprisals that were taking place and supported the policy that Lloyd George was putting forward a dominion status for Ireland.

I must admit that my approach to that debate was personal rather than political. I was not particularly interested in Ireland but I was definitely so in one of the speakers, D H Johnstone of Christs. To worship from afar was one of my escape routes from emotional frustration; I found it both satisfying and safe! Johnstone was eminently suitable for this role. He was tall, dark and romantic looking, full of Irish charm and a good speaker who could combine humour and seriousness. The next Irish debate that I heard was in the May of 1921 when, after various abortive attempts to find a solution to the Irish dilemma, Lloyd George finally made an offer of dominion status which, was to lead to the creation of the Irish Free State in 1922. Of this debate I wrote

> 'The subject was Ireland, the attraction TP O'Connor,
> a name in those days with which to conjure. I was not
> impressed, describing him as having "a shaggy grey
> moustache, greyish eyes, tousled hair. He spilt snuff
> all over his front and ranted a good deal, now up,
> now down, now thundering, now cooing and smiling
> expansively. Truly one sees all types at the Union but
> eloquence, particularly of the prevalent kind, is apt to
> leave one cold. D W J was rather subdued over it. I

think he felt that such oratory was hardly the kind to capture the Union.'

Interested as always in Prince Albert I also noticed that

'H.R.H. came in towards the end. There is a distinct sprinkling of white across the front of his hair and he can't be more than 21.'

Though less immediately pressing the British domination of India was also beginning to be challenged, and merited one debate, also in the October of 1920. Neither of the guest speakers interested me sufficiently for me to record what they said or even to remember their names.

In the two years during which I followed the debates, though my coverage was not inclusive, and I may well have missed some that were significant, the House was chiefly concerned with the domestic problems of reconstruction. In that the motions mirror the interest of the post war generation of students they have some historical value. Though they followed no very settled pattern nor order it is possible to divide them roughly into three groups, those that were of a more general character, those more immediately dealing with possible constitutional changes to meet a new society and a wide batch of motions that concentrated on the new in both industrial and political life. Examples of the first group could include the motion on 17th February that; 'Compulsory National Service is against the interests of Great Britain.' and that; 'Unrestricted freedom of speech is in the best interests of this country.' Next year they were debating that, 'In the Opinion of this House the Influence of the Press is pernicious', on which my comment was that it was 'killingly funny'. It is perhaps worth noticing that none of these topics attracted outside speakers. The outstanding debate dealing with constitutional issues was distinguished by the appearance of Hilaire Belloc and there had been a great rush on tickets. For once I jotted down the general

112

tenure of his argument on the motion that; 'The power of the Crown ought to be increased'. His argument was that Parliament had lost all moral power, corruption even threatened to touch the judiciary, we were really an autocratic people and a monarchic rule of some kind must come. Therefore it had better come gradually through the present reigning family. Belloc I described as

> 'a bulkily built short man with a very red face and spectacles. He sat with his eyes shut and his hand over his face most of the time. Ruth thought he must be praying for grace not to stop the speaker who followed him. It would be interesting to have known what Prince Albert thought of the motion. The House was so crowded that he got wedged in the press by the door for three speeches and when he finally made his way to the committee benches, sat down waving, his hands in the air with a gesture of utter exhaustion.'

Temporarily democracy seemed to have been open to question among the young men of Cambridge as next week the motion was; 'That Democracy as a form of Government has no future.' I found this another fascinating debate. Again partly due to the opportunity it afforded of hearing a prominent public figure, Dean Inge. The impression I took away with me was that; 'he had the actor type of face but a bit frostbitten'. I could not remember anything of his speech except that Syndicalists, Anarchists and Socialists were not really democratic; hardly a piece of divine revelation.

Fascinating, though debates on the theories of constitutional might be they had very little relevance to the practical business of running the country. At the most they were an exercise in kite flying. Of far more practical concern were problems of industry and of clashing social conceptions. By 1919, when my interest in the Union first began, the prosperity and euphoria of the post war years had come to an end. It was no longer possible to ignore the problems that the nation had to face. The effect of an industry organized to win the war had been to strengthen the position of the labour force. Their good will had been too important to disregard; their co-operation had become vital. With the prosperity boom over, working people were determined to hold on to their new found status. The trade Unions seemed almost trigger happy to use their industrial muscle to gain better wages, shorter hours and even to control their own industry. This was particularly true of the miners who were bitterly opposed to their pits being returned to the control of their original owners. By the February of that year the question of the nationalisation of the mines was sufficiently topical for the Union to make it a subject of a debate. I found it a dull debate with no outside guest speakers to enliven it, but I found one speaker of some interest, not because of what he said but because he was Arthur Henderson's son, now up at Trinity. He spoke in support of nationalisation but I decided that it was more out of loyalty to his father's position as a leading labour politician than out of any wish of his own. I described him as

> 'little and rather cherubic and he stood the banter well
> but when he spoke her kept nervously moistening his
> lips. His discourse was muddled; it gave the impression
> that he had a good case to present but that it failed to
> emerge from his argument.'

In May the Union was seeking another solution to industrial unrest, weighing the respective merits of co-partnership and nationalisation. Again young Henderson spoke and again almost managed, by a slip of the tongue to score a home goal. Yet another solution was propounded by the historian and well known writer D H Cole who spoke eloquently but, to me at least, unconvincingly of the virtues of Guild Socialism. Clearly I prefer the man to his industrial philosophy. I thought him; 'attractive, youngish, dark with the lean and hungry look of one who thought too much.'

Apart from idealists of an impractical bent such theories had little appeal to practical men or the emerging Labour party. It is fascinating to trace their growing influence within the Union in 1921. At the beginning of that year, 21st January, the motion before the House was: 'This house views with appreciation the increasing tendency towards national ownership and control.' The first speaker, a Mr Richardson, was obviously entirely sincere in his advocacy but rather crude and unpolished in his presentation, suggesting something of a lack of social expertise. My comments on the debate were

> 'Richardson made some laboured and rather doubtful witticisms on women, then made a good speech. He always convinces me in his sincerity and reasoning, but he really should keep off original light humour!'

The next to speak, attacking, the motion was the younger brother of one of Ruth's friends, the supplier of our tickets. Him I described as speaking well

> 'in the conservative way, i.e. declamatory and calling the other side names. Ruth thought young Adams fatuous, but fatuous or not, he woke the House up. Maurice Dobbs put it to sleep again. With shining, face and sleek hair, he talked sound sense for half an hour with never a variation of gesture or tone. I was bored and my attention wandered.'

He was certainly a complete contrast to my somewhat conventional picture of a member of the growing Labour party. He was well groomed, well dressed and wore white spats, in every way the complete opposite of Richardson. Later he was to become an economist of some repute to all appearances an intellectual rather than a politician, though I never found him reachable.

The growing influence of what today we should call the Left had been marked as early as the November of 1920 when the House debated the motion 'That this House would prefer a Labour

Government to a Coalition.' Apart from the substance of the motion the debate was interesting because of the future of two of the speakers who took part in it. One was a future Chancellor of the Exchequer, though in 1920 merely a prospective Labour candidate, Hugh Dalton. I dismissed him as making,

> 'quite an able speech but a mass of platitudes, dragging in the League of Nations and in places displaying rather poor taste, for which I added censoriously 'he had no excuse being an old King's man.'

The other speaker to engage my attention was none other than Prince Albert. On him my comment was

> 'H.R.H. spoke wellish, but I really don't know what about.'

This was a pity. As a man who had fought at Jutland and who was to become George VI, his views on this topic would have been worth recording. In writing History omissions can be as significant, like Sherlock Holmes' dog that did not bark in the night, as some recorded fact. Had there been a stammer in the Prince's voice I should certainly have noted it, since when I wrote up any account of the evening's debate I tended to concentrate rather on the style and skill of the speaker than on the substance of his speech. By the April of 1921 whoever arranged debates was so far in sympathy with the aspirations of his Labour party members as to put forward the assertion that 'The political power in the immediate future lies with the Labour party.' Of Dobbs, who spoke first I noted, rather condescendingly, that he spoke well and was not so long and dull as usual. I was more interested in the main guest of the evening, Philip Snowden, a prominent Labour politician. Him I described as

> 'a peculiar looking man with a large rather protruding forehead, a sharp nose, bright eyes and thin repressive lips.'

I was struck by the impression he gave of possessing great driving power in spite of his habit of constantly clasping and unclasping his hands as he spoke. To me he seemed to talk sense, arguing that the Labour Party was no more a class based party than any of the other parties.

Though at the moment membership of the Union was confined to members of the university the same restriction did not apply to inter-college debates. As part of the social rapproachement that marked post war Cambridge between the sexes, Girton had its own debating society and in the March of 1920 we invited the Jesus debating society to join with us to stage a mock trial. Who was the moving spirit behind this innovation I had no idea but it was an event that I described as

'great fun. The court was arranged in the great bay of the Stanley Library and Dr Wingfield was the judge. The case before the court was the trail of Otanda (played by Betty Hoyle) on a charge of murder and theft. Theo Llewlyn-Davies and Kitty Snell defended and two Jesus men, Williams and Holman were the prosecutors, Williams was awfully good. He had dressed in a wig and gown, looking the part admirably and had a quick way of making points which were apparently pointless. Theo was very clear and sort of comforting to the defendant. She worked up a fair hypothetical case against Gerald Newmarket, the finder of the body. EEP was priceless. She was called as a member of the staff to give testimony as to Otanda's character and said that if she had a fault it was being too quiet and retiring. The applause of the audience was an eloquent witness to this piece of sarcasm. EEP then went on to say that these young things must have a confidant and that she had offered to lend her £50. The plaintiff then asked "Did your feelings not runaway with you?" EEP replied "The feelings of staff never run away with them," This was greeted by loud and prolonged applause from both sexes of the audience. Theo was good and clear but spoilt her last speech by mock resentment ... The verdict was not guilty and Dr Wingfield was heard to mutter "There was not enough evidence to hang a dog".'

Not all inter-college debates were so enjoyable and light hearted, The night that we debated with Downing at their invitation could only be described as sticky.

'A bus load of us were deposited at the college and my little group of friends huddled together, looking a little forlorn until coffee was served. The President bounded up, said we did not look as if we were enjoying ourselves, hoped we were full of speeches and produced a man, small and dapper, who solemnly fed us, talked to us all at once and led us to the Hall. This we found very cold, so he went back for our wraps. The debate was damned dull. Our little man, the shepherd, made a good speech which he had written out and learnt by heart. After that he stowed us in a bus and so we came home.'

Obviously a good evening was not enjoyed by all and my sympathy now, though not then, goes out to the poor young man who found us and speech making heavy going. But at least Downing kept up its reputation for good manners.

A couple of weeks later the roles were reversed. The Christ's debating society were the guests and Girton the hostesses. My interest in that debate was purely personal. D W Johnstone was a Christ's man and at the end of the debate I actually managed to achieve a momentary exchange of words as we were leaving the Stanley. During the debate I had forced myself to make a short contribution

118

though, as I did not include the motion in my account of the evening I have now not the remotest remembrance of what I said. I usually did try to speak at debates but to do so was pain and grief to me. Coming away as the crowd dispersed I attempted the removal of the chairs which he took from me at the same time asking, 'Did you see the account of our dinner in the *Granta* Miss Marshall?' The dinner in question was one that I had attended at the Eighty Club the previous week at which he had been present but where we had not met. To my disappointment my dinner partner had been a rather dull and married professor. Our conversation was short but 'I was rather bucked that he should know my name'. It was a promising, beginning and any other moderately socially competent woman would have seized the next opportunity to follow it up. Alas, alas I did not. Some few days after I saw my adorable Irishman walking towards me as I was making my way to King's Parade, I was seized with confusion and embarrassment. Did I smile or did I not? I was so desperately frightened of what I then called 'making myself cheap', so I dived in to a conveniently close paper shop and bought a *Granta*. Apparently he also wished to buy a *Granta*, or so I thought then. Looking back I surmise that that may not have been his only wish. I have said very little about my appearance but I had a very good figure and a not unattractive face. More embarrassed than ever and uncertain what a lady should do, I kept my eyes on the counter, pretended not to see him and dashed out. Like my attempts at skiing, later, the only thing I learnt to do was to stop. In my diary that night I asked the question, 'Can you cut a man you have not been introduced to?' Shades of the modern student that I could have been such a nonney! I did confess to feeling a fool afterwards. We had one more brief encounter a term later. I was having elevens with Ruth at Mathews when I saw him come in. Fortunately she had her back to the door and didn't. This time, as he went past our table I looked up and smiled. My reward for being so forward was a strained smile in return but he did not speak. Alas I was learning that the postman rarely knocks twice, particularly if he happens to be a good looking and charming young man.

My ego did however receive a considerable boost. Having listened to so many debates to my utter amazement I was given an opportunity to show to what extent I had benefited by studying the success and failures of a long sequence of speakers. I was asked by Miss Jones, who as History tutor had replaced EEP when she had departed on her travelling scholarship, to second her at the staff debate. In my own words;

> 'I was flabbergasted and immediately protested that
> the responsibility was beyond me. I knew that she
> thought well of my work but to be told that she had
> only consented to speak if she could choose her own
> supporters and there was no one she would as soon
> have as me: I was so clear headed and it depended on
> the first speakers to set the tone of the debate. As she
> added several derogatory remarks, I called them catty,
> but only to my diary, about the present state of the
> college debating society, and was looking to the debate
> to improve things I was doubly flattered and I said I
> would do the best I could. Having made the decision I
> was surprised not to be immediately overwhelmed by
> the task to which I had committed myself, that I knew
> would come later. At the moment my determination
> was to make a success of it, telling myself that it was
> an honour that I could not refuse and, in a sudden
> burst of new felt confidence, I told myself that there
> was no reason to suppose that I would be worse than
> most people, even though the opposing team was to
> be led by a formidable fourth year research student,
> Barbara Wotton, tragically widowed in the late war,
> better known today as Baroness Wotton and still as
> formidable. She had chosen Gwen Farquar as her
> supporter. Daunting though the prospect was it had
> its compensations in the shape of a couple of tete
> a tete consultations with Miss Jones in which we

worked out our plan of campaign and a joint coffee party between us and the opposing team. Little did I guess that Mrs Wotton would become an imposing member of the House of Lords. On Saturday the 26th February I had to face the ordeal which for one awful moment threatened to be as appalling as I had feared. I was to speak third after Miss Jones whom I described as killingly funny and Mrs Wotton who also, I conceded spoke very well. But by that time I really was not concentrating on her performance. My time was coming nearer and nearer. Then I had to get up and my first sentences were quite lost in my general weakness. However eventually I did hear my voice coming from somewhere and got on alright without my notes. I think I said nearly everything I wanted to say. I asked Joan 'Honest Injun' and she said I had managed very well. I hope I did. Anyhow I did not disgrace myself and Miss Jones.'

The immediate aftermath was an anti-climax. I got back to my room to find the fire nearly out and R, when I was still strung up and dying to talk about the debate, was interested only in having seen her current heart throb that afternoon. My bitter comment was; 'I hate people who are in love'. Next day however I had my reward when Miss Jones told me that I done nobly and that she was proud of her supporter.

This small personal triumph, marking my transition from being a listener to a speaker of the word is a fitting conclusion to what was only one strand that made up the many activities that filled my life at Cambridge during my second and third years. To listen to the Union debates was to be but an observer on the fringe of the university life which would have been a barren experience had not Cambridge much, much more to offer beyond the intellectual stimulation of the spoken word.

CHAPTER FIVE: THE SOCIAL WHIRL

To give the impression that work, together with an evening spent listening to a Union debate by way of relaxation made up the pattern of my life when I returned to Girton in October 1919, would be far from the truth. My second year was one of consolidation and of widening horizons. Cambridge had much to offer beside academic achievement and, with the energy of youth, I filled my days to overflowing. No wonder that entries scribbled late at night begin with the moan 'I am so tired' before I chronicled my doings for the day. Most of them were humdrum snapshots of college life, the ups and downs of college friendships, comments on lectures, records of the day's work etc. For instance, on 1st March 1920 I wrote with some satisfaction,

> 'Did eight and a half hours. Did my Time Paper
> because I am going out tomorrow.'

Next day I wrote

> 'Lectures etc in the morning. Did seven hours just by
> working after Hall. Went to Mr Perowne's tea party.'

As the term progressed and my social life expanded young men and social activities appeared more frequently, though for the most part during the week we remained largely inhabitants of a female world.

But mixed tea parties were always described. To me they were still red letter events if they took place in one of the men's colleges. This gave me both a sense of belonging to the wider Cambridge world and satisfied my curiosity as to how the other half, the masculine half, lived.

Such parties were strictly chaperoned by some unwilling don, or don's wife, who had been pressed into service. Often among my friends the long suffering Miss Dean. She must have had a very soft spot for young people and I hope she enjoyed them as much as I did. In my last year at Girton the rules were relaxed to the extent that we could have elevens or tea in a cafe alone with a man without first having to ask permission. This was liberty indeed. But the rule that demanded a chaperon for any entertainment that took place in a man's room, unless he were your brother, remained. Though inviolate not unbroken! Rumour had it that some students committed this enormity. Less reprehensible, though still breakers of college rules were students who went out after Hall without permission, coming, in furtively via the window of a friend, who conveniently lived on the ground floor. Such behaviour I considered 'fast', a word of disapproval in my vocabulary, though, looking back, I can understand the temptation to slip out and in again without permission, for to be back in college by eleven was irritating when it meant leaving an interesting meeting in full swing. Though an exit permit was required to attend meetings of Cambridge societies, chaperones were not obligatory except at Union debates or at dances and then some pillar of respectability was considered necessary to protect the virtue of students from Girton and Newnham.

Such meetings could be very pleasant social occasions as when on the 21st January 1920 I went to the Peterhouse History Society to hear a paper on 'Leaves from a Venetian Diary'.

> 'It was in a funny quaint reference library up at the top
> of the college' I wrote 'They gave us coffee first which
> was better in intention than execution. Abrahams was

president so he is obviously reading History.'

Abrahams' personality had intrigued me when I had heard him at Union debates. Now my verdict was

> 'I am not sure that I like his face near to. There is something sensuous, not quite that, but something I do not like.'

The 23rd provided me with a greater thrill. I had been brought up in the Liberal camp. Among my childhood memories was that of my aunt, my father's sister, chanting 'Stamp, stamp upon Protection', while my mother's nephew was the Liberal MP for Bosworth and a devoted follower of Lloyd George. So when Asquith came to Cambridge to open the Liberal Club I counted myself lucky to have secured a ticket for the meeting, at the Guildhall. Because the following episode gives the flavour of the hazards that the Huntingdon Road presented to Girton students when they wanted to indulge in activities after dark, I am inscribing my entry for the 23rd March in full. Apparently so many students wanted to attend that a special bus had been laid on to pick us up at 7.30.

> 'By 7.45 no bus had appeared. Hectic suspense. Finally we rushed back for lights, seized our bikes and decided to bike. It was an exhilarating rush down there in the dark. Elspeth and Helen were on borrowed bikes, and the latter had no brakes. We passed people who had started before us and got there at 8.05pm taking about ten minutes over the journey. We arrived with trembling legs, at least I suppose they were but the trip was so exciting. There was a Long queue stretching, right round to the back. However we got places in the crush. The place was packed. Mr Glover Lowes Dickinson, looking like a Mongolian devil and Mr Gaskoin looking, like a lifeless image, were there on

the platform. Just near us was Swan, the captain of
the Cambridge boat. There was a great shouting and
clapping when Mr Asquith and the committee came
in. Proceedings were started by Mr Morgan of Trinity.
Then Asquith spoke. He had a semi-confidential
delivery, not stirring or inspiring, and he looked just
like a benevolent Father Christmas. He was remarkably
like his caricature with a thick fringe of white round
his head. He talked a good deal of scandal in a "of
course I wouldn't say anything about anybody for
worlds" manner. He told a rather cutting story about
Mr Balfour whose name was greeted by such rapturous
applause that he looked rather discomposed. He is the
new Chancellor and I thought it rather bad taste to
tell it here ... He talked a lot and said little. Evidently
Liberalism is (1) Free Trade, (2) Complete Home Rule
for Ireland, (3) non intervention in Russia, (4) no class
politics. It was all very well but he did not lay down
a definite programme. He talked of "the practical
application" but never got near it. I don't think he has
any inspiration of leadership left and I don't think he
will get in at Paisley. To the Liberal cause he will be
more of a hindrance than a help. I almost wonder if
Labour is better. I have joined the C.U.L.C. Perhaps
next term I will join the L.U.S.S. and try them both. I
really don't know!!!'

Whatever my reservations I continued to be interested in Liberal
activities though whether this was because I enjoyed going to the
meetings or because politics fascinated me I'm not sure. Possibly, like
most motives mine were mixed. It was a sign of my growing social
self confidence that I went to the dinner which the Eighty Club gave
at the Lion on 13th March. It was the first time I had attended a
function of this kind and as none of my particular friends were among
the Girtonians who went, I felt rather lost. I was lucky in my dinner

partner as Runciman took me into dinner. Rather condescendingly I described him as 'a good looking boy who rows fourth in the third Trinity boat, so we discussed the races etc.' For these I had not lost my passion and, whatever the pressure of work, the Lents saw me on the tow-path. My diary always contains full details of each day's results. To have a ready made topic of conversation eased my awkwardness and with something of a schoolgirl's gusto I enjoyed the food, writing

> 'It was a long dinner but very good. I feel full yet, a
> sort of solid substratum, unlike the feel of college
> food. Then we drank to the King. It was most thrilling.'

The speeches that followed I found less so, describing most of them as dull and not over convincing.

> 'It is fairly easy' I wrote critically 'to present a good
> case for the government if one only takes one side
> at once. The trouble is they will never keep the same
> position for two days.'

After the speeches came the ritual of signing menus which I designated as 'quite fun' having collected some from men whom previously I had only heard at Union debates. One comment that I made may have been of some slight historical interest namely

> 'that the applause that greeted Asquith's name was
> much greater than that which greeted Lloyd-George.'

One of the advantages of being up at Cambridge was the opportunity to see in person some of the leading figures of the day. Today the TV has made them not only household names but household faces. We take this so much for granted that we forget that it was only through the written word and the still photograph that the politicians could make their impression on the mass of the voters. To see the famous in the flesh was a bonus. So I was delighted to have the opportunity of seeing as well as hearing Sir John Simon when he addressed the Liberal club on 30th April. He seems to have met with my approval.

> 'He has a clear cut pleasant face, almost bald with a fringe of fine grey hair. When he talks he sways to and fro a little with a backward curve. His figure is slender. Like so many of these great lawyers his voice is a little disappointing, quite pleasant and cultured but with no swinging eloquence and hampered by a tendency to get high as he works up and ends in a squeak. When he wants to be humorous on the other hand he speaks a key lower. I don't know why? He was fairly lucid on the liberty of the subject, ie. John Hampden but otherwise very vague. All the Liberal speakers I have heard are; they won't run down the Coalition except covertly and they haven't much programme which they can produce or dare produce, and so are rather up a lamp post.'

One proof that my interest in Liberal policies was genuine was the fact that I made the effort to attend a Liberal Club meeting on the May of that year to hear the report on the Commission of Ireland and Constitutional Reform that had just been published. Like the poor they are still with us; Anglo-Irish relations still wait to be resolved and the House of Lords to be reformed! As I read these political extracts in my diary the more I appreciate the old saying that 'The more things alter the more they remain the same.' However enlightening, or otherwise the meetings that I attended were, my involvement at least marked another step forward in my Cambridge experience. I was, very tentatively beginning to play a part in the wider male dominated world of university life in that I attended business meetings as well as more glamorous occasions. When Runciman, now secretary, proposed the nomination of a student from Newnham or Girton to the committee and then suggested Grace Rattenberg as being very capable and living in London being the only Girtonian there I felt it encumbent on me to second the nomination and squeaked out a tiny 'I will' as if I were at the altar. This at least was a tiny advance into publicity.

Politicians however were not the only persons of note whom I had the opportunity of hearing. On May 6th 1920 I heard Lord Hugh Cecil preach at St Edwards. I duly noted the heads of his sermon and rather less respectfully described him as

> 'grey with a grey moustache and the air of a superior shop walker' adding 'I mean no disrespect but the type'.

Alfred Noyes, who came down to read his poetry to the English Club got more favourable treatment from me.

> 'He was not what one would expect. A trifle nervous perhaps in speaking, with a humorous kindly face, rather blunt and English, not very poetic looking. He had gold rimmed glasses and was going slightly bald. He read his things well with perhaps more effect from tone than emphasis. He did the usual Highwayman and Lilac Time but what I liked better was the Lord of Misrule and the Legend of Drake. In his poetry what I like is the combination of colours and the feeling for the past. Not a deep poet nor tragic and yet effective. He writes as it were with a brush while over him hangs the glamour of the good old days.'

I rather suspect that this was something I shared with him despite a couple of years' training to become a professional historian.

My other, and indeed more numerous diversions were of a more personal and frivolous nature and centred more round young men and the emotions they aroused than the fascination of politics or the impressions made on me by the great and the good.

Not all my close friends were so inclined. Winnie Lumb, my working partner, never took part in these frivolities. Neither did Helen Harvey and I regret to confess that these filled far more pages in my diary than did the activities of the Liberal club and similar interests. This was not necessarily true of Girton students as a whole. Though there were only some 160 of us in residence, we were split up into small groups of friends and what went on outside them was speculation and rumour or supposition rather than knowledge. It so happened that Fate decreed that I had friends in both. Winnie, my working partner showed little interest in my young men and was inclined to take life seriously. Helen Harvey, then in her second year and also reading History, was a person of great warmth and charm and wide interests, a delightful companion but someone who seemed to have no room in her life for men. Her great friend Jessie Belfield who lived next to me in Bear Pits was, in that adjective that I discovered I worked to death when describing anyone or anything that gave me pleasure, was 'nice' to me. I might easily have been sucked into that group and so missed much that Cambridge had to offer and which I definitely needed to experience, had it not been for Ruth the neighbour on my other side, who had an outgoing personality and great vitality. She had not particularly wanted to come to college and, though she worked hard, she was determined to enjoy herself. I think she would not quarrel with my statement that she enjoyed male company and collected young men with considerable aplomb. The other friend to draw me into Cambridge was of course Elspeth who opened doors to academic functions that would otherwise have remained closed. Both were among my earliest friends and, as my account of my first social blossoming when the Americans descended on Cambridge demonstrated, it was through them that I began to explore the social scene.

When I returned to Cambridge at the beginning of my second year the scene had changed and the pattern set by the Americans vanished with their light hearted presence. This meant that if we did not wish to retreat into a female community new friends had to be sought and new points of contact established. That I was able to do this was initially due to Elspeth. The Giles were uniformly kind to me and I was flattered and thrilled when I was asked to dinner early in the term to meet some young men afterwards. By now I was beginning to feel less overawed by the prestige of the Master's Lodge though young men, who joined us after Hall when we played games until 10.10 were not very interesting and proved to be but ships that passed in the night. More interesting were the glimpses behind the scenes of academic life that connection with Emmanuel brought me when Honorary degrees were to be conferred on three naval heroes of the late war, Admirals Jackson, Heyes and Maden. Elspeth asked me if I would like to watch the procession from the gallery. It was most impressive. First came the Chancellor, Balfour, resplendent in black and gold with a page bearing his train. I described him as

> 'a well built man with grey hair and a thick moustache.
> His little page went to the dinner at Trinity last night,
> refused ginger beer, drank champagne, smoked a
> cigarette and survived it. The young hopeful comes
> from Eton and is, I think called Dugdale.'

I wonder if in later life his career lived up to its early promise. More indiscreet was the gossip that Elspeth passed on to me that

> 'the Princes wrote home and told the king that they
> were going to sit on each side of the Chancellor.
> George wrote back telling them not to be fools but
> sit among the audience which they did! With student
> exuberance the three admirals with the red of their
> doctorate gowns worn over their naval dress and their
> hats adorned with little black velvet were seized and
> chaired. Next was the turn of the Generals, Trenchard,
> Bying and Robertson. The first two were likewise
> elevated but Robertson marched unperturbedly on but
> in vain. He was caught from behind and shared the
> fate of the other distinguished fighting men. Having

apparently learnt their lesson the Princes came last after the crowd had gone. "Albert wore flying uniform and looks better than he did at the Union" was my personal comment.'

What afterwards proved to be the core of my social life, came like the source of a mighty river, from quite an inconspicuous beginning. On the 6th November I wrote

'Have just come back from a free dancing lesson in the Corn Exchange. A list was put up on Wednesday asking who would like to go. Ruth and Joan made me put my name down and Joan went too. It was as far as I could see a dance; no one taught us anything. First we stood in a clump near the door. Then a few were introduced and we started. Then the men came in without an introduction and on with the dance. By means of sitting and looking wistful, for we had no programmes and no numbers I got a partner every time!'

Summing up the evening I declared

'It was quite nice but not thrilling. I don't know that I care about going again. It might not be so nice.'

Next week I did not put my name down and as Ruth did and Elspeth had gone home I spent a lonely evening. It was fear I suspect that had prevented my chancing my luck again. I was not and never had been a naturally good dancer and my chances to practice had been largely confined to what in my diary I called 'the dancing'. On this particular Girton activity my memory is a complete blank though in my diary I allude to it again and again. From these entries I gather that it must have been a college all feminine affair.

After this diet of female partners my panic at the thought of facing with a MAN an ordeal which I might have the mortification of failing was understandable. Luckily next week I changed my mind and plucked up my courage to make a second trial of its attractions. This time things must have gone better as I wrote on returning

> 'I went to the dancing club tonight and did enjoy it though I hadn't expected to because I thought the men stodgy. Actually they weren't bad in the dancing. Several were tall with moustaches and danced well. Several asked me twice so I felt quite bucked. I had a partner for every dance and so was quite happy.'

By the end of term the dancing class had been reorganised into a regular club with the title of *Vingt et Un* which met every Thursday during term. Apparently its original members must have numbered 21. Technically we were not members but guests. How we women were selected I never knew. Each week a notice would go up on the college notice board saying that the following had been invited for that Thursday. I can only assume that those of us who had volunteered to act as partners in the original classes formed a nucleus but I never discovered if we were invited individually or whether the secretary had had a list of semi permanent names. All I know is that had my name been omitted I should have felt humiliated and scorned. Fortunately it never was.

Though *Vingt et Un* had not the elaborate trappings of a college ball it had a formality that might surprise the modern habitué of the Disco. Though tails and ball gowns would have been out of place as a matter of course the men wore dinner jackets and the women simple evening dresses. Two of my favourite ones I can still remember. Best loved of all was the one I described as 'perfectly lovely, white georgette, cut on Grecian lines and it suits me perfectly'. I fancied my figure, and judging by my photographs not unjustly. I was high waisted with long slender legs which were hinted at rather than revealed under the soft fall of my skirt as I danced. I had small feet, only size four and good ankles. My other favourite dress was a delicate rose pink that was the result of impulse buying, probably from a catalogue where I had seen and purchased a

> 'slip of a crepe de chine blouse. It is the quaintest thing, with only buttons on the sleeves, which is only quarter length, a rose petal in colour and hardly more substantial. I don't know what good it will be to me but it is certainly worth the money and anyhow I love it.'

My mother's creative dress sense came to my rescue. She completed it with a slip and full tulle skirt. It made a pretty dance frock. One of the thrills of *Vingt et Un* was to don one's finery and then move to the music of a small band. Fashions in dances, like so much else in the twenties, was changing. True we still danced the Valetta but the old square dances were soon dropped. Attempts at the Lancers ended in chaos; no one could remember the figures. The waltz remained a favourite as one dreamily drifted alone in a man's arms but the more energetic fox trot and military two step were increasingly popular. So were the new tunes to which they were danced. 'The Yankees are coming' and the jingling lines of

> *'Katie, beautiful Katie,*
>
> *You're the only G-G-G-Girl that I adore*
>
> *When the moon shines over the C-C-Cowshed*
>
> *I'll be waiting by the K-K-Kitchen door.'*

We waltzed to the dreamy strains of 'In a boat for two, gliding along with you, while the moon shines in all its glory', or the ever popular 'Whispering'. But of all the tunes that bring *Vingt et Un* most vividly back to me none has the spell of 'O Sole Mio'. I love it still

134

and had I ever been forced to chose eight discs to console me on my desert island that would have been one of them.

Looking back I can see how much I owed to *Vingt en Un*. It was much more than the source of pleasure and excitement as I dressed in my finery, piled into the taxi with Ruth and Joan, Soulie and Susie, wondering how the evening would go. It was the core of my social life outside the college walls. There I learnt to adjust myself to female friends and to live in a female community; in itself an art for which I shall always be grateful. *Vingt et Un* gave me my first experience of exploring my relationships with men unhampered by my family's protective observance. It was as if I stood on the banks of the river of adult experience, gradually wading deeper and all the while questioning whether I ever should, or ought, to take the plunge and swim. Looking back, as someone of my age must do, I cannot think that having been brought up mainly with boys helped me to understand men any the more easily. Adolescence had come in between and it was from that I was now struggling to be free. I still had an incurably romantic view of life and was still adolescent enough to try to crystallise it into verse despite the fact that I never progressed much beyond rhyming couplets. In the February of 1920, just as I was approaching my twentieth birthday I was still naïve enough, but also self conscious enough to recognize my position, writing

'I have come in contact with men, some I like, some
I don't. Yet I would stand well with them, think on
them, dwell on them.'

Then I burst into my verbal credo,

'Yet one thing I know

That I cannot spend my treasure so

One must keep oneself in hand

135

And aloof from lightness stand.

All that is the best of me

I must keep inviolate, free

For him who one day will come

And of my life make up the sum

And yet I still would please

Lightly laugh or gaily tease

Just to drink of flatteries balm

Must I then my true self harm?

Oh I know, I know so well

I have things I cannot sell.

Yet within me there is strife

For the pleasant things of life.

Then my willpower I must use

If myself I would not lose,

Keep my thoughts all fancy free,

Give woman's heart no liberty.

Since I was not born to please

Men with true unconscious ease

Let me never bend my will

To achieve my object still

Books will still suffice for me

So I keep my spirit free

I am unworthy, that I know,

Strive I, work I, ever so

And yet Oh man, who ere you be

I keep myself unstained for thee.'

It was in this spirit that I went each week to *Vingt et Un*, gazing with romantic thrills and hopes at the very ordinary young men who partnered me there. What, I wonder, will be the reaction of the modern Girton student of nearly twenty to my heart searching? Sex was something that distinguished male from female, cows from bulls, dogs from bitches. I knew the facts of life but there was no TV then to portray the performance, no novels, or at least none that came my way, to give explicit descriptions of the sexual act. Had there been I should have been horrified and disgusted. Love was still the gentle pressure of an encircling arm in the waltz, or the tender kiss of the betrothed in the moonlight. Had one of my partners attempted to kiss me without honourable intentions, and by this I meant matrimony, I should have thought him a cad and that I was somebody for whom he had no respect. Of all the men I knew at Cambridge no man ever did. Looking back I am not surprised! It is a tribute to the standards of my youth that promiscuous behaviour was confined to such women who invited it; those recognised as 'nice girls' were treated with well mannered propriety.

Vingt et Un was itself becoming more formal as it emerged from its chrysalis dancing class origins. Regular members and their guests had begun to know one another. Men and women no longer congregated in separate groups each eyeing one another. An entry for 12th March recorded the change that was taking place. They had programmes. It is alright if you know people but I rather liked the adventure of no programmes. However I was booked up before the first dance and so felt quite happy. Then came my account of the evening.

> 'Had four with Wandesforth – heaven knows why
> because we don't dance very well together and have
> very little to say to one another. Later in the evening he
> said he didn't know many people there, so perhaps that
> explains it!

Dear Pryor-Wandesforth: I can see him still in memory's eye. He had won an MC in the war and with his gleaming golden hair and small moustache was the epitome of an English gentleman with perfect manners and not much conversation, he was the most reliable but not the most exciting of partners. His cousin Wilfred Pryor, with whom on that occasion I was lucky enough to have three dances, was my main heart throb during, the second year. I confessed that

> 'I like Pryor the best. I think he is so graceful and
> playful without being silly or ridiculous and quite good
> looking too!'

Later I confessed that I thought I was falling in love with him. Perhaps it was necessary for me to indulge in such fantasies, fantasies that would have been satisfied if he had danced with me often and paid me small flattering attentions, so adding that touch of romance to give a final spice to the evening. At least I can commend my taste if not my commonsense; Wilfred Pryor was tall, dark haired with a dark moustache and charming caressing manners. Also he was a good dancer so that with him I did not have to worry about the steps or my feet. Alas love's young, dream, like so many of its ilk, was indeed the substance of which dreams were made . By May I was disenchanted:

> 'I don't like Pryor, horrid man. He never danced with
> me until no. 12 and he danced with those beastly
> Newnhamites the whole time. Pig!!! I must say we had
> two on end but I don't love him any more and soon
> I shan't like him. Men are fickle, fickle, fickle, much
> more than women!'

Meanwhile I consoled myself with the fact that I had the long vacation in which to get over my hurt and when I returned to Cambridge in the October now a third year, I wrote

> 'I had the last extra with Pryor who to my amusement
> I find bores me a little now. Alas he is off to China
> next term so to my utilitarian sense he is not worth
> cultivating now.'

So that is that. These little passions are very amusing when over but at one time I quite ached over him. It is a consoling thought to realise that one does recover pretty soon. I do not know how many of my friends indulged in 'these little passions' and were either hurt or exhilarated by them. Some I know did but nowhere could we have found a more pleasant, courteous and safe set of men on whom to practice our social graces than our hosts at *Vingt en Un* and I shall always be grateful to them for many hours of valuable experience not too dreary bought.

Another bonus that *Vingt en Un* bestowed was that door to even more pleasures to share with the men who had become our friends. When Pryor asked me to tea in Peterhouse I was doubly thrilled, thrilled because it was Pryor but thrilled too because I had never had tea in a man's rooms before. Everything was very correct as the long suffering Miss Dean was also invited to chaperon the tea party. His rooms were at the top of stairway D, right under the eaves, tiny but comfortable. I described the afternoon as 'a nice peaceful interlude,

139

not thrilling' then with a lapse into schoolgirl values I recorded that I had been given crumpets, chocolate cake and chocolate biscuits. Such tea parties were well conducted affairs owing to the presence of a chaperon. this was not always easy to arrange. On one occasion I remember that an elderly clergyman had to be pressed into service. We in our turn asked the men back to have tea at Girton. These too were necessarily well behaved but when Ruth's parents came to Cambridge and so could act as a more indulgent chaperone, Ruth managed to cram eleven people into her room. 'It was great fun' I wrote, 'I enjoyed it immensely'. That was in February when the weather made outdoor junketing impossible but in the May term, with the Backs in all the glory of Spring, river picnics took pride of place. They are among my most favourite memories.

The Cam might not be very wide nor impressive but it was an essential part of the Cambridge that I loved. To walk through the Fellows garden at Clare, to stand on its graceful bridge, to sit on the bank at King's and watch the punts with their white flannelled men pole gracefully by and, most pleasurable of all, to lie oneself stretched out on the cushion comfort of those lazily moving punts as our escorts manoeuvred their craft towards the peace of Granchester. Even here though the formality observed was al fresco it was nonetheless imperative. No member of the university would have appeared unless correctly attired in white. Nor on the river would he ever man any craft but a punt or canoe. Only townies ventured on the Cam in a rowing boat wearing a suit. In such matters I was quite definitely a snob, if indeed it was snobbery and not loyalty that made me proclaim that I belonged to the university and not the town. Even so it was hardly a commendable trait. I remember now with shame in my fourth year dodging an invitation to go on the river with a research scholar with a working class accent who was later to enjoy a most distinguished career, because I knew that he could not punt and would not be wearing the regulation white. There were other rules of etiquette to observe once Cambridge and the Backs lay behind us and the peaceful reaches of the Cam lie entrancingly ahead. On our way to this Eden we had to navigate our craft through Byron's pool where men bathed in the nude. Naturally we averted our eyes and the pool was deep enough to avoid embarrassment. But when a head appeared with a face that was familiar did one smile or tactfully look the other way? True there was nothing to be seen but we knew what lurked beneath the concealing waters. So in general the head turned away and with blank faces we drifted on.

Often we carried a picnic basket with us and anchoring at some favourite spot, maybe Paradise, we disembarked, spread out our cushions and boiled our kettle on a methylated stove. As the waters of the Cam were not of the cleanest it was essential that the water for our tea was well boiled. Once, when the stove had proved uncooperative or slow or ran out of fuel, the consequences were dire though not disastrous. Perhaps I was lucky to escape with an upset tummy! The first paper of my Tripos Part I was on Monday 31st May and on the Sunday a group of us decided to relax by going on the river rather than indulge in a last minute swat. It was my belief then, and has also remained so, that it was more important to face an examination with a clear mind than to acquire some last piece of half digested knowledge. A touch of desperation is a useful spur to prick the adrenalin to flow. So Ruth, Joan and I with Adams, Sampson and Francis Perowne agreed to meet, unfortunately however Adams and Sampson had quarrelled with Perowne, while Galetly and Mathews who had some of the food arrived late. However eventually we did all meet and found a spot where we decided to picnic. It was not a good decision as the thick grass hid patches of cow dung and some of the cushions were soiled. Nor were we successful in finding the right place for our supper when we landed at Paradise, as our first choice smelt. I did not say of what. However, though there was still a strained atmosphere I had one consolation; the food was good, including fruit and cream. The fact that I rarely omitted describing the fare when I ate out must, I suspect, have been a reflection on the Girton diet. The return at least was cool and peaceful as we drifted back to the strains of Ram's gramophone. As always the magic of the river worked.

> 'All day' I wrote, 'I had forgotten it; it has only been an unbelievable thing at the back of my mind; too remote to worry about. I am so tired I think I am sure to sleep to-night.'

Even through those three hectic days of Trip the river remained our oasis of peace. One of Ruth's many young men put his punt at our disposal and in it she and I lay relaxing after the ordeal of two three hour papers each day. Then on the Thursday came my 'first day of release', as I called it. The morning I spent with Elspeth shopping in Cambridge and indulging in a leisurely elevens. Then I cycled back to college, changed into what I described as my white frock and with Ruth set out again for another river picnic with two other men from *Vingt et Un*. We punted up to The Orchard, where we had tea. Coming back we anchored at Paradise and, like children released from school, played noughts and crosses on Ruth's shoes. Then came the usual rush to get back to college, as we had neither exits nor a chaperone and so were forced to refuse our escorts' invitation to take supper with them. On Sunday I was back on the river again, this time with Joan, Perowne and Ram. We punted up beyond Byron's Pool, had tea and then moored in a creek half hidden by a tangle of brambles and roses overhead. Ram and I lay stretched out in the punt but Joan, released from the pressures of Trip ragged about with Perowne until his landlady's cushions fell into the water.

> 'It was perfect coming back. The sun came out
> and made all the reflections green and peaceful
> and everything was so quiet and still with here and
> there the sound of a gramophone drifting, over the
> water. We had a dreadful scurry back. Didn't leave
> Scuddimores (the boathouse) until 7.45 and had to get
> back before 8pm to sign.'

The climax of these river jaunts came when the members of *Vingt en Un* invited us all to a grand picnic. Our procession of punts foregathered at The Orchard where

> 'tea was spread on long tables and we all sat in deck chairs like a school treat. We ate and talked quite fluently under the influence of tea. I being near the table managed to secure food with very little trouble. After about an hour, when we had all been finished some time, the men suddenly rose to their feet. I thought it was time to go but fruit salad with thick cream appeared instead. So, though fairly full we all ate that too. Then we did go. It was great fun coming back. All the punts, five in number were lashed together, and we drifted down steam, mostly into the right bank, to the sound of two rival gramophones. Everyone laughed but no one misbehaved and Lawes took photos from the bank. Then about 6.15 the punts broke up and I got into Hall in time for the savouries. I enjoyed the party even more in retrospect. Everyone was so nice and behaved so well, no raging, so that it makes a calm oasis and a pleasant change.'

My mother, who was coming to Cambridge for May week was due next day so, though the thrill of the races still lay ahead, when the river would cast a different spell over me, for that summer my picnics were over. Nostalgically Rupert Brooke's Granchester summed up for me the magic of the river. A magic which emotionally I tried to record after reading his haunting lines

> 'The thrilling sweet and rotten, unforgettable unforgotten river small.'

> 'It will always bring back to me the lower stream and the lazy banks, not effaceable, not forgotten until all things are forgotten. Because of this Granchester

means a poem to me because its lines hold for me
the key to the door where the old sensations lie, put
away in rosemary and lavender but no rue. The river,
coming back at night along the Backs, with the half
dusk falling cold. Do you remember?'

An emotional outpouring, yes, but one that sums up for me the magic of those river picnics so long ago.

Less emotionally exhausting was the fact that at Cambridge I was able to indulge my fondness for the theatre. This was one of the few areas where the town and gown both had something to contribute. In the twenties the commercial theatre flourished and its life blood had not yet been drained away to London. The great actors of the day still went on tour, either before the London opening or afterwards, and a town like Cambridge was sure to attract good companies with the latest London successes or long established favourites like the D'oily Carte. When we could scrape together the money or spare the time we went to the theatre, an activity that included those of my friends who never received invitations to *Vingt et Un*. The contribution made by the gown, if I may so describe the dramatic efforts of the members of the university were of even greater interest. I use the term members of the university deliberately. There were three such theatrical societies, Footlights, the Marlowe and the ADC. All had their membership limited to members of the university. This meant that, as in the days of Shakespeare's England, the entire cast was male. Looking back I find in my diary no hint of resentment at this exclusion but rather admiration at the skill which the female parts were portrayed. My long apprenticeship to theatre going had sharpened both my interest and my critical ability and I was quick to appreciate the high standard of excellence achieved by all three, from the high drama of Renaissance to a skittish soubrette in a Footlights' show. But of all the performances that I saw no one had quite the magic of *The White Devil* at the Marlow. Perhaps its magic was still more enhanced for me because I had had very little opportunity to

144

see anything but modern plays, opera and musical comedy. Perhaps in this long extract for 13th March 1920 I may still be able to convey the standard of excellence reached by theatrical societies of Cambridge in those immediate post war years.

'It was splendid. First the music weird and wailing, so that it seemed to be tugging at one's heart strings instead of those of the violins . The acting was wonderful; so consistent to the Renaissance type, all a trifle aloof and remote from life and yet the passion real enough to make a very perfect picture all in harmony. The man who took Victoria looked beautiful. He had small regular features and eyes that almost filled with tears. His acting was splendid. I had rather seen it so done than by a woman. It gave the air of the haunted pageant of passions long ago. His voice was good, like some boy singer before it had broken. So round and clear it was, so that one could see why the Duke must love her. He was excellent too. I heard his name was something king (Sieveking) and that he had bought the New Cambridge to publish his own poems in it. A versatile youth with a big nose too: the rudder of the soul. He too was handsome and wore his clothes well. He died most excellently too, with screams and death gurgles complete. Faminio died magnificently too, like a Renaissance villain true to type, with too long a speech and yet he saved it by not gesticulating or twisting in agony. I must speak of the scenery. Practically all the effects were got with curtains and lights; there was no attempt to produce conventional street or rooms though we got the effect of the latter absolutely. The whole thing was magnificent and I enjoyed it to the extent of weeping at the end, and my legs, they hardly seemed as if they would lead me down the stairs safely.'

The Cambridge dramatic club concentrated on contemporary plays but, when I went to their performance of *The Great Adventure* in the following May week, I was surprised to discover that some of the players who had so impressed me in *The White Devil* were equally at home in modern dress. Lubboch, who had taken the part of Ludivico, took the leading role, a performance I rated as

> 'Simply fine. In fact I quite loved him, he was so
> unaffected, almost childish and so loveable. A.S. Seely
> as Janet Cannot was a masterpiece. His voice I should
> recognise anywhere. I have seen him now as Louka,
> the Moorish girl in *The White Devil*, and he has always
> the same voice. All the time he remained a woman with
> little tricks and mannerisms. One realised that she was
> just the wife for him. H. Bishop was lovely as the suave
> lord, who tries to smooth everybody down. Bishop has
> a trick with his hands of throwing them out somehow.'

He too had been in *The White Devil*. Paget who had played Flaminio in it had only a small part in *The Great Adventure* but even so I thought his one of the outstanding performances. After reviewing these in some detail I added

> 'I was interested in that collection of young men.
> Lubboch got a First in his English Trip; as he had
> a play every term he is no fool. Some day I shall
> chronicle my collection.'

Alas I never did and wonder now what happened to all the youthful theatrical talent that had so impressed me. Later many names prominent both in the theatre and on TV first discovered their potential while up at Cambridge but I do not remember among them the names of the men who were strutting the boards in 1920. Footlights was probably more prolific but criticisms of their May Week show do not figure in my diary, partly because it was so popular

146

that tickets, were hard to get, and partly because the pressure of everything that had to be crammed into so short a time. Footlights was squeezed out as being merely a musical revue.

In addition to the shows put on by the three theatrical societies there were occasional ad hoc productions presented for a particular purpose. Perhaps the most distinguished of these was the performance of a Greek tragedy played in the original Greek by the Classical Society. I was privileged to see one of them. It was for me a unique occasion when in the March of 1921 I saw a performance of Orestes. Rather to my surprise the House was only half full. It was an experience I enjoyed though my one year of Greek for Little Go was no help in understanding the dialogue. Rather to my surprise, as I recorded

'After a while the Greek ceased to trouble me and became natural. It was so beautifully spoken and the cast had such topping voices.'

The actor who most impressed me was Burden of Corpus Christi who played Clymenestra and whom I described as looking

'perfectly beautiful in a long gown of red and goldy stuff and some sort of head dress. He had a most beautiful voice and I shall long remember his first appearance in the great doorway, framed in stone, standing, out against the black curtain.'

In all these performances women, not being, members of the university, were excluded but on two theatrical occasions Girton students were invited to play the female roles. The first of these was when it was decided to put on a performance of *The Fairy Queen* in the Lent term of 1920. I was inclined to damn it with faint praise considering it

'good I suppose but I was not thrilled. The thing

lacked vim and was incoherent, the acting for the most part mediocre. The colour and staging' I admitted 'were very good but that did not appeal to me.'

Nevertheless it was something of a breakthrough, though of this I seem to have been unconscious, in that three Girton students took the female leads: Eileen Thomas was Hermione, Helen Lehmann, the sister of the celebrated actress Beatrice Lehmann, Helena, and Ruth, Hypholyta. The other occasion was when during May Week of that year a special performance *One of Comus* was given in the gardens of Merton Hall. It was graced by the appearance of Squire, the poet, and a leading literary figure of the day. He played Comus. I found him impressive adding

> 'I don't know what he is like in real life. Today his arms and face were burnt a deep brown, his wig was black and tousled. His eyes, darting and fierce were the only points of light. His acting was brutal and impassioned – very good. It must have been difficult to recite yards of Milton in a natural way. Dennis Arundel the attendant spirit, struck the right note from the very first. He was wrapped in a sky blue cloak that covered him except for his legs and arms, while a golden wig shed long hair over his shoulders. His diction was perfect and his actions beautiful. Later he came back dressed as a shepherd in a tiny white tunic that left one arm free. I have never realized before how beautiful a man's figure could look. The fair skin, the snowy tunic and the falling hair stood out against the green of the garden and borrowed a magic radiance from the sun.'

With so much to offer in the way of distractions ranging from the fascination of contemporary politics provided by the Liberal Society, through the glamour of the Bump races, the weekly frivolity of *Vingt et Un,* the idyllic pleasure of the river to the feast of theatrical entertainment, both commercial and amateur, it is surprising that so much could be squeezed into a day which, except at the weekend, was still dominated by work. It was no wonder that my diary so often repeated the refrain

'I am so tired too tired to write anything except through a mist of weariness. I have had a perfectly hectic day.'

If all work and no play makes Jill a dull girl at least that taunt can never be hurled at me. Somehow I found time for both. Perhaps the most valuable lesson that Cambridge taught the aspiring student was the self discipline of managing to get the most out of life, of-organizing energy and time, of accepting the fact that pleasure was but the icing on the cake. It is on that cake, to complete the picture, I must concentrate: frivol as I might, I must never forget that in 1920 I had to sit Part I of the Tripos.

CHAPTER SIX: GOING FOR GOLD

However valuable in the art of living, and even educational in that sense of the word the knowledge acquired by way of lying lazily in punts poled by white flannelled young men, or dancing, with them at *Vingt et Un* might be in the future, in 1920 they were merely the icing on the cake. In the May of that year I sat the first part of my History Tripos and as the fateful month drew near my horizon was dominated by the need to work if I were to attain that standard of academic excellence that was the reason why I was at Girton. My results in the Mays examination at the end of my first year had been gratifying but academically unimportant because they were not part of my final degree. With the results of Part I, I should have to live for the rest of my life. So, because I was never any good at last minute cramming, I had to map out a programme of work and stick to it. It was not always easy. In February I confessed

'I found it very hard to do my seven hours because the spring was so glorious outside. The air smelt of scent and the sun was so warm and hot so that Stubbs seemed unusually dry.'

For the information of the uninitiated, Stubbs was the standard collection of medieval statutes, charters etc, all essential for my paper on Medieval English History. It was not my favourite reading. As trip drew nearer the pressure of revising grew heavier so that by the beginning of May I was moaning 'So sick of revising it makes me wriggle all over'. Not only had I to revise the two new courses I had studied in my second year but also the three studied in my first year. It was like juggling with five balls at once. About my sixth paper I could only pray since the Essay Paper was not only unpredictable it was also considered vital in the determination of one's class. On the Saturday before the ordeal had to be faced I wrote

> 'It is a hopeless feeling that now there is no time to repair the gaps in one's knowledge and one wonders whether the questions will let you air the knowledge you have or present a hopelessly blank wall.'

Perhaps one of the bravest and most sensible decisions I have ever taken was to have the courage to be true to my conviction that it was more important to be physically rested and mentally fresh than, like a capon, crammed with last minute information. So I went on a pre Tripos river picnic and sleepily and happy I got into bed.

For the next three days life was an odd mixture of pressure and normality; an ordeal which I survived more easily than I had expected as my diary demonstrates. For so important a milestone I think it worth to be quoted verbatim.

> 'Trip. I was called at 7.30. Had my bath and got dressed. Went to chapel and half wished I hadn't. It made it more impressive. Choked over my breakfast but ate it somehow and went into the bus pretending to rag. We went in and settled down. Then I got my paper, realized that it was not quite double Dutch. I wrote 23 pages including blanks.'

Then came the almost casual entry, considering that I had to face another paper in the afternoon.

> 'Had lunch and tried to get tickets to Footlights but failed as the queue was so long and I had no time. Went to join Ruth in Adams' punt. I am sure Adams said Dorothy today but I can't pretend I mind. R. says that tomorrow the punt is to be moved into a Creek. I said "to suffer smells in King's rather than get into bad odour at college I thought it sounded rather good."'

As a friendly gesture Adams had put his punt at our disposal to relax between papers, but to be seen so doing even in these exceptional circumstances, would not have commended us to college authorities so we thought the privacy of a side creek more discrete. At least I returned to the examination hall refreshed and commonsense was rewarded in that I confessed "I quite liked the Early Constitutional paper" but nobody else did and so I am afraid I might have done it badly. At tea EEP said they were all looking reproachfully at my back.'

During these three days we candidates were treated almost as sacrificial victims, pampered to prepare them for the kill. In the morning a fresher called us with the unknown luxury, an early morning cup of tea. When we returned they revived us, or consoled us, with a generous tea.

Obviously I had myself well under control. Next day writing

> 'I felt quite calm and tranquil, even the faintest tremor seemed to have gone. I did not like the Economic History paper much. I knew it but it did not thrill me. The Medieval European in the afternoon was disappointing, not really hard but in trivial outline and not in the detail which we had mugged up. I felt disappointed and did not do it very well. In the

evening we had the chicken and ham that Mother had sent us sitting in Woodlands under the pines. It was so lovely and remote.'

I was equally unenthusiastic about Wednesday's papers.

'The Later Constitutional was vile and we thought it would be our best. The contents question had no labels and so I did not know them and did the rest of the paper mostly on Political Science. We all loathed it but it really wasn't as bad as that. The essays were beastly; all on queer things. This was daunting for it was popularly supposed that when it came to a decision on class it could make all the difference between a bottom and top second, or a top second and a first. The subject which I finally chose was "That democracy divided communities into individuals and brings them together again as mobs". I wrote six pages and spelt psychology, "physcology" but I think the substance was pretty good.'

My final summing up of the examination in its entirety was

'On the whole I have neither liked nor disliked the papers. They were easier than I feared and I am afraid I did them too factually, never had time to treat my facts philosophically and I hoped that is what the examiners want, being men.'

But at least it was over. It was lovely to think that, all one's work was done for at least a month. At last I was free to enjoy all the delights that May Week had to offer: young men, river picnics, *Vingt et Un* and all the excitement of the bump races, concerts and the May Week performance of the A.D.C.

These delights were given an additional glitter in that my Mother was coming up for the last few days of term; her first visit since Armistice and my first opportunity to parade before her my hard won social aplomb. How far I was successful in this I am uncertain, as she confessed herself amused by the half protective, half humorous manner all my friends displayed towards me. As Cambridge is always packed for May Week I had some difficulty in finding suitable rooms for her and for my young brother, five years my junior whose health having broken down after measles, was now with a tutor at Swaffham. My mother having arrived the night before, we went to collect him from the station, I observing, with sisterly candour

> 'He is much improved, not so messy looking and
> better mannered. Some day he will be rather nice I
> think. We then went up the town and had elevens
> at Mathews. William with great glee ate seven cakes!
> Mother proceeded to buy him a new hat and tie and
> me some white gloves. We then went back to our digs
> and had strawberries and cream.'

It was a full day, typical of May Week. In the afternoon we went to the performance of Comus, which I have already described. This ended at 4pm and we then went on to the Races, they in a special bus and I on my bicycle having collected Joan, whom I wanted my Mother to meet, Having watched the first races from the tow-path in honour of my family we crossed on the Grind to the Ditton Paddock: which I described as 'very nice, rows of little chairs by the water's edge and a big marquee with tea in the background'. The introductions over we went to have tea William acting as courier. Then we took our seats on the bank waiting for the second division. The evening ended with a concert at King's to which the ever helpful Adams had originally asked Ruth and me and had then politely extended the invitation to my mother. The mad rush that followed to fit in this final engagement was so typical that it is worth a mention.

> 'I had a mad peddle back, spent three minutes

gobbling, down some meat and potatoes then flew
to dress. It was then 8.05 and the taxi came at 8.20.
Joan came to help me while I scrambled into my white
Greek dress. When we arrived at Adams' room he was
still in his blazer, so we sat round and talked while he
made a sketchy toilet in the other room to the tune
of a gramophone. We sat in the gallery and had a
fine view of the people sitting below, every one was
in evening dress and the man flitting to and fro with
programmes. The concert was rather over my head but
I loved the sensation. I felt that here was a new side
of Cambridge, all these young men, so immaculate in
their white fronts were part of something in which I
too had a share and they were clever, taken all in all.
The diversity of them wrapped me round. We were
here tonight to hear them sing, but here in the Hall
were athletes, thinkers, speakers, writers, all part of the
one whole to which in sentiment at least I belonged.'

The next day I thought slightly less eventful though looking back I
should consider this a somewhat misleading statement. In the morning,
there was, as usual on special days, elevens at Mathews, this time to
introduce my non frivolous friends, Helen Harvey and Winnie Lumb
to Mother and William. She liked them both but William was bitterly
offended that they took so little notice of him. Then we paid a visit
to the Fitzwilliam Museum with which my brother, somewhat to my
surprise was thrilled and indeed wanted to re-visit the next day. Then
back we went to Mathews where we lunched on soup, salmon and
salad, coffee and cakes, a repast which I commended as 'very good'.
Was this the greed of youth that made me record so meticulously the
food I ate or a reflection of that provided by the college? Certainly
in my scheme of things good food was an important ingredient. To
look into the future so it remained and even in old age it is a pleasure
still to be enjoyed. I then dashed back to college to change from a
cotton dress into my navy jumper and skirt before we all went to the

races. It was a typical May pageant, whose flavour once again I tried to recapture, writing

'We saw all divisions go past. Poor King's 2 & 1, with Adams' at bow sunk on being bumped. It was rather hard lines. They were sunk every night except the last and he had invited his fiancée up to watch the races! In the second division there was a mess. Emma (Emmanuel) bumped and had her rudder broken with the result that each boat automatically bumped the one in front. We had gone up to the top part of Ditton Paddock where we had a view of the Plough Reach. We saw Lady Maggy (St. John's College) came round with Queen's so close on their heels that they were bumped just after rounding the corner right under our noses. That removed the remaining two boats from the action while behind came Cats (St. Catherine's). Then there was a general bump with the rather ludicrous result that Cats rowed the course in solitary state from Ditton Corner. As the First Division came up Lady Maggy stopped in front of us. I was pointing them out to Mother, fluttering my race card and getting generally excited when Sanderson (*Vingt et Un* partner) turned and grinned broadly and pointed us out to Francais (another member of *Vingt et Un*).'

The next day followed a similar pattern with elevens at Mathews, then lunch, after which I mounted my bike while they were to follow in a taxi. Alas I ran into another cyclist and buckled my front wheel. The incident is not of itself worth recording but the comment that I made in my diary has some significance.

'I was shaken and to crown it all he was only a townie. I could have survived it better from an undergraduate.'

I might not be a member of the University but I was certainly a student snob! The races over, my mother returned to her digs after putting William on the train to return to his tutor while I deserted my family and went to *Vingt et Un*. Saturday was devoted to social occasions and sight-seeing, doing the round of Clare, with its marvellous Fellows Garden, Trinity and King's. As usual we had elevens at Mathews where I spotted Jack Hulbert, his wife and brother Claude, and commented on the length of his chin. We then had lunch at Emmanuel with Elspeth and the Giles' before returning once again to the races with their usual excitements of bump and personalities. Then after a hectic rush to change in more formal clothes; in the twenties one did not go a theatrical performance in the equivalent of jeans, we went to the A.D.C. performance production of *The Great Adventure* which I have described previously.

Sunday was our last day. We went to King's chapel in the morning then out to Girton for lunch after which I had arranged for them to meet EEP.

> 'Of course she forgot' I wrote tolerantly. 'Finally I found her sitting peacefully on the lawn. When she saw me she gave a clutch of dismay to her head, started up and grasped me by the arm and hurried across the court. She was perfectly charming, when she sent me up to bring down a book that she wanted to show me and there on her mantelpiece was the note Mem. 12.40 Miss Marshall. Dear old EEP.'

We finished the day by going to an organ recital at King's

> 'The candles looked lovely gleaming through the door of the chapel: we were in the anti-chapel where only a few candles burned. All the same I was rather bored and let my thoughts wander. I'm not musical and its only function for me is to provide a key to the door

of my fancies. When the music plays I let them out to play too.'

So ended my second year a Girton. Next day we returned to Old Hutton.

Then came the agonizing wait until my results came. On the day that it was due both Mother and I were equally strung up. We had arranged with Helen to wire us as soon as the lists were up but to our strained nerves the wire seemed so slow to arrive that we began to think that Helen had, in some way, made a mess of the operation. In these days I do not think that there was a telephone in the village. Certainly our only quick contact with the outside world was to send a wire from our nearest Post Office from which a wire could be sent. That was over four miles away so the wire was brought up by a boy on a bicycle, who received a delivery charge of 6d for his pains. In the end we set out to meet him which we did about a mile from the house. Mother opened it, said a II.1 and handed it to me. I felt a moment of blankness. It would not be true to say that I hoped for a First but, buoyed up by the exaggerated opinions expressed by my friends, equally it would not be true to say I had not. We turned and went back. I felt nothing, not even relief, only a shaking all over and a vague temptation to cry. Next morning I woke with a sense of relief. Bed seemed more comfortable because I had got my II.1. I talked all day about it and did nothing but read *A Houseful of Girls* as a rest to my brain. Then letters came and my sense of achievement was boosted by the news that old Winnie and I had got II.ls; the rest, all my potential rivals had II.2s. There were no firsts. A fortnight later I was back at Girton for the 'Long'.

Like so many Cambridge labels this was misleading. The Long was a short term: a kind of hyphen between the second and third year, carved out of the Long Vacation. Its purpose was to break the heavy load of new work that faced the Third Year student taking Part II of the Tripos. When I arrived a Cambridge station instead of the usual scrum, taxis were easy to come by and the college seemed quiet and deserted. My friends from the year senior to mine, had disappeared for good and I missed Helen and Jessie. Absent too were the new friends I had made in the freshman year below me. The Long was not, if my memory serves aright, obligatory. Joan, with whom I had become increasingly friendly, had not come. Elspeth was not in residence and Winnie was not there. So I felt a little lonely and lost, in addition to feeling awkward about receiving the congratulations on my II.1 from quasi rivals who had done less well. In fact that first week, before Ruth joined me, things, as they say in the north 'turned out better than like'. Susie Wotton, Joan's cousin and her friend Rosalind Hilliard, took me under their wing, asking me to jugs and wandering round Woodlands with me. With so few distractions I worked solidly, trying to break the back of my new courses. It was a formidable task. These were (a) modern European History from the sixteenth century onwards; (b) the theoretical side of Political Science, a study of schools of thought, intellectually far more taxing than acquiring a knowledge of the actual structure of contemporary governments, which had been the major content of the Political paper in my first year and finally a special period. In the main the Cambridge Historical school concentrated on outline courses, designed to provide a picture of historical development of the western world since classical times. After a lifetime of teaching there is much to be said for this approach. It provided the backdrop to whatever specialist aspect one studied. The special period of which there were several from which to choose, was to provide the elementary use of original material in interpreting a limited slice of History. My choice was limited by the fact that for most of them a good reading of a foreign language was essential and this I had never managed to acquire. There was only one subject in which the sources were almost entirely in English and this was *The Whigs*, but I was not attracted by it and would have much preferred *The French Revolution* but the Whigs it had to be. Though I could not guess it then this was the first milestone in my academic career. Had I not been deflected into a study of eighteenth century England by my linguistic deficiency *English People in the Eighteenth Century, Eighteenth*

160

Century England and *Dr Johnson's London* would never have been written. Of such small incidents are the direction of a life so often the consequence. This has been my experience again and again. All I can say is that Fate has been very kind to me.

I was not however feeling grateful to Fate or anyone else as I struggled with my workload, writing

> 'I hate the Long. My days are monotonous and filled
> with stodge. I am tired and brain bound.'

I had some excuse for feeling thus. Lectures were few and most of the day devoted to private reading. Breaking new ground as I struggled with the problems of Cavour or to unravel the intricacy of the Eastern Question, trying to digest so much new and varied material was exhausting so that I was moaning that so many new fields to conquer left my brain tired after some six hours. The same complaint that I was dreadfully tired is scattered over my diary's pages so that I began to wonder if I needed a tonic as I did not think that a healthy person of my age should be mentally depressed. Truth to tell 19th century European History never held much charm for me. Finally I decided to go for the Whigs, as I elegantly put it, writing

> 'I am starting SHELBURNE. He seems a bitter sort
> of cuss but promises to be interesting.'

If uninspiring, the Long was a necessary evil. When I returned to Old Hutton it was with the foundation built sufficiently firm to base on it my vacation reading.

Nor was the Long without its minor pleasures and relaxations. One's nose could not always be in a book or one's thoughts centred on the state of Europe. Cambridge contained shops as well as libraries and having cycled in for a lecture, on a Saturday of all days, I shopped. My purchase was a Macintosh,

'a greeny thing, double breasted. I don't like it very
much. Still I THINK it looks quite smart, better than
my old one. It was 45/s. There was a dream for £5
rubber and silk in grey and navy. Then we had lunch
at Buol's. They do one well for 2/—. After that went
round Heffers. I spent three quarters of an hour there.
It is a fascinating place but demoralizing.'

For the information of the uninitiated Heffers was, together with
Bowes and Bowes, the most splendid of book shops. When I found
it demoralizing it was because it tempted me to buy books I could
not afford or to read books for which I had neither the time nor the
need to read.

If my impression of the Long was somewhat dreary the
impression was not totally fair. Though the University was officially
'down' in its lack of organised activities the Cam was still there and
the days long and sunny, Elspeth and Ruth decided that I ought to
be taught to swim. So far all my efforts to do this had been quite
ineffective, which indeed throughout my life has sadly remained the
case. Long after my Girton days lay behind me, when enthusiastic
young men offered to teach me, whether it was in the Cape Rollers
at Fishock or in the splendid baths at Prague, I took it as a tribute to
my figure, but I never expected their efforts to induce me not to sink
after three strokes to be crowned with success. They never were. But
in 1920 my friends were hopeful. After all had they not got rid of my
Lancashire accent? The lessons took place in a little back alley off the
Cam that had been artificially widened and where I would be within
my depth. Above all it was quiet and secluded. After several attempts
however I confessed

'I don't seem to get on any further. Just now and then I
get a feeling of power but it goes very soon.'

It was ever thus! Far more enjoyable was a notable river picnic, undoubtedly organised by Ruth, our companions being her latest swain but whose initials, G.S. mean nothing now to my errant memory and Mr Ram, a constant *Vingt et Un* member. At the beginning he punted while Ruth and G.S. sat together. I found it rather dull as I tried to make myself as unobtrusive as possible, but later things improved. It was too late to light a fire and Ruth had forgotten the milk. So we landed near the Orchard and while they went to forage, Ram and I ate up the chocolate in their absence. Eventually we had tea and my comment looking back was

> 'It was a nice party. G.S. had a refining influence that
> saved us from getting giddy. After tea we drifted home
> in the sunlight which is always the best part, content,
> with tea inside and mellow evening light out. It is the
> quintessence of Cambridge.'

More hilarious was the time that Ruth decided that it would be fun to take out a canoe and for me to learn to paddle. As I well knew

> 'I had no right to be there being neither efficient nor
> a swimmer. Ruth was both. Taking our tea we took a
> canoe and went. It was lovely drifting down until we
> anchored, tied to a tree and fed. Then it began to pour
> with rain. Finally in a fine spell we set out and tried to
> paddle but showed a surprising aptitude for the banks
> and two punt loads of men that were harmlessly sailing
> amid stream. By the end I was going rather better
> but by then it was pouring, so Ruth paddled in good
> earnest, I doing my best to second her. We arrived at
> Scudemores like drowned rats. He only charged us 3/-'

Scudemores was the boathouse we had patronized. The occasional tea party with the Giles' concluded the available social activities. I imagine Mrs Giles found a supply of young females a help in entertaining Emma men up for the Long. It was nearly over and

I was looking forward to the peace of home and the Westmoreland countryside.

Doubtless the work I had done while I had been in residence was important but a more important milestone was the fact that I had begun to envisage an academic future for myself. After a coffee party with EEP I stayed on, as I wanted to discuss the possibility of staying up for a fourth year. EEP in my words was

> 'very nice, said I could always teach, or get an administrative post, but if it was not vital to take a paid job I could concentrate on research permanently, if I shaped well at it. She said I had a bent towards scholarship and I think I agree with her. I feel it would solve so many problems if the money holds out.'

I had been worrying about making a career that would mean my being away from home for much of the year because I was conscious of how much my companionship meant to my mother. Now I should have something to do. If my bent lay that way

> 'it would be useful, though perhaps it would be a disappointment for me never to do something in the world but there I doubt my abilities, but not with my books. Somehow I think this solves things. In the winter we could go to London or elsewhere and in the summer stay at Old Hutton. Perhaps in that my life would get too narrow and peaceful. I don't know. Still it is an idea and Fate does not let people stay too long in one rut unless they resist her with glue.'

Two days after this encouraging conversation the idea of an academic career had taken root.

> 'They say that a man who knows what he wants gets it. Here is what I want is to get a university job and to marry Vignoles.'

Then with a sudden descent into reality I added

'that is I don't want it exactly as I don't know him but somehow it suggests itself to me as my loadstar.'

Vignoles had been the head of house in my brother's house at Sedbergh and, seeing him in the famous run, I worshipped from afar. My sentimental attraction was at least sufficiently alive for me to have discovered that he was now at Magdelene and I may actually once or twice caught glimpses of his red head as I cycled into lectures. Maybe, with those flashes of prudence that I sometimes showed, I realised that it was emotionally less painful to dream of being married to the hero of a dream than to agonize over the fact that wretched Wilfred Pryor seemed to prefer to dance with the Newnhamites rather than with me.

That was the last significant entry that I made before returning to Old Hutton and the freedom of the long vacation. It was like returning to a different world and being reincarnated as a different person. I was returning to a world I knew and a home I loved: to a village where I was not an aspiring student but Miss Dorothy, where I knew all about everyone just as they knew all about me, or at least as much as interested them, for in a village no secrets are hid. I was exchanging the excitement of a river picnic on the Cam for the joys of cycling over hill and dale, picnicking beside clear becks chattering as they ran over the grey stones that made their bed. Then as a climax consuming a huge home baked shilling tea at some small inn before facing the long ride home and I was at peace. Once again my mother had become the centre of my life. Important too were the long visits that her great life long friend Elizabeth Preston paid us. Indeed so much had she become a member of our family that she had become an honorary aunt, Auntie Biddy. She was in many ways a most interesting, if occasionally in my eyes a wrong headed one. She had a distinct predilection for the esoteric, she was always trying to pierce the veil of the unknown. She had a small statuette of 'the Buddha' as she used to say in her rich Irish voice. She was a theopolist and belonged to some equivalent of a Women's Free Masonry. Among her other accomplishments she could cast horoscopes and when I gave her the relevant details of Girton friends quite unknown to her it was often surprising how accurate her delineation of their personalities were. Perhaps my most haunting memories of her are when some evenings in our lamp lit parlour she would sing Hebrean Love Songs in a deep throated voice that almost seemed to caress the words as she sung them. With her love of Ireland, she was born in Armagh, and her interest in Irish legends she persuaded us to go with her to the Glastonbury Festival, as it would now be called, sponsored by the Clarke family, hence the location, where Rutland Boughton's new work *The Immortal Hour* was to be performed. It was a curiously informal occasion, though important enough for George Bernard Shaw to come down for it. That is the only time I saw the great man in the flesh. The venue was the scruffy little village hall. The music was provided by a piano, generally played by the composer, who, when he disapproved of the rendering of a particular passage, thumped hard to drown it. The audience sat on hard chair's and the whole thing was reminiscent of a village concert, all that is except for the magic of the setting and of the music which I tried to capture in the following two extracts.

'Tonight we went to *The Immortal Hour*. It was one of those things hard to put into words, so that I sat with wrung hands, waiting for the curtain to fall and end the strain. The note was struck from the very first; grim Dalua towering high in his black robes and peacock plume, as he stood silent with folded arms, while the green leaves danced elfishly round and the spirit voices called somewhere in grim mystery of the wood. Etain herself was like a blown blossom, as fragile and as fragrant, with her green dress and mistletoe bound hair. She drifted away at Dalua's command, Echochine came out of the greyness: Echochine in his hunter's

garb, the follower of dreams and visions and the
eyes of a seer. What need to recount it all with the
ever growing sense of destiny until Midir lures Etain
back to the Lordly Ones, the Shee, while the kingly
dreamer falls dead at the touch of Dalua. There was
a moment of silence. Then came the applause, which,
dying down, gave Langley, erstwhile Dalua, the chance
to appeal to the audience for a contribution to the
funds which had produced this magic on a shoe string
budget despite the generosity of the Clarke's. I lost
my heart to Johnstone-Douglas as Echochine. He had
a strong, lean face framed by a dark wig and lighted
by intense blue-grey eyes. His acting was magnificent;
that of a dreamer who is yet a strong man torn with
anguish. Langley as Dalua was all pervading and Gwen
Francon-Davies made an elfin, elusive Etain.'

The other members of the cast, as far as I know made no
permanent name for themselves on the London stage, but, as I wrote
in the January of 1987,

'to the modern generation she is no stranger. It was the
beginning of a great career'.

My own enthusiasm for *The Immortal Hour* was no flash in the pan.
On the Saturday afternoon we went to the matinee.

'I wondered how I should like it the second time. It
is always the most critical. One has not the freshness
nor yet the familiarity of an old friend. At first Dalua
seemed less impressive and I wondered. Then, as it
went on, I gave myself up to the charm of Eoehaid
and Etain till the first act ended. Today it was the
second act that proved my undoing. The first I was
calm but the second carried me away. It was Eochaid's

re-creative beginning 'where the water whitens mid the shadowy rowan trees' 'and 'The laughter of the Hidden Folk is terrible to hear' that upset me. The terror of his voice and face and eyes was so dreadful. The Midir came, tall with gold burnished hair and lordly mein. 'I am a green blown leaf' sang Etain 'and you are the wind from the south' In vain Eochaid tried to break the enchantment; Midir divided them. 'I cannot come to you' he strained to say. 'I cannot hear your half forgotten voice' came the feary voice of Etain as, with her hands in Midir's, she drifted away to where the Feary Ones were singing 'How Beautiful they are, the Lordly Ones, who dwell in the Hills, in the hollow hills. Dark grew the stage as Eochaid laid his crown on Etain's vacant throne. We were told that last time he laid his wig there too but a mistake in the lighting saved the situation; this time he gave it a fugitive touch. In the starlight came the dark figure of Dalua. Eochaid faced him 'Give me my dream' he said. 'Give me my dreams'. Dalua stretched out his hand and Eochaid fell dead at his feet while in the distance the Feary chorus died away. By this time I was weeping, great drops that welled and felled one by one until, under cover of the applause I could blow my nose.'

The *Immortal Hour* was not the only by Rutland Boughton opera to be performed at Glastonbury. He had also composed two others on the Arthurian legend, *The Birth of Arthur* and *The Round Table*. With neither of them was I much impressed but, before I tear myself away from my Glastonbury memories fans of Gwen Francan Davies might be interested in my description of her performance as the enchantress Nuime,

'She was wonderful in this part. Her gestures were uncanny, queer crooked things made by pale slim arms

and hands, while over her shoulders the long green
hair fell and her dress, like reeds, quivered in the wind.'

Later, when I was working in London I saw her in what I think must have been her first Shakespearean role as Juliet, while her Romeo was an unknown young actor with an unforgettable beautiful voice. His name was John Gielgud, a product of Ouds. I wish he had been a member of the Marlowe or C.U.C. when legitimately I could have included in this Cambridge saga, tribute to his genius, but I have digressed too long already and must return to my role as a third year student when on 8th October my vacation ended and back to Girton I came. Sad though I felt at leaving home I was beginning to look forward to the new term and all that it might bring. I was greeted by a newly decorated room which I described as looking topping now, with newly painted walls and my new rugs. It has quite an affluent look and very by bright and clean. As a third year I could have moved to what were considered more spacious and desirable quarters but I was fond of my room, it was convenient being so near the portress' lodge and I saw no reason to move. So for the last two years I stayed happily in Bearpits which two years ago I had viewed so disconsolately with its austere welcome as a freshman facing the unknown. Now it was my home and it was I who

'talked a little to the freshers at the At Home. I didn't
want to go but felt it was a moral duty and quite
enjoyed it and stayed to the end of dancing.'

So virtue was rewarded; as I often find that it is.

Each year seems to possess a certain quality of its own. The First Year is fragile, tentative, the Second a time for growth, the Third one of robust fulfilment. I enjoyed my Third year. I belonged to the Establishment, a person of some importance to my juniors; someone whom my tutors were taking seriously as a possible future scholar. All this was very reassuring. I had my own circle of friends with only one serious gap in it; Helen Harvey, a year senior to me had gone down. My pattern of life was by now a familiar one. Lectures, essay writing and hours of reading filled anything up to eight hours of the day but, because I kept to a steady programme there was time to fit in other activities. It was in my Third year that I had became an enthusiastic attender of the Union debates and a loyal supporter of the Liberal. As at the same time Ruth decided to join the Conservative Club politics produced the subject for future argument. Her choice of party was more of the milestone in her future than mine as eventually, though not in Cambridge, it led to her meeting with the man she very happily married. My more immediate emotional interests were centred on *Vingt et Un* and when I received my invitation to the first dance of the term I was considerably relieved, it would have been awful to have been dropped and my social life would have been shattered. fortunately no such terrible fate overtook me and for the remainder of my time at Girton *Vingt et Un*, with its descriptions of my partners and the ups and downs of my fortunes appeared with monotonous regularity in my diary including what, in the phraseology of the day I described as my G.P. (Grand Passion) on Pryor. So it is fitting that I should record the last *Vingt et Un* before he departed for China.

'My dance with Pryor was a mad one because they threw down balloons from above and then he went careering round trying to hit them. It was the last *Vingt et Un* of the term and after we had danced to John Peel and sung Auld Lang Syne we cheered him. The Laws and I chased him with our balloons – it having gone down it was a lovely weapon of attack. I behaved thoroughly badly. Well he has gone now. That is something definitely over, even though it never began. I am sorry. He was just what I wanted in a man "a gentle man and strong" (to quote from Jeffery Farnol's popular romantic novel *The Broad Highway*) always courteous, considerate and English enough to make it a matter of course. He was a standard by which I might well measure other men and I am glad to have known him. It was a madcap dance but in the end we said goodbye quite seriously and that is all. I feel a little sad now though the ache went a month ago, but he was so well worth knowing and I never knew him. Yet *Vingt et Un* won't be quite the same next term.'

How young I was and how guileless. Why I have included this pathetic revealing episode is because it illustrates an approach to matters emotional that is totally unaware of sex as a potent factor in human relations. My information on that subject was purely clinical. Merely to know that babies are not found under gooseberry bushes or brought by benevolent storks can at best be described as negative knowledge. *Vingt et Un* was little help here. I never experienced even a surreptitious kiss and would have felt insulted if I had. To be kissed by a man who had not 'honourable intentions', by which I meant matrimonial ones, was to be held cheap. A student of Girton today who during three years had never been kissed and who never expected to be must either be singularly and repulsively ugly or qualify for a place in the *Guinness Book of Records*.

Though my social activities were an important part of my Third Year they were merely the embroidery on the solid fabric of work. With Part I behind me Part II began a fresh chapter in my academic life. My subjects, my lecturers, even my Director of studies were new. EEP was snatched away from Girton by the distinction of being the first woman to be given the Albert Kahn Travelling Fellowship. When she returned to England it was not to us but to the London School of Economics that she went, though she still kept up a close connection with her old college. Her successor was Mary Gladys Jones. Like EEP she too was an old Girtonian. Both in style and appearance both women were very different. Miss Jones, or 'the Jones' or 'Emma G', as she came to be nicknamed, was the older of the two by nearly nine years. EEP was born in 1889 and Emma G. in 1880. The former had been clearly marked out for an academic career having carried off several distinguished scholarships and prizes before being appointed as Director of Studies in Girton in 1913, in 1921 becoming a lecturer. Miss Jones' earlier career had concentrated more on the craft of teaching. She had taken a course in pedagogy and the London University Teachers Diploma in 1909 and had been head of the training Department at both Cheltenham Ladies College and Alexandra College Dublin before taking up the Girton appointment.

With such a background she was in every way fitted to be an excellent tutor and director of studies. She was more formal in manner than EEP, and did not immediately charm in her casual, friendly way, but no one could have been a more responsible capable tutor. In her own way she had quite as much to give her students as her more glamorous friend and I became devoted to her. I owe her much and was indeed lucky to have had two such wonderful women to shape and influence my early academic life. Winnie shared my admiration for her and she, in her turn gave us unstintingly of her time so that after a particularly interesting tutorial, in which I flattered myself that I had made a good impression on 'the Jones' Winnie and I continued to discuss the points she had raised for another hour. So encouraged were we that

> 'we are quite decided and determined to get Firsts next
> year. So much so that I shall be very disappointed if
> we don't.' In conclusion I added 'I really feel that she
> likes us. Indeed I have believed opening up herself to
> a seemingly intelligent audience. When we asked her to
> what was in essence a "working jug" she came at 9.30
> and stayed until 11.00. She gave us a most valuable
> coaching and is a dear woman.'

I never had any reason to retract this opinion.

I had three new courses into which to get my teeth. In the Long I had concentrated on the nineteenth century in European History and had only nibbled at my special subject, The Whigs, and the history of political thought. My first lecture in the new term on the Whigs turned out to be better than I had expected. It was not a subject that initially had inspired me. Winstanley I described as

'Thin and ugly with a big voice, very clear in his
lecturing and may be good in creating his atmosphere.
Should like to hear more before judging,'

My instinct had been sound. He was an excellent lecturer, devoted to his period so that gradually the Whigs turned into fascinating people playing their part in the political drama of eighteenth century England. It was a period in which I began to feel at home. I wish I could say the same for European history. It was a vast period to cover and it was not until later in life when the role was reversed, in that I was the lecturer, did I find any understanding or grasp of its persons and problems. This I must lay, regrettably, at the door of my lecturer, Mr Reddaway. He knew too much and had known it for too long. He was dull and uninspiring and, as he had already written the standard text book that covered much of it, his lectures had nothing to add to it. Because Girton students did not cut lectures I attended. Political theory I found the most intriguing, the most difficult and most stimulating and we were lucky to have among our lecturers, Graham Wallis, author of *The Great Society* and an outstanding person in his own field, who everyone wanted to hear when he came to Cambridge. As we had had another lecture at II at King's so a typical Cambridge scene ensued

'Imagine the scrum. Everyone struggling to get their
bikes and the stream of people going through Trinity
St. At the corner of which two vans obstructed the
way. The lecture was in the Hall at Magdelene which
literally overflowed with people, law, economics,
history of all grades. He is a grey haired and
moustached man, rather an untidy, kindly face that one
may come to be very fond of. At first I thought he was

going to be entirely above our heads but the latter part was more intelligible, all about Social and Biological Heritage.'

Full though my Third Year was, the pattern of my days had by then been fixed and to describe again that pattern would be needless repetition. To me the men with whom I danced week by week, or how many hours work I did day by day and with what comments and the grades by which it was rewarded, though important to me, would add little to my purpose to leave for future generations a picture of the Cambridge that I knew in the twenties. So I shall confine myself to picking out any events which will add something to that picture. The 51st anniversary of the founding of Girton was marked by an old students dinner, of which I wrote bitterly

'They offered everything twice – as if it would deceive old students. Afterwards there were speeches, very dull. We clapped Kitts so much that she blushed and drank toasts in lemonade.'

Here alas I failed to make it clear whether it was the Mistress or the students who drank the toast in so abstemious a manner. Otherwise little that was new seems to have caught my imagination that Michaelmas term. What was a perpetual feature of Girton life was the struggle to keep warm in face of the threat of miners or railwaymen going on strike and our precious scuttle of coal being threatened. One entry described how I was

'Writing this by firelight after having washed up my jug things. It seems a shame to waste the warmth when coal is scarce and the weather cold. A handful of sticks make quite a blaze to see by.'

Later in the term I indulged in a poetic picture of Woodlands in Winter, which to Girtonians may bring some nostalgic memories

'All the trees were white with frost; underneath the leaves were brown. Silence reigns everywhere. All the boughs are grim and bare save where the freezing hand has frozen dreams that come from wasted lives, now as dead as the leaves.'

After which I indulge in puerile reflections on life and death – all part of growing up in Cambridge! Do the students of today still chew their romantic philosophical cud as they wander round Woodland?

Cambridge would not be Cambridge without the occasional rag. The one that I remember best and with the most pleasure, partly because I was involved in it myself was the Pavement Club. The initiators of the club decided that the pace of the modern world was too much for them: what they needed was a time for meditation. They also decided that the most fitting place to experience this would be King's Parade. Accordingly I think but, as I have no precise date, cannot be sure, the First of May was deemed suitable for the first meeting of the club. The rules were simple. The members sat peacefully in groups blocking the entire road and played such simple games as Happy Families to the fury of the traffic that they obstructed. It was crazy and peaceful and the idea took on. An advertisement appeared inviting the members to a grand picnic lunch to be held on Parker's Piece (a large open space) at one o'clock. Joan and I decided to go. There were swarms of people of all sorts. Men with stoves and baskets and even one dressed as a baby in a pram and wheeled by a man dressed as a nurse. The sun came out as we crossed the grass. The Quntgua was drawn up on a lorry playing *Whispering* faintly but valiantly. The crowd pressed tight round the sitting youths and soon fragments of food were hurtled through the air. The president got up and shouted a speech to the effect that last week the Club had obtained a name for good behaviour and had aroused admiration everywhere. This week it was a beer garden; if this continued. Finally we saw two other Girton students, Molly and Eileen with food and we bravely sat down with them on the edge of the throng which soon swallowed us up. The party next to us were cooking sausages on a primus stove and further along others were eating fruit salad and cream. We were ill provisioned and our frugal buns tasted rather dry. One group were dressed like women, another, preferring a more, genteel existence were playing chess. Then the band played God Save the King and the Club began to break up.

There was an aftermath to our daring exploit in taking part in a University Rag. Kitts put up a notice asking any student who had taken part in the Rag to report to her. I felt aggrieved.

'Why on earth' I wrote, 'couldn't she either have vetoed it before or leave it. As we only sat and ate a bun I would not feel it was very reprehensible.'

We felt honour bound to report our misdoings. It was in some ways an amusing interview.

'Joan and I had some difficulty in getting our faces straight before we went in. Kitts was prepared to thunder but Joan, with her quiet dignity and air of presenting a reasonable case to the reasonable person pointed out that our particular participation only took place at the second meeting of the Club on Parker's Place. Kitts admitted that that was a difference but that at our age we ought to have had more sense. Since some of the First Years had sat down in King's Parade and as Third Years we ought to have set a better example. There was a pause until Joan broke it by saying in a very social voice "There were 100s there, literally 100s and to sit down seemed the obvious thing to do." With that Kitts dismissed us, saying she was sure we had not been misbehaving ourselves.'

I think Kitts must have been more amused than she let us see, as usually when Joan went to see her it was to arrange such things as
176

quiet Sunday afternoons. For Cambridge the joke was almost over though the Pavement Club did make one final flurry at the end of May Week. This took the form of a stream of bikes, the members went both to Newnham and Girton and sat on the grass after cycling round the court. This I missed as I was in Cambridge but later saw them sitting on the sacred grass before the Senate House, their bikes piled high. Finally the leader, garbed in a John's blazer, a kimono and a motor helmet climbed into the Greek urn and made a speech. It ended with the Club joining hands and dancing ring-a-ring of roses on the grass. Then they all cleared off before the proctors had time to arrive. How very young male students can be. At one of the May Week shows I cannot remember which, but I think it was a revue put on by the C.D.C. someone composed a catchy song the refrain of which was '*I'm going to join the Pavement Club in King's Parade*'. Distinctly out of time I can sing it still and when I do I can see again the carefree students who took life so lightly in the days when I was young. Would so peaceful a gesture amuse their modern counterpart. I have a feeling that they take themselves more seriously now. And who would find a Girton student sitting on a pavement with a young man when now they share a college.

At the end of the Lent term, the night before I came down, I summed up the situation as

> 'It has been a good term, heart free and a lot of work done in spite of my pleasure gadding. I don't feel very worried about Trip. By the end of the vac I shall have covered my periods pretty well I think. I hate to think that college is nearly over.'

Already however I was beginning to hope that the May Term. which started on 18th April, might not be my last. EEP earlier had been encouraging about my possibilities of doing research and Miss Jones, as ever, was helpful. Within a week of getting back I went to see Miss Firth, the Newnham Director of History to discuss my coming up for a fourth year. She said I ought to come up in the Long. I won't. I don't want any more work after this for a while. For me Trip would start on 30th a mere six weeks ahead, and I refused to contemplate my future after that. Life was becoming a procession of 'lasts'. The 20th May was my last *Vingt et Un*, the 23rd my last lecture, on the 25th I finished revising my set books. By the 26th I had only a few political science notes. and a bit of European, after which I considered my preparation to be complete. Before Part I the river was my receipt for dealing with tension to my catalogue of river picnics, chronicled before, I will add two more to complete the picture. The first one on the 21st

'It was a perfect day, all hot and sunny the trees were so green. I wore my sky rocket dress. At the Orchard we had large beakers of lemonade and fruit salad with lots of cream. Just after that Alfred (my friend Soulie's current male admirer) dropped the pole on her head and jumped about saying "Does it hurt much? Do tell me. I'd rather know" while I paddled furiously a Yankee retrieved the pole. Meanwhile poor Soulie was choking back tears while he proceeded to comfort her. I never realised that the pole was so heavy and we kept going into the bank so they had to paddle . But apart from that they retired to the front of the punt and left me to cover myself with water which I did. On the Saturday before Trip started once again I resorted to that sedative for pre examination nerves, the Cam. The weather was not propitious. It was raining and for most of our picnic we sheltered under a tree playing the gramophone. However we consoled ourselves by having a really splendid meal in my room instead of the uninspiring fare provided in Hall. It consisted of chicken, ham, salad and new potatoes. It was good, particularly the potatoes. These luxuries were followed by coffee and cream.'

As I said earlier I had not only an understanding mother but one who was located deep in the country where rationing was considered an unnecessary infringement of the farming community's right to sell to whom it wished. Hence the supply of butter and the occasional chicken so appreciated not only by me but by my friends. Perhaps it was this early experience that convinced me that friendship was often cemented by good food and that when with age, or even maturity, few things are as pleasant as to wine and dine with congenial friends and to toss ideas to and fro as we linger round the table. As a student food by itself was sufficient; an appreciation of wine came later. On that occasion I confessed 'I am too full to go to sleep but I'll try.'

The account of the Tripos examination was singularly bare and matter of fact. The night before I had written

> 'I don't feel a bit like it and can't believe it is really here.
> We have our special period tomorrow. I hope I can
> do it. I feel rather tired. It is just 10pm so I shall go
> to sleep. I have done nothing all day but lounge about
> and rest. Betty Simon asked me to their sing-song in
> Honeysuckle Walk after Hall which was rather nice.'

At least it had been a relaxing, if rather aimless day and I had not clogged my mind with last minute revision but had conserved my energies: advice which, when the role was reversed I gave my students. My description of the ordeal was extremely laconic and took less than half a page in my diary.

> 'The papers today, my special period were dull but
> safe. I feel a safe II.1 and even rather pleased; perhaps
> I shall not be when the results come out. I felt very
> tired but after Hall the blessed sense of leisure that
> comes after strain was glorious and the sun shone
> on Woodlands. But I am tired now and don't like the
> thought of tomorrows papers.'

My fears were justified.

> 'I didn't like the papers so much today. The modern
> European was sort of queer and the political science
> not what we had expected. Winnie had not liked it
> either.'

Apparently the essay paper, believed to be so important in deciding class was, in my words, beastly. So, summing it up I wrote disconsolately.

> 'I did so want to get a First. Now I know I can't and at
> the same time know the extent of my longing. I expect
> I'll get what I got before.'

It was possibly a trifle disturbing that the second day of the Tripos for History students coincided with a state visit of the Prince of Wales to the university. The examination, as a consequence, started early at 8.40 and the atmosphere cannot have been much help towards our concentration. Certainly, papers or no papers, we intended to see this famous young man.

> When we came out I met Joan and we careered round
> to find a gap in the crowd to see him. First came the
> cheers, not very prolonged, then the car which was
> past almost before we had realised it. We just saw an
> ordinary boy with a sun burnt face which showed up
> the almost goldness of his hair, and doing a peculiar
> sort of salute. Winnie and I then went to Buol's and
> had lunch, fillet of whiting, in the middle of which
> there was a cheer and we rushed to the window,
> bending double over some quite strange people
> and we got a good view of H.R.H. coming out of
> King's the crowd was almost all undergrads and they
> pushed round the car, quite orderly but they pushed
> it and bumped it and the attendant policemen right

round. There was no pomp and ceremony. According to Elspeth, who always had inside information on university occasions in contrast to the Prince of Japan, who prefaced his visit with stacks of requests, all the Prince of Wales stipulated was (a) an open conveyance, (b) not to wear funny clothes in the street, (c) time to smoke a cigarette after lunch.'

It was back to the examination room. After so much rushing round and bending double in the middle of our hurried lunch that we could tackle a paper at all staggers me now. What a wonderful thing is youth!

Then came the festivities of May Week. Would it I wondered be my last or would I achieve a fourth year? For the last few days I put my hopes and fears behind me. There was the usual rush to fit in everything, a C.D.C. performance of *Charity Begins at Home*, a special showing of the film that had been shot while the Greek play was being performed, and the Girton Dance, which by now had become an institution. Then came the waiting time.

The results were due on 18th June. We were staying with my Aunt Clara at Blackpool and had arranged for the wire to be sent there. All night I had had broken sleep, murmuring, as I finally dozed off 'suppose it's a II.2.' Not that I really thought that but I thought I ought to prepare myself. Next morning my mind must have gone almost blank. Perhaps it was my mother's skill in organizing a shopping expedition that temporarily absorbed me and which made us late for lunch. So when I saw my father standing at the street corner and waving his arms wildly I thought he was merely trying to hurry us up. My aunt was a great one for punctuality. The wire had almost slipped my memory when my mother asked

'Has the wire come?'

In an excited sort of voice back came his reply,

'A first class, a first class.'

Mother asked dazedly

'Is it a joke?'

But Daddy had been waiting an hour to catch us. All I could say in what felt like a half strangled voice,

'I'm so glad. I'm so glad'.

Daddy told me that Winnie had only got a II.1 and I remember being very sorry, almost dashed as we walked along the street. It was not until we sat down to lunch, salmon and parsley sauce and peas, that I began to realise and, for once I could hardly eat my food. I felt half sick with excitement. It was so much the fulfilling of my wildest dreams. Looking back it seemed to have been achieved with so little effort, so little worry. I hadn't over worried and not been a slave to my books but had my pleasures too. I could have done no better if I had.

CHAPTER SEVEN: A CAMBRIDGE FIRST

A Cambridge first is a golden key that can unlock doors which without it would be extremely difficult to force. I was soon to have practical proof of this in the shape of Kitts' congratulations with its reassuring message that, 'she was glad to see my name among the First's and thought it would be alright about the Cairns.' This was a College Studentship awarded for a year to a student doing research in Economic History which, in 1922, included what today would be considered social history. The award would be of double value. It was an honour conferred by Girton and a very useful financial help to my parents in continuing to support me at Cambridge for a fourth year. It. was the first contribution I had ever made and one which, though they were no longer as pressed for money as they had been when I went up to the university, they were still glad to have.

The next step was to find a suitable subject. Hopefully I had already been considering this before I had gone down in June. By then I was set upon an academic career and though my hopes of a studentship were still nebulous at least both EEP, who had returned from her travels, and Miss Jones had been encouraging. As soon as Trip was over she sent me to see Dr Firth, the Newnham Director of Historical Studies. To my surprise I found myself agreeing to look for a medieval subject on the grounds that it would be more limited in its scope and 'not beyond my experience of life, which I feel anything modern would be'. That was on the 4th June. On the 7th, when I went to see her again, we, or rather she, had narrowed it down to the economic position of women in the 15th century if there was material enough. In choosing a subject theory and practice are very far apart. Ideally the student prospective researchers are already committed to working on a topic of their choice. This having been approved the search for material begins. In practice the reverse is often true; possible material is located and the student is left to turn it into a thesis. To spend days and weeks looking for material is frustrating when it is insufficient to be the basis of a serious study. For me to have persisted in looking for a medieval subject would have been a great mistake. It would have demanded two skills that I did not possess; my Latin was weak and, as was rapidly to be made clear to me, palaeography was a skill for which I had no aptitude. Fortunately the decision was taken out of my hands by Emma G, doubtless in consultation with EEP. When I returned to Girton in the autumn, 8th October to be precise, I was informed that the County archives had recently acquired a mass of local government papers, mainly for the late seventeenth and early eighteenth centuries. As nobody seemed to know much about their contents I had better see what I could make of them. In this I was to be joined by a research student from Newnham, a graduate from Liverpool, by name Miss Hampson. She proved a pleasant enough colleague, rather quiet and reserved and quite definitely not a prospective candidate for *Vingt et Un*. But our relationship never developed into a close friendship and there was a slight strain between us as our work progressed and it became more and more difficult to divide our available material into the basis for two theses. I think she felt, and with some justification, that where our interests conflicted. as a Cambridge graduate mine were more likely to take precedence over hers. My first reaction to working among

184

'uncatalogued, un-worked and dirty manuscripts' was unenthusiastic.

We were to do our research under the direction of a Mr Salter of Magdalene, where we went to see him together. He did not seem a very formidable figure. In the entry I made that night I described him as

> 'a darling with fair hair and moustache and red cheeks, affable and obliging and rather nervous. He played with his fingers continually and laughed a lot. Said he did not know much about the subject and would be interested in what we unearthed "don't you know".'

In my own mind I promptly christened him Mr Saltena the principal character in "The Young Visitors" once so popular in the twenties. I wonder does anyone read it now? The first task that he set us was to write an essay without consulting any of the authorities on the work of the magistrates in our period to test our background knowledge of the period.

My assignment was to describe the working of the Poor Law prior to the legislation of Charles II. What was even worse he wanted it in by Saturday. Though the very first A that I got from EEP had been on the Elizabethan Poor Law that had been three years ago and by now such knowledge as I had then had disappeared into the mists of time. So Miss Hampson and I went on strike, saying that it could not be done. This unexpected task had to be fitted into a busy social programme. When I had returned to college this is something I had not expected. I was not looking forward to the new term. Helen and Winnie had gone. So had Joan Bedale with whom in my third year I had become increasingly friendly after my beloved Elspeth had been stricken with a strange disease, which in the light of subsequent knowledge I think must have been leukaemia. She was not yet an invalid but had decided not to go on to Part II of the English Tripos. So I felt bereft of friends writing sadly the night I returned

'For half an hour after I had put my room straight I
could have wept with desolation and resigned myself
to a lonely year. I must get to know new people and
tomorrow see Miss Jones and get to work. I shall have
plenty of time for it. I shall be alright but one's self
does seem so important.'

My gloom was not prophetic. Soulie Wotton, my next door
neighbour in Bear Pits, and I became increasingly good friends. Also
Ruth, who through illness had not been able to sit Part II of the
Tripos, came back for another year. With her arrival the following
evening life resumed its old familiar pattern as we had jug together
and gossiped. The old pressures returned. Somehow I had first to do
some background reading and then write Mr Saiteria's wretched essay
before Saturday. It was not easy. On Wednesday I had an elevens and
a tea party, on Thursday I had got involved in the meeting of some
society, while on Friday there was the first *Vingt et Un* of the new
term. It was business, or rather pleasure as usual.

As a preliminary to writing my essay I tackled Miss Leonard's
standard book on the early Poor Law. Next day I was congratulating
myself on having got that out of the way when I discovered that
in my haste I had skipped a hundred pages in the middle; not an
auspicious beginning. However before I went to bed that night the
draft of the essay had been finished and I wrote,

'I hope it is alright because I think it would make poor
Mr Salter uncomfortable to pull me up.'

I need not have been so concerned over his feelings; Mr Saltena
had the upper hand. Having said that the main part of the essay was
good

'He proceeded to fling various things at our heads
that we ought to have read, including a man called
Vives of whom we had never heard. He then said I

had a different opinion from his over the spelling of separate and he was inclined to think that his was the correct version. He also observed that it was usual in Cambridge to add a final 'e' to Magdelen College. He dashed about the room a lot and flung things at our heads, not literally, and got generally excited, telling us the old, old story of the bottoms falling out of the Girton cabs. Apparently he had never heard of the Girton bus that had replaced that ancient means of transport.'

It was fortunate that we were not left solely to the ministrations of Mr Saltena. In the twenties very little was done to prepare the prospective researcher for the task that lay ahead and because it was not drilled into me from the beginning, things like the correct foot noting technique still give me trouble! I was however given invaluable advice from EEP on how to arrange and structure my material into an acceptable thesis. Though she was now a lecturer at the London School of Economics she came to Girton at intervals to take a seminar for Miss Hampson and me. It was both a joy and a thrill to see her again and to find her

'Just as EEPish as ever and looking much younger than before. She had coffee with us and she is just the most adorable thing that ever was; full of wit and vivacity and with such a childlike joy in her own charms. In the seminar she was very capable and showed us just how to set about things.'

I owe her a great debt of gratitude. What she told us then is still the method that I use when I have a book to write. Like her lectures this advice was deceptively simple, concrete and practical. As our preliminary examination of the Cambridgeshire Quarter Sessions papers had already suggested that the main business of the justices of the peace was to administer the Poor Laws, the first task that she set us was to make a bibliography of books on this so that we at least knew what had already been written on the subject and its background. Once a nucleus of material had been accumulated and related to this wider background it should begin to be possible to delimitate the scope of our more detailed research and to know on which points it would be necessary to concentrate the search for further material. By the end of the first term I realized that the focal point around which the business of the Cambridge Justices' business revolves was the act of Settlements and Removal, which determined the responsibility of which parish was responsible for the individual pauper whose case was being considered. This in turn involved questions of bastardy, of vagrancy, of relied provision of work and workhouses, of parish administration and contemporary opinion. In essence I now know what I was looking for and how to classify each new piece of evidence that I unearthed under its appropriate heading.

Writing a thesis, as I was to discover, is like trying to complete a jigsaw, when you have to start by hunting for the pieces and have only a vague idea as to the final picture. It is frustrating, wearisome and occasionally very exciting. Here again EEP's advice was invaluable and eminently practical. Each new bit of evidence must be copied onto a separate card and its source meticulously entered. It is then placed under its appropriate heading which in turn dictate the structure of the final thesis, each heading providing a chapter. At last it is possible to see the wood for the trees and the path through them. It is also time to begin writing chapter by chapter and not necessarily in their final order. That can be decided later; the great thing is to have something concrete on which to build and not merely a floating mass of ideas in the head. Last came a piece of advice that was to stand me in good stead for the rest of my life. It was to buy a typewriter and to THINK on it. This proved an immense saving in time and trouble in the days, probably already half forgotten, before the invention of the Word Processor, when the only way of either putting in or taking out unwanted or misplaced material was the laborious method of scissors and paste. Typewritten pages were easier to handle and easier to read than handwriting, particularly mine. So I bought myself a small portable Corona thereby saving eyestrain and temper.

Would I had followed EEP's advice as meticulously as it deserved. Research is a slow business. Too often I was apt to forget that more haste can so easily mean less speed. There is a thrill in finding new material, none in copying it until both wrist and brain are numb and the careful dating of each scrap of paper with full details as to its source seems the last straw. As I was to discover when I came to write and wanted to use some extract and was unable to trace its source without infinite time wasting trouble. With my typing it was once again a case of being in too much of a hurry to bother about perfecting my technique. I did not persevere until I could touch type and to this day my typing is the despair' of any publisher with whom I have dealings. My ability to spell, despite the heroic efforts of my form mistress long ago, is decidedly erratic. Obviously Nature did not intend me to write books but Fate, in the shape the Cairns, decided otherwise. My failure to notice spelling errors in others may have been some consolation to my future students but it can hardly have improved their literacy.

The only other technique with which it was considered necessary to equip us was a course of lectures on palaeography given by Mr Jenkinson of the Record Office. It was more than lucky for me that my subject did not require such specialised skills to interpret my material. Quarter sessions records and parish registers mercifully were written in English and in everyday script, for I soon found the subject beyond me. Many are the moans in my diary such as

> 'I have a book on Court Hands which I think is going
> to drive me mad' and a few days later 'I have been
> struggling with English Court Hand. As soon as I have
> learnt B, I have forgotten A. It is awful.'

Nor had Hilary Jenkinson, apart from the fact that he was some sort of a connection with Joan, anything to recommend him to me. I described him as

> 'not very good looking or thrilling and he never lifts his face from his notes.' To me he remained 'that wretched man', doubtless an unfair label as even I had to admit that 'he was a noted scholar in his own field.'

Far more capable of both appreciating him and profiting from his lectures were two other mature students, both of whom later enjoyed distinguished careers. Helen Cam who had recently been given the Pfeiffer Fellowship and who therefore consorted with the dons rather than with us lesser fry, I already knew slightly and we attended Mr Jenkinson's lectures together. I suppose we cycled in, that being the usual Girton method of transport for the student lecturing community and Helen was never a person to stand on her superior academic status as the holder of so prestigious a fellowship. But we never became more than friendly acquaintances, though whenever we met at conferences in after years, she, in spite of her international reputation as an authority of English medieval history, was always the same unassuming person whom I remembered from my Girton days. The other member of our lecture group was a Mr Schofield with whom I somehow became acquainted. I think he came from a northern university, though I am not sure of this, and I think he was lonely and would like to have been friends. But I did not encourage him for reasons of which I am now ashamed, when our paths crossed again and I discovered what a kind, courteous and helpful person he was. Alas Cambridge had turned me into a snob. He had suggested taking me on the river and I thought it unlikely that he was adept with a punt pole and would appear in regulation flannels. In short people might believe I was being escorted by a townie and that was unthinkable. He at least must have benefited from Mr Jenkinson's lectures. When next we met in London it was in the MSS Room of the British Museum where I found him in control.

190

Thus armed I slowly began to acquire the skills of my craft and work out an appropriate routine. Mr Saltena took us to the County Office where the Quarter Session records, that were to be the base of our research were kept and I was introduced to the University Library which was still housed in the old Senate House. My first impression was

'It is a maze and nobody knows where anything is!
Two officials were very helpful. I fell in love with the
librarian. He got up when I came in and went out and
had a dark interesting face.'

It soon became part of my life. There were little tables interspersed among the stacks where one could spread out one's papers and read or write in peace, in every way a haven of tranquillity after the crowded Seely Library of my undergraduate days. In addition it could be a cave of treasures. I suppose somebody knew the principles, on which the books were arranged and catalogued and gradually left to my own devices I acquired a general idea of where the books that I wanted were likely to be. I raced through the easily accessible academic journals, commenting on the paucity of articles that had any bearing on local government in my period. Then I turned to standard eighteenth century authors, writers like Eden whose state of the Poor with its factual local detail was a treasure house in itself. As I did so it occurred to me that it would be interesting to compare his ideas on the causes of distress with the evidence I was beginning to turn up in the Quarter Sessions records. In other words I was beginning to see the wood for the trees and find a path between them. What is more I was doing it alone; no one was telling me what to read. Rummaging among the stacks, Looking for one book, often I would find another, of whose existence I, and probably no one else, had any previous knowledge. The fact that the stacks were open must have helped many people to seem erudite when they were merely lucky in turning up new sources. Meanwhile the County records provided me with both solid ground on which to base my thesis and also a fascinating picture of things as they really were in eighteenth century rural Cambridge. It was not long before I was writing

> 'I thoroughly enjoyed doing the records. I don't know
> how they will turn out but they are most amusing.
> Already I am beginning to recognise as old friends Mr
> Stevenson, Gent. Treasurer of the County and John
> York, Keeper of His Majesty's House of Correction.
> The county hierarchy is beginning to take shape. I can
> hardly think of anything else.'

No wonder that I felt a new excitement and exhilaration.

Little of this was due to Mr Saltena, who I suspect found directing two young women a potentially embarrassing task. For instance on one occasion

> 'when I left for lunch, leaving my beautiful notes
> spread out on the table, in my absence Mr Salteria
> came in and left a book. I think he chooses a time
> when we shall not be there. Beastly man.'

So far he had not proved a very helpful director of studies but looking back I can see that it may have been better to be neglected than over directed. Inexperienced we might be but at least we had time to grow and freedom in which to do so.

When he did condescend, or dare, to put in an appearance at least it was a flamboyant one. On another occasion, when perhaps he intended to make one of his visits expecting us to be absent he was foiled.

> 'I had stayed in working when I had intended to go
> out. It was as well I did. About twelve there was a
> knock on the door and in walked Mr Saltena. He had a
> waistcoat on and over it a woolly one, over that a coat,

192

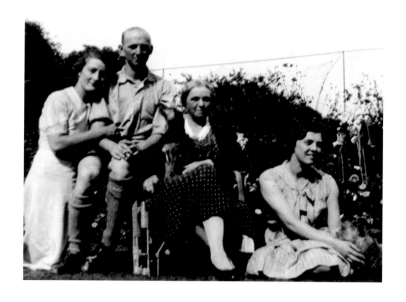

From R-L: Dorothy, her mother, her brother William, and his wife
Winnifred (kneeling).

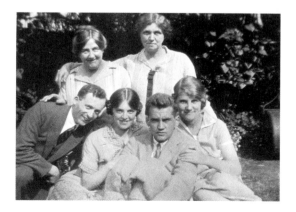

L-R top row: Bridget Preston, Dorothy's mother
L- R bottom row: Friend, Dorothy, Desmond Preston, "Dabbott".

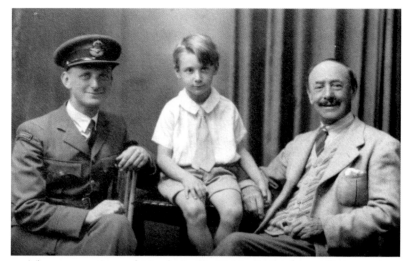

Three generations of Marshalls: David Marshall, his grandfather and father.

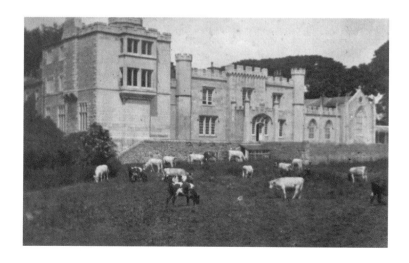

Leighton Hall, Carnforth- Dorothy's father's school in the Lake District.

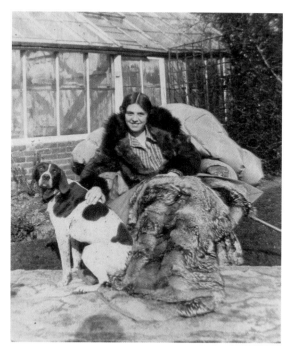

Dorothy (in furs) at home in Old Hutton, Kendal with her favourite dog.

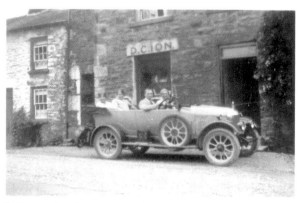

Dorothy's first and only car, a "Bullnose Morris", in which she changed gear to the tune of "Onward Christian Soliders!

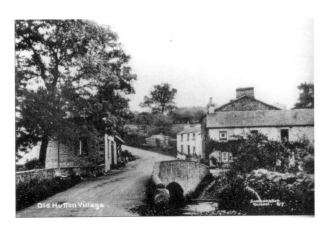

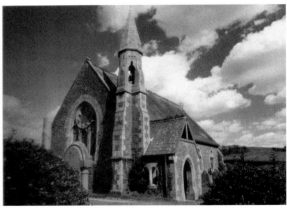

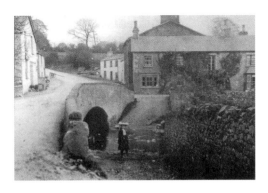

Images of Old Hutton,
courtesy of John Parker

196

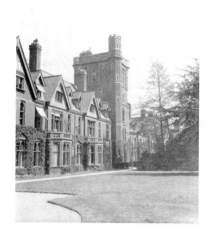

Girton as it was in 1918 (when Dorothy first saw it).

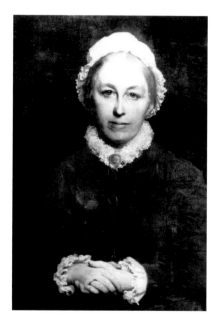

Emily Davies, Founder of Girton College, Cambridge (from a portrait by
Rudolf Lehman 1880)

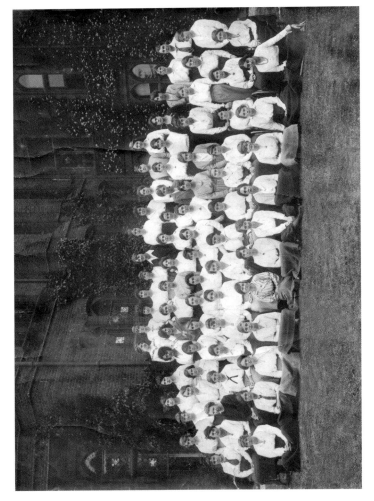

Dorothy's year at Girton - 1918 (see names opposite)

First Year Students 1918
(maiden names in all cases)

Back Row
1. D. Marshall
2. R. Corder
3. E. Giles
4. S. Wotton
5. M. Charlesworth
6. B. Roll
7. D. Hatt
8. J. Shuter
9. A. Stephen
10. M. Church
11. A. Marshall

Second Row
1. R. Stern
2. C. Horlock
3. H. Lowenthal
4. E. Pedley
5. D. Dear
6. D. Alcock
7. W. Trenholme
8. G. Wright
9. E. Thompson
10. K. Snell
11. G. Farquhar
12. V. Pembroke
13. L. Dowler
14. A. Evershed
15. M. Dyson
16. S. Cooper

Third Row
1. J. Bedale
2. N. Jolliffe
3. G. Burnett
4. G. Maclean
5. C. Layland
6. E. Curtin
7. D. Stanton
8. L. Frankenburg
9. G. Lanfear
10. N. Simpson
11. S. Mann
12. N. Williams
13. M. Laws
14. B. Trevelyan
15. M. Brown
16. E. Robinson
17. E. Deane

Fourth Row
1. C.P.Jones
2. E. Binns
3. B. Smith
4. J. Lawrence
5. W. Lumb
6. J. Wilson
7. M. Bough
8. R. Hillier
9. T. Rose
10. M. Cam
11. G. Harker
12. R. Cooke
13. R. McMillan
14. I. Shields
15. R. Rowland

Front Row
1. H. Yates
2. H. Murphy
3. E. Walker
4. M. Ball
5. S. Hartley
6. M. Coates
7. P. Bill
8. P. Brock
9. R. Whitehead
10. C. Jones
11. M. McGregor

Supplied by D.S. Dear 1945

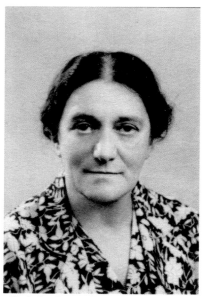

Gwladys Jones, Dorothy's tutor for her last two years at Girton.

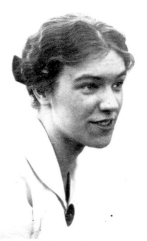

Eileen Power, Dorothy's tutor for her first two years at Girton.

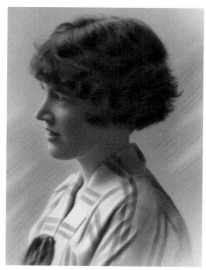

Elspeth Giles.

200

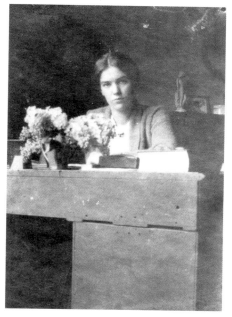

Eileen Power (Dorothy's inspiration, guiding light and lifelong role model) in her study at Girton.

Eileen Power "posing".

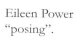

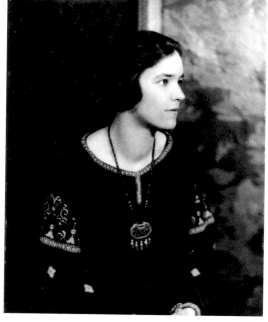

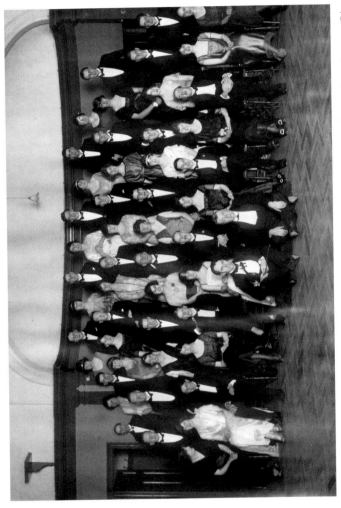

"*Vingt et un*", the dancing club that afforded Dorothy much harmless delight during her time at Girton.

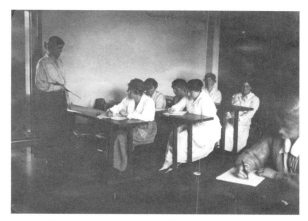
Honours history class Girton (circa 1918).

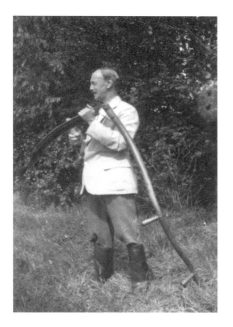
John Marshall with scythe.

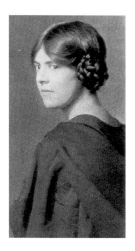
Dorothy as an undergraduate.

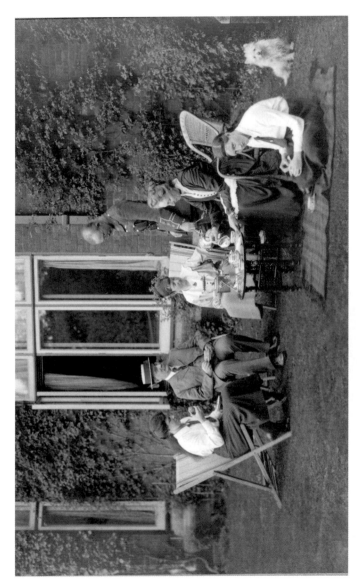

The Giles family at tea, with Dorothy's great friend Elspeth (centre) (Emmanuel College, Cambridge, 1920s)

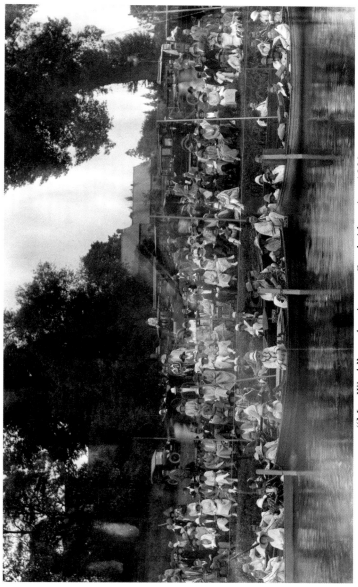

"May Week" on the river at Cambridge circa 1920.

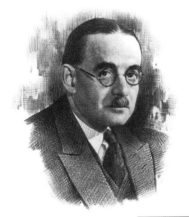

Professor Harold Laski of the London School of Economics. A leading left wing intellectual of the day.

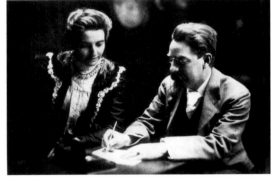

Beatrice and Sydney Webb, famous social historians.

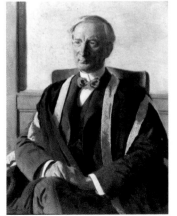

Lord Beveridge, whose famous report laid the foundations for the Welfare State.

With thanks to the London School of Economics for their permission to include these images.

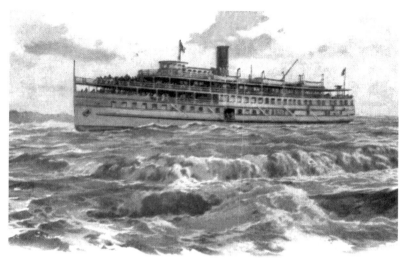

"Shooting the Rapids"

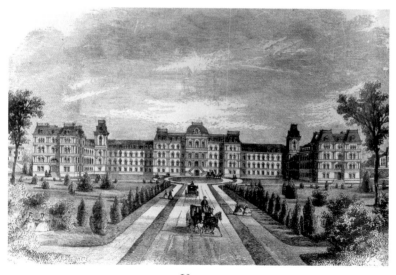

Vassar.

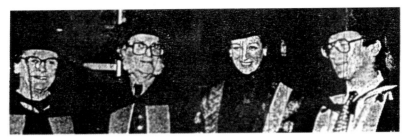

From L-R: Dorothy, Norman Nicholson (the poet), Princess Alexander (Vice Chancellor) and Robert Fesk (journalist), at the award of Hon. D.Lit, Lancaster University, 4/12/84. Nelson Mandela was also so honoured but was still in prison in South Africa at the time.

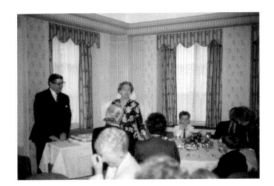

Dorothy at Claridges, addressing her guests at her 90th birthday party (March 1990).

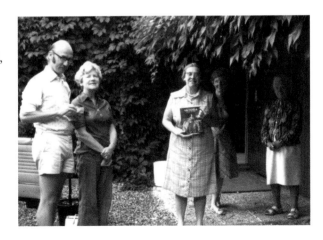

David Marshall, Joy Farr, Dorothy with her 'Victoria'. Behind her are Joan and Joy's mother flannel bags and a flat tweed cap. With his red face he looked just like a country yokel. He inspected our work but did not offer many suggestions. He seemed rather impressed with my tidy notes. Indeed they are in very good order and I can turn up anything as I want it. It was more than he was with my spelling. When he asked about Mr Jenkinson's lectures I gave him my notes. "Why spell archives with an extra e" he queried. Then he met Tynonet for Tironoin and I thought he was going to say "my dear girl". That was his attitude but he refrained from the actual words, merely asking me what I meant and carefully correcting it with a pencil. By that time I was laughing helplessly and saying he should never see my notes again. So when he met coonology for chronology he supposed he had better not correct that.'

From this interview I could only suppose that his knowledge of spelling was superior to his information about the Poor Law. His casual attitude towards his responsibilities was more than compensated by the meticulous care and sympathy that Miss Jones constantly provided. That 'darling woman' I called her in my diary. With her I could talk over not only problems immediately connected with the work I was doing but my hopes and dreams for the future.

It was not only my future that was at stake. In the autumn of 1922 the future position of women in the university was also about to be decided. Since the previous year the battle had been going on between those members of the university who wished to extend its privileges to the women's college and the diehards, mostly non resident, who were bitterly opposed to it. To them the fact that women from Girton and Newnham were examined by the university and that the results of the Tripos were classified on an equality with the men was concrete enough. Control in every detail was in male hands. These opposing views finally crystallised in two Graces, the name for the formal acts of the Senate. The 20th October was the day of destiny when the Senate voted. My own reaction to that momentous occasion is reflected in what I wrote that night.

> 'Today seems another chapter in Girton's history closed. Today the Senate voted on Grace I, which would have given nearly full membership of the university to us and Grace II which merely conferred titular degrees. When I went down to the library this morning everything was quiet. I met Elspeth for 11am and at 11.30 the voting was just beginning. At 11.45 we finished and I walked down with her to Emmanuel and as I came back there were crowds of undergraduates all running to some rag and some undergrads on a cab, one with a red nose was speaking and the rest were hurrahing. I went round by Rose Crescent, feeling small and forlorn and somehow in a hostile country. A little later I heard the crowd moving. Apparently they had an effigy and coffin and were holding a mock funeral and had intended to stop the Girton bus, but it had been warned to change its destination so they were sold.'

> 'By tea we had heard that the voting had gone steadily against us. I put on my red dress the better to face any situation. Then after Hall Mackenzie-Harper, Ruth and I had coffee together. At 8.40 we went along to the Stanley, where Kitts was to announce the news. As she entered we all stood up and remained standing. She was obviously upset but awfully plucky. We had lost Grace I by nearly 300 votes and won titular degrees by nearly 600. She said we were to sit still and smile. Some of us, though not her, would see the thing through. It was a setback and that was all. She said that all through she had never heard real complaints about

her students and that our behaviour had been all that
she could wish. She tried to understand the attitude
to those titular degrees. I don't quite understand what
she meant. Then Theo Rose (the senior student)
got up and said how much we all appreciated what
she had done for us and how much we wished that
degrees might have come while she was still Mistress.
We clapped and stamped. Then Kitts thanked us and
the tears were not far off her voice; for my part, I
felt choky. Finally she said something about being
wanted on the telephone and charged out – to her
room I guess to have a good cry. Poor Kitts. We went
up to McHarper's room and sat in the dark by her
window. Nothing happened, though we had heard that
a torchlight procession was on its way. Then I insisted
on jug. It is *Vingt et Un* tomorrow night and I almost
dread it. What has hurt me the most has been the
attitude of the undergrads. They defeated the motion
at the Union by over 200 and were rather beastly to the
Girton cyclists and taxi. I don't think I think much of
men!'

There was a postscript to this condemnation. Next night, on my
return after the dance I wrote that the men

'were awfully nice. They never said anything beastly.
Hardly anyone said anything at all.'

The failure of Grace I was a bitter blow to the generation of
Girton women who had fought so long and so gallantly for the right
to become full members of the university. They had to wait until
1948. By then many of them lay dead on the battlefield, believing
in victory but not seeing it. To alter the metaphor they were like
Moses seeing the promised land from afar. But to my generation,
more empirical than idealistic in their attitude the passing of Grace

II, which secured titular degrees, reinforced the maxim that half a loaf is better than no bread. Perhaps the equally old saw that 'a bird in hand is better far than two in the bushes' is more equal and the granting of a titular degree was more like a slice of bread than half a loaf. The people who suffered were the Girton and Newnham dons, the tutors and directors of studies women like Emma G. In practical terms the situation gradually improved. It was the non resident 'Old Guard' who had been determined to keep the women in their subjection while in the running of the day to day administration of the university the male dons more and more came to regard their female counterparts as colleagues. As a result de facto more and more frequently women began to play a more active part on committees of various importance as the years went by. The barriers came down but the Senate House was still male holy ground.

To ex-Cambridge students the titular degree was an immense boon. The majority were still destined to be absorbed in some branch of the teaching profession and to have no easily recognised professional label was a serious handicap, particularly with regard to the non academic world. Though the initiated knew and recognised the value of having attained a good class, or indeed any class, in the Cambridge Tripos, to the less well informed a BA was something they knew and respected. Though I had begun to cherish the hope of a university post I never contemplated becoming a Cambridge female don. This was not so much due to humility as to the fear of disillusion. I had had four years, on which the memory concentrated on all the happiness they had brought. I did not want that memory tarnished by the work-a-day business of earning a living. Whether I become a school mistress or was lucky enough to secure a junior lectureship in a London college, or at one of the newer provincial universities now I could put the coveted BA after my name and wear a gown. For all practical purposes the word titular need not exist. It could safely be ignored. To me this was of special importance. Cambridge in 1922 had also instituted a new degree for which, after three years' supervised research and the production of a thesis deemed worthy of publication, conferred the title of PhD standing for Doctor of Philosophy. This title had been imported from Germany. My father had been a PhD of Marburgh. Now I could hope to follow in his footsteps. The PhD supplied a useful rung in the academic ladder between the BA or MA and the D.Litt, the doctor of Literature. It was a definite encouragement to research in the older universities that previously had been missing because the step from the BA and MA was not, as it was in the newer universities, gained by further achievement but merely by survival and the willingness to pay the necessary fees. An MA, with the rights that the title conferred belong automatically to any male member of the university of four years standing who complied with the regulations. To me the PhD arrived most opportunely. I had already become involved in research. Now I could register for this new degree and provided at the end of three years I could produce a thesis considered by the examiners to be worthy of publication would gain the coveted title. In the twenties the PhD were still a select band. The new degree was possibly slightly suspect, as a foreign importation, and we were not thick on the ground. To be able to call myself Dr Marshall was a distinct advantage in applying for a lectureship. My dream was coming another step nearer and my future career beginning to take shape. With this carrot in front of my nose I worked steadily and happily and with growing self confidence. Looking back, to alter my metaphor once more, I took to research as automatically as a duck to water, I had found my pond.

To continue the analogy I was a newly fledged duckling, benevolently watched over by my academic mother, EEP, and my foster mother Emma G, with my father Mr Saltena, drake like, showing occasional interest. For the most part I swam happily practising the lessons they had taught me. There were ups and downs. Some days I went hungry, lean hours of frustrating search so that I described sadly as

> 'I spent the morning champing round the library and finding very little, the afternoon in the County Hall doing even less.'

Ten days later I was still complaining

'I got very fed up with work today; none of the books
I found were what I needed.'

My remedy was the supposedly female one of cheering myself up
by buying two pairs of shoes at bargain prices in a sale, a suede pair
marked down from 40s/-d to £1 and the other reduced from 50s/-d
also to £1 which I described as

'a mad orange brocade, lined with kid and with real
leather soles.'

No wonder I felt more cheerful. In the main however, I was
making steady progress both in accumulating material and in using
it. I would suddenly stumble on an unexpected find of documents,
suddenly unearthed at the County Hall. One typical haul I described
as

'ugh! they were dusty and dirty, a mass of odd papers,
indictments, recognizances, lists of juries and all
wrapped up in what seemed to be odd wills. I found
one rather nice account of some charity money but
nothing else thrilling. The only ones in our period were
about 1734 to 36 and some for 1754. I wonder where
the others are. I shall ask if we can root around. After
lunch I went to the library and couldn't find a thing I
wanted and the Middlesex Quarter Sessions stopped at
1709. I was very fed up and depressed but took myself
in hand and told myself to study what I had got
already and going over my notes I find I have quite a
lot of odd facts collected. I have been arranging some
of my headings.'

A few days later

'I decided to start writing things out under headings. I can think better on paper and I want to find out how much material I have. I think I'll start my vagrant soon and collect for the workhouses.'

In coming to this decision I was putting into practice EEP's advice not to indicate that I had made up my mind how to deal with vagrants per se but that their final place in the thesis to be was still undecided. Not until the bare bones of each prospective chapter had been assembled could I guess at the ultimate shape of whole. The growing awareness of what would be is one of the great fascinations of writing as the rapprochement between the writer and the material grows, so that intuitively a sixth sense develops. Instinctively one approach is right, another wrong. By the beginning of the May term, when EEP was on one of her flying visits to Girton, I handed over to her what I described as 'my poor halting manuscript'. When I took it to her room

'she was asleep with her hair half down. Not many people would have been so pleased and sweet at being disturbed.'

The result of this perusal was encouraging; if I put my back into it and it grew into a book she thought the London School of Economics might publish it. With her sanction I made an application for a scholarship at LSE for the next year and felt that my academic future, like my thesis, was beginning to take shape. Meanwhile it was my last May week and I intended to enjoy it.

To suppose that my fourth year had been devoted solely to work would have been far from the truth but the tempo had changed with changing circumstances. I was no longer a frightened fresher but a senior of standing, sure of myself and of my own position. In other ways too I was under less emotional pressure in that my closest friends had gone. Elspeth was a semi invalid living at home, Joan was teaching in London. Of my old group only Ruth remained in residence. Instead I had a wider circle of friends. There was nobody about whom I felt possessively jealous and my long suffering diary was no longer littered with introspection and bad poetry. This new found tranquility did not mean that my non academic activities had lost their charm, merely that familiarity had made them less exciting. *Vingt et Un* continued to be the centre of my social life. If it had packed up I should have lost contact with most of the male company to which I had become accustomed. So I was definitely relieved when I knew that it was to continue. How long it would do so I was doubtful, I had heard a disquieting rumour that on the 21st October there were only 23 members. As only a few were regular in their attendance, this was hardly a viable number for a healthy club. When I returned for the Lent term the situation had definitely improved. On 27th January I wrote

> '*Vingt en Un* was quite fun tonight. They have 27
> members and are starting a waiting list. We had
> biscuits with the lemonade. Mr Standen told me how
> P.W. got his *D.S.O.* Most of the officers at his battery
> were killed and the men ready to bunk and he kept
> them there fighting the gun and when it was over three
> ammunition dumps were on fire and he and another
> man put them all out.'

Pryor-Wandesforth was a cousin of my mourned Wilfred Pryor and a typical ex-army officer, a perfect gentleman with very little conversation. He even looked the part, shining fair hair, I think his eyes were blue and he had a small military fair moustache. Over the three years that I was a guest at the club he was one of my most faithful partners. I rarely had less than two dances with him and I knew as little about him as I did at the beginning. We remained friendly social acquaintances at a small talk level though at the last meeting of a term he could indulge in what amounted to something very like school boy ragging. Perhaps that was typical too.

Looking back over the abyss of time I find it difficult, even with the help of my diary to recreate my attitude towards men. Though I was rarely a wallflower I longed to be the favourite choice of my own favourite partner and I was puzzled at my failure to do so. Physically I had much to offer. I had a beautiful figure, large brown eyes, soft brown hair that I wore in earphones and a good complexion. I wore pretty clothes, my mother saw to that, and I was far from dumb in that I enjoyed good conversation and the cut and thrust of an argument. With hindsight I think the one vital ingredient that was missing was that sexually I was totally un-awakened and must have exuded frigidity from every pore. I was a romantic, my mother, who had a deep rooted aversion to sex, the result of her own unhappy marriage, had taught me never 'to hold myself cheap' and though I new about sex in a sketchy sort of way emotionally it was not a fact of life. Indeed I remember being very puzzled when reading Tom Jones, to improve my eighteenth century background, I found Tom attracted to a woman because, though she was not good looking, she possessed alluring breasts. What I wondered had breasts to do with being attractive to men; it was all very odd. In the same vein when I read Pamela I observed that

'It was no longer amusing now and becoming
sentimental now that they had fallen in love.'

By this time I was indulging a sentimental relationship with my own cousin Don. His people were missionaries in India and he spent much time with us during his vacations; he was an undergraduate at Reading. We had become 'kissing cousins' slightly to my mother's disapproval, but I never got beyond the stage of holding hands and kissing and writing to him frequently. It was indeed no more than an affection that I felt for him and that is as far as my sexual experience went.

How far this was true of my fellow Girtonians I have no means of knowing. Within my own circle of friends, sex as a physical experience was not discussed and those members of our college community whose conduct did at times suggest a closer knowledge of such mysteries were regarded as 'fast'; not a desirable quality in a nice young woman. This did not mean that we were not interested in the heart throbs of our friends, indeed my diary is full of much comment on them but they were for the most part merely transitory romantic attractions, by which some people did get hurt though in two cases to my knowledge *Vingt et Un* contacts led to marriage. Because sex was not discussed I did not realize that one of my own friends must have been a lesbian, though whether practising or not I cannot hazard even a guess. At that time, and indeed for years afterwards I doubt if homosexual meant anything to me and of lesbians I had never even heard. Yet I must have had some latent curiosity as I went to hear what Maud Royden had to say when she came to lecture at Cambridge. In the twenties it was daring for a woman to express in either print or on a public platform a subject so taboo. The title of her lecture was The Relationship Between Men and Women and does not seem to have offered me much illumination. I described her as

'Not a bit as I had expected her to be. She was little dark and going grey, dressed in a mustardy apricot and had a quiet, forceful delivery. One thing she said I liked, the longing for home expressed by Christ in "Birds have nests, foxes have holes but the Son of Man has nowhere to lay his head." She did not say much in ideas that was new to me. Probably being a mixed audience she couldn't, and though she said one must direct and not repress the sex impulse she did not say how. Perhaps again she couldn't there. I wish I could talk it over with a nice youth like Don.'

Meanwhile, again with hindsight, I may not have been as devoid of the power to attract men as I believed, the trouble was that like the magnet in Patience I 'set my heart on a silver churn' instead of the iron and steel that would have provided me with willing victims. In other words the men I fell for were not the men who fell for me but there were others who did who failed to appeal to my romantic soul. Here is one example

> 'Soulie and I had notes from H.T. and D-- (will not disclose his name as, for all I know, he may still be alive) asking us to go as passengers in the Cambridge University Hill Climbing Club on Saturday, in his 30 HP Vauxhall. Luckily I am going to the Rugger and rules won't allow it. Anyhow, I was rather amused, but why did I please him by listening so sympathetically to the tale of his own experiences for I don't like him and never want to dance with him or see him again.'

He must have been persistent, or I short of partners for in subsequent accounts of *Vingt et Un* his name appears regularly and though I cannot confirm this my recollection is that he asked me to the Trinity Ball for the May week of 1921, but I had not a night to spare and had to make do with a performance of Princess Ida, a rather iconic substitute! I seem to remember him as rather a spotty youth but I longed to be invited to a May Week Ball even so.

Earlier in my *Vingt et Un* career there had been other men who enjoyed my conversation and the quality of my mind, at least I suppose they did, but who, because they were not Pryor, I ended up by avoiding them as far as I could. At the mature age of 22 I was however beginning to show a little enterprise in securing the partner I wanted, so at least I was learning.

Apart from *Vingt et Un* my university interests were if not harrowing, at least shifting. The Union debates no longer were the fascinating occasions that I once had found them. So it was only when some speaker who interested me came down as a guest speaker, did I exert myself to secure a ticket. When Ian Hay came down on the 9th May I was interested sufficiently to make the effort. Only my generation will remember him now as a popular novelist. Wilfred Owen has grown in reputation and Rupert Brooke has enjoyed a revival, though less as a war poet as a poet killed in the war but in the twenties it was not until the play 'Journey's End' that people were ready to face the memory of the blood, tears and sweat of the trenches. Ian Hay wrote in a lighter vein. My verdict on the debate and on him was

> 'The debate was not very good but Ian Hay was very good, rather in a lecturing manner but very funny and convincing too. He is a tall slim man, just getting bald, with a dark moustache and rather dark eyes.'

My involvement with the Liberal Club activities too was waning. This may have been due to the fact that I was less dependent on it for a contact with the male sex. *Vingt et Un* supplied that but my personal politics may have been partly responsible for my switch of loyalties. In the early days of the split in the party, members were still inclined to belong to the Asquith camp, my cousin Willy Edge the member for Bosworth was a devoted follower of Lloyd George and after a long conversation with him, which I found

> 'frightfully interesting, and he more than half converted me to Lloyd George, though I did not show it. Mother thinks he'll be in the Cabinet next Election if L.G. is returned and gets in and would take me as his secretary and I do hesitate between that and my history.'

It was a choice I was never called upon to make: L.G. went into the political wilderness and my cousin followed him there.

Though I did not realise it at the time I think that subconsciously I was beginning to outgrow Cambridge at the undergraduate level. The novelty, the excitement and the thrill had gone. So too had some of my agonized uncertainties. I had fewer close friends; of my old group only Ruth remained in residence. They had been replaced by a widening of the circle of what might perhaps be best described as friendly acquaintances. Only Soulie I regarded as a person whose friendship would last beyond my Girton days and in our friendship there was no emotional strain. As a fourth year, as I have already said, my own position both in the eyes of my fellow students and in my own, was more secure and so I retreated more into the life of the college. Instead of discussing young men and the state of our emotions I drifted into discussions that revolved round ideas with students like Grace Rotenberg and Margery Dyson, whom I have only lately discovered was the daughter of the Astronomer Royal. I cannot remember being interested then in the social background of my friends. It was only when I came to assemble my memories of my Girton days that I thought it might be interesting to consult the Girton Register and distinguish how many distinguished men had daughters at Girton. Helen Lehmann was a second year in 1918, the less well known daughter in the annals of the Lehmann family that of Beatrix the actress and Rosalind the novelist. Beatrix I never met, Rosalind was a first year in my second and she I never know either. We moved in different sets but even to me she stood out in her year. She was a strikingly gook looking young woman. I am not sure if I approved of her. Indeed I must confess that I did not. She was all sophistication and it was rumoured went to men's rooms unchaperoned! From hearing a recording many years later as a castaway on a desert island I got the impression that her memories of Girton were as different as chalk and cheese from mine. Helen I liked. As a second year she was kind to me and I remember her with affection. What is more surprising is the fact that I remained so ignorant of the lineage of my very dear friend Helen Harvey. Her father, the Rt. Hon. William Harvey, had been Governor of Bombay. It was not that she was reticent in talking of her family, she was proud of them and of her mother, who had married young and must have been a very beautiful woman. She conveyed the impression to me that they were an interesting, unpredictable set of people, as indeed she could be herself but there was no hint that I can remember of lineage or power in her background. Politicians' daughters too were thick on the ground. Walter Runciman's daughter and the two Simon girls were my contemporaries. Perhaps this lack of interest sprang from the fact that Cambridge was of the offspring of distinguished folk, accepting the same social code and speaking with the same accent, Girton escapes this particular form of snobbery. How right my particular friends were to insist that I must get rid of the Lancashire accent that had been the legacy of my years at the Park School, Preston. Unlike today academic women were supposed to have academic voices.

It was these memories that motivated me to consult the Girton Register to find out the composition of my first year, though tactfully I have not identified them here by name. The clergy, solicitors, public servants and doctors seem to have predominated but among these groups there was a sprinkling of journalists and writers. Quite numerous were the entries who referred the reader to see *Who's Who* for further details. To balance these some students came from families engaged in trade or manufacturing or farming. Perhaps these, from the point of view of the social historian, were the most significant in that here were families breaking new ground, advanced and radical enough to believe in education for their daughters. Running through them in alphabetical order their fathers were a farmer, a linen draper, a cocoa merchant, a rubber merchant, a worsted spinner, a manufacturer from Bingley, a farmer from Oxfordshire whose daughter had been educated at Oxford High School, a jeweller's daughter, educated at Haberdashers' Aske, a millers representative from Mosley and a sugar broker's daughter who had been at the Abbey School, Malvern. Her father must have been a wealthy man, probably there may have been a West Indian estate somewhere in his background. As a contrast next followed a postmaster's daughter, a Co-op manager form Keighley, an assistant secretary to Bass and Co., and from Burton on Trent, then followed a shipbuilder, whose daughter had also been to Malvern in this case to St James. Sandwiched between him and an East India merchant a Brewer, also from Bass and Co. Finally a gold and silver merchant and a yarn agent from Darwen brought up the rear of this conglomerate procession. Linking this latter with the mass of parents who belonged to one of the professions came a few engineers, the details pertaining to them being too vague for me to know quite what place they occupied in the social hierarchy. In addition there were a few parents about whom no details were given. Presumably they were men of private means and no distinction.

Apart from the weekly frivolity of *Vingt et Un* and the excitement of the Lent and May Week races, which continued to retain my loyalty, my day to day existence seemed singularly devoid of any special events in which I took part. When at the beginning of the Michaelmas term King George and Queen Mary came on the 14th October to open the new Institute of Natural Botany I voted it

> 'a very dull proceedings. He looked quite nice, she
> is well preserved – with starch – and Princess Mary
> prettier than I had expected.'

Occasionally there was an amusing rag. Conon Doyle was billed to lecture at the Guildhall on 'sex equality after death, spirits in everyday life and materialisation'. I had had a busy day and not gone with Soulie. I stayed and had a peaceful jug. When she returned she told me that the hall had been packed to overflowing. Then at 9.15 an obviously prepared notice had been put out saying that 'Conon Doyle had failed to materialize'. The whole thing had been a rag and I congratulated myself on having escaped a fruitless wasted evening, adding to my account of this non event 'As usual they suspected Caius'. What I should have been sorry to have missed was the A.D.C. production of a burlesque pantomime, Aladdin, which they gave at the end of term. It was a display of Cambridge undergraduate wit and humour at its very best, though I doubt if anyone outside that charmed circle would have understood its jokes and allusions. Denis Arundel and Harmar of King's wrote the music. Arundel played the princess himself, while Paget cleverly managed to give the impression of a principal 'boy' in the pantomime tradition in spite of his sex, while Caius supplied the policemen in the persons of Bevess and Bishop. In one very characteristic scene of student satire the action centred round the election of a Professor Greek who had been made up to look like Sheppard of King's, by now very much a Cambridge institution himself. The whole production I described as 'awfully good'.

Though I was less enthusiastic about such intelligent relaxations as the Union debates and the political societies rather to my surprise I developed a new interest in Rugger. This I owed to a visit from my brother who insisted on our going when he came to visit me. We placed ourselves in a good position in the centre of the Grandstand and waited until the teams ran out. The match was between Edinburgh and Cambridge. Here is my account of the match.

> 'For the first half hour I thought William would have had convulsions at my attempts to understand the game but I then mastered it sufficiently to fill me with a sense of pride. By the end I found myself muttering in a quite professional manner "you fool, you fool" when someone fumbled the ball. There was just one thrilling moment when Saxon got the ball and scored a try and the scrum half, who I think was Styles of Pemmer, converted. He was always in everything and played awfully well. I thought him the best man in the game. Edinburgh played simply toppingly in combination. Their forwards spread over the field like a net; they were both sure of hand and sure of foot. Gardiner, our back, was quite efficient. I distinguished also C.D. Cook the three quarters. The score was 5–14 against us.'

So thrilled was I with this new experience that I insisted on Ruth coming with me to watch Cambridge play the Old Merchant Tailors. Partly from nostalgia and partly because Rugger was, like the Lent races, an integral part of Cambridge life. I described by that much over used adjectives 'topping' and for the benefit of posterity listed the Cambridge team. They were:

Back	F.A. Gardiner (Pemmer)
Three quarters	R.R.J. Saxon, R.H. Hamilton Wickes (Peterhouse), S. Cook (Cats), D.B. Cook (Pemmer)
Half backs	D.P. Thres (St John's) and H.P. Styles (Pemmer)
Forwards	R. Cave-Smith, G.S. Conway, A. Carneigh-Brown, H.K.P. Smith, W.W. Wakefield, A.D. Ross, T.R.K. Jones and C.D. Ryder.

In fact I had been bitted by the bug and during the Lent term went whenever I could drag a friend along with me, afterwards making critical judgements on the play. When Cambridge played the United Hospitals I remarked condescendingly,

'I thought passing working in conjunction was better this time. Some of the forwards were very good.'

Then followed some individual commendations such as Saxon who 'was in fine form'. My final verdict however was

'we won about 30 to 18. It wasn't a very thrilling game but I loved it. I do wish my friends were not such mugs in the way of going to things. I must go next Wednesday if I can.'

Re-reading my diary I was struck by the unconscious way in which I wrote 'We' or 'Our men' when describing the game. Though the University only regarded me as a titular BA, Cambridge was in my blood and was mine. In my mind I belonged and in my heart I always shall.

My time of residence was nearly over. On the 11th May I went to my last *Vingt et Un*, a prospect that I seem to have viewed with very little emotion writing

> 'I don't care a bit except that dancing is over forever
> except for the Girton dance.'

Even though my mother was coming up for the last few days of May Week I was suffering from a feeling of anticlimax and May Week had lost its flavour. I confessed to a

> 'fit of jealous blues and greens. Ruth has been asked to
> the First and Third Trinity ball and I do wish someone
> would ask me. I have been fighting with horrid
> thoughts.'

I had to comfort myself with the reflection that

> 'my thesis is progressing slowly, about three pages a
> day it sounds awkward but I think it is taking some
> shape.'

This however failed to produce a more cheerful frame of mind for my diary continued

> 'I do wish Verity would ask me to Pemmer. He is going
> without a partner I think and I do want to go to one
> May Week ball. But of course he won't. No one will.
> However the bitterness is well nigh past.'

Like Cinderella my despondency was premature. I too went to the ball.

CHAPTER EIGHT: THE LONDON SCHOOL OF ECONOMICS (LASKI AND FRIENDS)

The invitation was as unexpected as it was welcome. Often throughout my life I have found myself quoting or more likely misquoting as I have never taken the trouble of checking, which has become part of my mental philosophy, the lines with which Gibbert ended his translation of classical Greek dramas;

> 'the end men looked for cometh not. A way there was that no man sought. So has it happened here.'

They certainly applied to a farewell tea party that. Ruth was organising for the 20th May. The evening before I described it as

> 'a large and impossible tea party; P.W. Sturton, Verity Humphries and Graham. It's going to be a mix up'

Like most of my suppositions my forebodings were not fulfilled.

> 'The tea party' I wrote 'went off quite well. It was a little stilted perhaps but as it was the last time we were likely to see each other it was decided to commemorate the event by the taking of photos and then the party

sorted itself out into separate groups. Ruth had
Graham. He is quite impossible. They had a parasol to
themselves, and no one tried to steal him!'

Who the proffered Graham was, or why he was impossible I
no longer remember. My taste in men was not the same as Ruth's,
who always had some young man in tow, some of whom I definitely
liked, especially Adams and Sampson, but of others, who, as they
may be still alive, shall be nameless, I definitely thought were not
people with whom at *Vingt et Un* I cared to dance. Sturten and Verity
drifted towards Soulie while P.W. inevitably sat down beside me. So
did Humphries. I do not think that I had met him before. If I had
it must have been a mere 'ships that pass in the night' encounter
but he plainly interested me because I described him in some detail,
unconscious as yet that he was to be my Prince Charming.

> 'I liked him. He was rather like a good looking red
> Indian; American blood perhaps. Privately I nicknamed
> him Nap because he reminded me of the hero in Ethel
> M. Dell's now never read, or even remembered novel
> '*The War of an Eagle*'. He was not talkative but had a
> nice smile. As he and P.W. stayed until nearly seven
> they cannot have been too bored.'

I did not however expect our paths to cross again. My mother was
coming up for my last May Week, which as every Cambridgite knows
is in June and my brother, now a young man of 17, was to join us. It
was for his sake that we were to go to Fenners to watch the cricket
match between Sussex and the University. It was just as we were
about to set out when Soulie assumed the role of Fairy Godmother,
bursting into the Girton waiting room with a 'Dorothy, you lucky
devil. Humph is looking for you to ask you to the Caius Ball' a
piece of information that she had just got from a mutual friend. I
don't know how Cinderella felt but my knees 'went all of a dither.
It seemed unbelievable.' My problem was, how was I to give him

the opportunity of finding me in a way that would appear decently accidental. Meanwhile I had to go to that wretched cricket match, sitting there wondering and questioning. It was not until I was cycling back to college that fate relented and I had my chance. I saw Nap in Trinity Street and slowed up, feigning ignorance as he caught up with me saying "I have been looking for you all morning. My partner has just got engaged and feels that she ought not now to come with me to the Caius Ball. Could you? Would you? It was not the most flattering of invitations but if I had not been his first choice I had been his second and his first had been made long before we had met at Ruth's opportune party. So I threw my dignity and the tickets we had bought that night for the Beggar's Opera, to the winds and accepted. As I rode out to Girton I kept singing to myself 'oh it's shocking, the way my heart is rocking.' I had obtained the summit of my desires; like Ruth I too was going to a May Week ball. I could look the world in the face.

The last few days of that memorable term were too full and I too exhausted to write my nightly screed. On the 22nd June I left Girton for good and, as I sat in the train, decided before the memory faded to resume my neglected diary confessing that it was an experience that I had enjoyed even more in retrospect than at the time. Perhaps a first ball is always a strain, particularly with a partner who is almost a stranger. Had it been with my cousin Don, for whom I was beginning to cherish romantic notions, it would have been different. As it was I did not know quite how to conduct myself or what to expect. I was still woefully naïve as this verbatim account of that memorable evening will illustrate. Even now I blush a little as I read it.

> 'Nap was awfully nice and danced well, particularly in
> the long spin after we had had hours when my energy
> distinctly flagged. That at least is one handicap that
> I later overcame: learning can be an embarrassing
> business.
>
> 'At number 14 on our programme we paid a visit to

First and Third Trinity which they were holding in the
Guildhall. It was very bright and noisy and full of light.
Newman's band are topping. I enjoyed that. At the
19th we went to Pemmer . At about 5.45 we had our
photos taken. It was a long ordeal. Then I danced with
Nap until 6.30. It was the nicest at them all. Then we
had breakfast in Nap's rooms which revived me. After
that he took me home. All the time he was perfectly
attentive and did look after me well. I hope he did
not find me too troublesome a partner, but it rankles
a little with me that he had not danced more with me
himself. This was unreasonable as I had danced ten
with him and ten with the rest of the party. I came
back looking quite fresh, lay on the bed for a minute
and then went fast asleep. Later that morning mother
and I had coffee at Mathews and coming back I saw
Nap. He was sitting on his cycle. He smiled friendly
like and called out that he was too tired even to lounge.
Somehow it made leaving very near and clear: I hadn't
cared much before. Now I realised I had gone past
Caius for the last time and seen Nap lounging there.
Caius had been pleasant in my life this term and it
hurt. I think my last vivid impression of Cambridge
will be that of Trinity Street in the half sunshine, and
Nap in a blue and white striped blazer, the colour had
run a little at the cuffs, sitting on his motorbike and
smiling at me. I am glad I had that one May Week
memory to take away.'

Another chapter of my life was over.

Leaving Cambridge did not mean that I had severed my links with
Girton. It had been decided that I should be registered for the new
PhD degree and Girton had helped to make this possible by the gift
of the Old Girtonian Studentship for the following academic year. It

was an honour of which I was, and always will be, very, very proud. In addition to everything else that Cambridge had given me it had transformed me from the nervous raw recruit of 1918 to the potential scholar. The thesis which I presented for my PhD afterwards made the basis of my first published work *The English Poor in the Eighteenth Century*. Had I been looking for a title for my biography then it might well have been *From School Girl to Authoress in Eight Years*. It was not a bad record and part of my everlasting debt to Girton and more particularly to Eileen Power and Gwladys Jones.

The next two years of my research was spent in London as a post graduate student at the London School of Economics. I had hoped to continue working under the direction of my dear EEP, who after the end of her travelling scholarship had joined the staff there in 1922 as a lecturer. She had other plans, telling me that I ought to work under Dr Lillian Knowles and that a change would be good for me. I should make contact with other minds and Dr Knowles was a fine scholar and an experienced director. As usual Eileen Power was right. I gained a great deal from my contact with Dr Knowles; nor did it mean that the Cambridge link was broken. She too was a Girtonian of an older generation. She was also a pioneer in the new field of Social History. She had worked under Archbishop Cunningham on his monumental work on *English Industry and Commerce*, then having been appointed to a Lectureship at LSE, had become Professor or Economic History. This was no mean distinction for a woman of her generation: she had gone to Girton on 1890. It was characteristic of her shrewdness and basic commonsense that she once told me that marriage and a career were perfectly compatible, a view not then commonly held, provided a woman had both a good husband and a good housekeeper! Presumably she had both; she also had a son who later became a distinguished scholar himself. As a director she had the unenviable job of seeing a weak spot and suggesting both that something was lacking and where and how the gap could be filled. Under her guidance my research made steady progress. The foundation of the thesis had been laid in Cambridge. Now came the time to put the pieces together, to relate and interpret my material and to make a coherent whole. This, as I discovered for the first but not the last time, can be a humbling experience in that it reveals how much still remains to be done. My work in Cambridge had largely been confined to an intensive study of the administration of the Poor Law in that county. Now under Dr Knowles' direction I was forced to ask myself how far the Cambridge authorities were typical of the country as opposed to the county. For this it would be necessary to find other Quarter Session records. There was also the question of the urban poor. Did they fit into the general pattern? All this meant that long days in the Reading Room of the British Museum as I hunted for new material without which my thesis would not be complete. As a research student I had been given a reader's ticket and the Round Room became my second home. This privilege I enjoyed from the autumn of 1922 to the end of 1984 and by now I must be one of the oldest relics of my generation of readers still alive. In 1922 my mother and I found a temporary home in a furnished flat in Belgrave Road and from there I would catch a 24 bus from Victoria Station, stake a claim to my favourite seat, and work steadily until lunch time, reading, copying extracts until my hand ached or hunting in the massive catalogue to chase up some source that Dr Knowles had suggested I ought to consult. Research had become a way of life which in the main it has been until London bustle and London libraries became too expensive and too exhausting for my ageing energies. Lunch I took at the Plane Tree in Great Russell Street. It has long since vanished and I pay tribute to its memories. The word coffee shop in its modern meaning had not yet invaded the English language and I suppose the Plane Tree would have been described as a Tea Shop as it was not important enough to be described as a restaurant. It served a very good two course lunch for a very modest price, and as the British Museum did not make provision for the inner man, habitués of the Reading Room used to foregather there.

Apart from the British Museum my academic life in London centred round the London School of Economics. It was a modern utilitarian building in Boughton Street, just off the Aldwych. Its aims were, compared with Cambridge, also utilitarian. People who enrolled there were not interested in acquiring the social graces. They looked to obtain power by other means. There were no age long traditions, no ancient buildings to dictate a formality of behaviour to the crowds of students who swarmed everywhere, decanted as they were into corridors rather than streets as lectures ended. Here social intercourse was not likely to be prohibited owing to the lack of a formal introduction. Nor did there seem to be any distinction between the sexes. It was a free for all but not one in which I played much part. As a research student I occupied the middle ground. I was neither 'fish, flesh nor good red herring' and my degree did not entitle me to equality with the teaching fraternity. I do not recollect the term don being generally used there. Had it not been for the late flowering of a submerged Cambridge romance, apart from Dr. Knowles my experience would have remained largely impersonal.

The *deus ex* machine who most unexpectedly rescued me from my island of isolation was the man who had so stimulated my romantic interest when we had attended the same lectures in my first year, Kingsley Smellie. Though I did not flatter myself into thinking that I was as important to him as he was to me never the less, with that curious personal chemistry that occasionally attracts two people to one another I was conscious that he was equally aware of me. But, because in the twenties well brought up men and maidens did not speak to people to whom they had not been introduced, the attraction went no further. Even in the conventional twenties I do not doubt that more enterprising men and maidens contrived to circumvent such difficulties but in Harry Lauder's words 'He was shy and so was I. We were both the same, but he got bolder and bolder on the journey coming home.' Alas we were never given that opportunity. So in the time when we attended the same lectures we never crossed the abyss of convention and gradually my romantic fancies wandered elsewhere, to the Americans in my first May Week, to Wilfred Pryor and again to that distant romantic looking figure

Denis Johnstone, though the fact that we only exchanged a few words at the Girton debating society was due to my timidity not his. I was still too deficient in the art of discreet encouragement; I could hook my fish but lacked the skill to land him. In my third year I saw very little of K.S. We did separate special subjects and he faded from my thoughts. Via the grape vine of the academic world I heard that he had taken a brilliant First and had been appointed to a lectureship at LSE, but had not expected that our paths would cross as I was so seldom in the building except when I went to a tutorial, nor did I give the matter much, or indeed any thought. That we did meet was due to chance or fate. I was just leaving a tutorial when we came face to face on the landing outside Dr Knowles' room. This time he took the initiative which as a lecturer on his own home ground he was entitled to do and said rather diffidently 'I believe we used to go to the same lectures at Cambridge.' I cannot remember how I replied and, because of the gaps in my diary, I have no corroborative evidence on which to draw, but I must have been sufficiently encouraging for the attraction between us worked and he took me under his wing forthwith. It did not, as in the best romantic novels, develop into a romance, though more than once it hesitated on the brink. Whether this is something I regret or not I have never been quite sure. For the next four years, as our friendship grew I pondered often as to whether he would finally ask me to marry him or what I would say if he did. Outwardly he was no longer a cripple walking with two sticks but I am as sure as one can be that sexually he was as inexperienced as I and those false, legs, one he told me was amputated just below the knee and the other above the ankle, might have been an inhibiting factor for both of us. But he had a lovely mind, courage and much kindness so who knows. But when I heard last year that he had died at the age of ninety I was sad. Somehow I had thought him dead long ago, for by then we had drifted apart. Had I known that he was a widower and blind I would have got in touch with him again and, too old for love making I think we should have enjoyed each other's company.

It was through him that I began to take some part in the life of the school. Having been there for a year he had made many friends and I was adopted into this circle. At his invitation or suggestion I came to evening meetings at the school. Without his backing I should never have got to count as friends people like Vera Anstey, Ginsberg or Barret Whale, whose sister afterwards became a colleague of mine at Cardiff. I doubt too if I should have had the initiative to attend the meetings of the Research group, Let alone attend the meal in the Refractory that proceeded it. As much social as academic it brought me into contact with new and lively minds. On one memorable occasion the past was linked to the present when Maurice Dobbs and Kingsley Martin were the guest speakers. The former I thought 'very affable' adding with some surprise 'he really is married'. My surprise would have been dramatically greater had I known, according to an interview in the Sunday Times with Philby, not long before his death that it was to Dobbs, by now a Cambridge don, for help in making a contact with a Russian agent in Paris, though Dobbs was far too discrete to appear to be involved personally. When from the gallery of the Union I had regarded him from afar I had been bored by his dull competent speeches and amused by the contrast between his elegant appearance and his socialist views. Now I know how much more than socialist views it had concealed. The subject for discussion that evening was the Press and Public Opinion. At the moment I was more interested in the other speaker, whom I still described, as relics of Cambridge days as 'Martin of Magdelene'. I had come across him by name only because he had been involved in the production of the Fairy Queen in which Ruth bad played Hippolite. I never remember him speaking at the Union debates. If he did he had made no impression on me, and I had never expected him to blossom out into a brilliant journalist and future editor of the Manchester Guardian. The impression he made on me as a speaker that night was

'He is very good. Far more original that Smellie but very conceited. I don't really like him and he is very cocksure. Men are clever though and assured chiefly the latter. Though Dr Knowles today alluded to clever women like yourself I did not feel myself in the same category as Martin in spite of my criticism of him.'

If Smellie was conventional in his behaviour, gossip that circulated round the school implied that Martin was not and that he had refused to marry the woman with whom he was living believing that matrimony was an infringement of personal liberty, though I believe that later he did succumb and marry. LSE itself was supposed to be a hot bed of socialism and advanced thinking. The conversation at table before the meeting was certainly a contrast to what one supposed to be the conversation at the Girton High Table. But as I was never admitted to that holy of holies who Knows!

In the twenties the LSE could claim to be the power house of constructive socialist thinking under its Director Sir William Beveridge who, in his report did so much to lay the foundations of the Welfare State. Among the older generation two names stand out, those of Sidney and Beatrice Webb for the massive work that they did on the administrative history and framework of English Society, linking their description of parish and county with constructive criticism for the future. Another great luminary in the LSE's sky was H.R. Tawney. I had heard him lecture during my last term in Cambridge and afterwards was privileged to meet him through the good offices of Miss Jones. My financial future as a research student was uncertain though I was hopeful that I would be given the Old Girtonian. However should this not materialize, EEP suggested that I should also apply for a scholarship at the school. Accordingly Miss Jones asked him to coffee and included me in the invitation, it was not I thought a great success confiding to my diary

> 'I felt an awful gawk. He's nice I think and kind but I
> feel he knows all I know and more about the Poor Law
> and I fear I shall not get a scholarship there.'

Unlike the elegant Dobbs, my memory of Tawney is of a shaggy man, shaggy moustache, shaggy eyebrows and shaggy clothes but of benign countenance and a man with many friends. One story that circulated among the junior staff was that during a stay in hospital an exasperated nurse was heard to describe her patient as 'That dreadful man. His bed is always covered with books and he won't let me wash him.' Unlike Cambridge the School was a world in which men and women were equal. Indeed gossip asserted that the ultimate control, even of Sir William was in the hands of the redoubtable Mrs Mair who, like Bunty pulled the strings.

To live in the world of famous people is always interesting, though the personal contact may be small and gossip a substitution for knowledge, but with one star in that galaxy, with a peculiar brilliance all his own, Harold Laski, I had a personal relationship. This I owed to Smellie, who was a protégé of his and who, I suspect would have approved of me as a future Mrs Smellie, though this is pure surmise on my part. In Freda, Laski was blessed with a delightful, charming and cooperative wife. It was the practice on Sunday afternoons to keep open house for anyone to drop in in addition to their distinguished invited guests. It was a wonderful opportunity sometimes to meet the famous and always to be assured of brilliant conversation. Once when I went, to my great grief I heard that Paul Robeson had been their guest the previous week. I hope I did not abuse the privilege too often, but if I did I was never made to feel unwelcome. Certainly over the years, both as a research student and later when I was in London, I went frequently enough to be familiar with the general pattern of conversation and to hear more than once Harold's best stories. Freda must have heard them ad nauseam and I never ceased to admire the role she played in their double act skilfully providing her husband with his opening gambit. Plainly they were a devoted couple, and as many young people at the school, I was grateful to them for their kindness.

The two great interests in my life so far had been History and the Theatre. The other two, travel and wining and dining, came later. In spite of the pressure of work and so other leisure attractions I had found time to go to any performance put on by the ADC or the Marlowe that was open to the public. In addition when any specially interesting play or well known actor or company came to the professional theatre in the town I made an effort to see it. Even so theatre going had to be fitted in with so many other attractions that it must be classed as a minor interest in my Girton days. In London, theatre land with all its allure was only a short bus ride from our flat unlike Hutton where my vacations were spent. In London I could indulge my old love of the theatre. Here again the Fates were kind. Just as in the person of Smellie I had one contact in LSE so in Cyril Phillips I had a contact with the theatrical world. Since the days when I had first known him as a subordinate member of the management of the Birmingham Repertory Company he had not only dug himself in but had become Sir Barry Jackson's business manager and London representative. It was the heyday of the Birmingham Rep and in the October of 1922 it had brought the 'Immortal hours' to London where it ran until the April of the following year. For six months it played to packed houses, having caught the popular taste, though few people remember its music now with the sole exception of The Fairy Song, 'How beautiful they are, the lordly ones' which occasionally appears in musical programmes on the BBC. Barry Jackson had brought the original cast when I had seen it in Glastonbury to London. Gwen Francon-Davies as Etain took London by storm with her elusive, magic charm and a star of the English stage was born. I was a devotee of The Immortal Hour and, as free tickets could be had for the asking saw it I do not know how many times. On one red letter evening Cyril took me behind time scenes and we had supper with her after the show.

> 'I found her charming. Not a bit like Etain but quite
> unaffected, rather pretty and friendly. She asked me to
> go round any time.'

A subsequent venture by the Birmingham Rep. was less successful but also momentous in that it heralded the first appearance on the London professional stage of an actor who also was to become a star.

238

The play was Romeo and Juliet. Gwen Francon-Davies was Juliet and Romeo John Gielgud. Perhaps because it was put on at the Regent, an old theatre not in the West End but near King's Cross, the London public had been prepared to trail out there to see *The Immortal Hour* but the management miscalculated when they thought they would be lured there to see *Romeo and Juliet* even with Gwen Francon-Davies as the bait. Had it not been for Cyril and free tickets I doubt if I would have gone myself. I was deeply moved by it, writing afterwards:

'They both seemed so pitifully young. When all was done and over she seemed to have achieved womanhood still untouched, unsexed but half awake and Romeo loved more as a poet than as a man. Neither of them had the slightest idea of life; that is why they killed themselves so easily. Gwen Francon-Davies was not altogether satisfying in the more dramatic scenes. She lacked weight, she remained a child. But the balcony scene was beautifully done, and coloured ribbons at least saved her from the charge of being "a pert young lady in her nightgown". Romeo I liked. He was young and untouched too with a charming voice and a slightly derisive laugh. He played the part effeminately, but the text gave some justification for that. So I felt Romeo might have looked to do the things he did. He was so coldly, youngly desperate when he heard of Juliet's death, so very young. Heyho. But Shakespeare had no idea of a curtain. I do deprecate his habit of winding things up after all the interesting people are dead. I suppose as a child I should have liked it; Elizabethan audiences must have been more childish than we are. Judging by Shakespeare's characters they wept more easily than we do. At least Romeo and Hamlet did.'

After this excursion into literary criticism I added that I must go again. When I did so on 3rd June I was too late to be able to reassess Gielgud's performance. He had left the cast, why I do not remember it may have been because of illness, but Romeo was played, at very short notice by Ian Swindley. It is a name that few modern theatregoers will remember but I have always considered him the most convincing Hamlet I have ever seen, and after being inspired by Stoney I collected Hamlets whenever I could. But as Romeo I preferred Gielgud. Ian Swindley was a more mature Romeo, both more passion to and more desperate in the tragic scenes. But what remained in my memory was Gielgud's smile of boyish bravado when he heard of Juliet's death 'Tush, thou are deceived.' His Romeo was a destiny blown boy.

By the June of 1924 my mind was more focused on the future than on the present. My thesis was finished and my student days were nearly over. The time when I must earn my living was very near. I had no doubt as to what my career would be. Though my love of the theatre, intensified by my second-hand contact with the London stage via Cyril, still held me in, so that I was hopefully writing plays myself, until success came my way, a more gainful way of life was necessary. I came of two generations of teachers and it was almost automatic that I should become one too. In spite of my secret aspirations to become a playwright I was content, and more than content, to follow the family tradition.

Confiding in my diary I declared by credo

> 'I want to teach History as a whole, to make my pupils care for it. After all it is a fine thing to teach History. I think it is the finest of all subjects if I prove worthy.'

My First together with a prospective Ph.D. enabled me to aim high. Ably backed by a wonderful testimonial from Miss Jones I applied for vacancy at Wycombe Abbey.

> 'I hope I get that,' I wrote, 'I should like it. Near

London, nice country and awfully nice for mother. I
see that Sheffield and Exeter both want lecturers. I
shall apply there too.'

My chances of the latter were slim. The post war scarcity was
over and there were too many young men in the market. To be a
woman was still a disadvantage. However I had been asked to go to
Wycombe for an interview. I washed my hair in preparation for the
ordeal, repeating once again

'I do so hope they will have me. I am so tired. I want
to be settled.'

Of the interview I remember very little, merely an impression that
it was friendly and civilized and that the setting was beautiful. I felt
that they were considering me favourably. Had I gone to Wycombe
Abbey I should probably have remained a teacher all my life had not
fate once again stepped in with a more exciting prospect.

While I was pondering on my future, Vassar College, one of the
oldest, if not the oldest of the great Ivy League American women's
colleges wrote to Girton saying that they had a sudden freshman
bulge and, as this was for one year only, they were considering
appointing an English woman to lecture on European history for
that one year. My luck was in. I was a prospective PhD at a time when
English PhD's were in short supply, particularly female ones. I was
uncommitted and in Miss Jones I had a staunch ally. My parents put
no obstacle in my way. Indeed my mother seized the opportunity to
accompany me and see America. If she had not I doubt if I should
have been encouraged or would even have contemplated it. The link
between us was very close and I knew how much she depended on
me, not in practical ways, she was far more efficient and had far more
enterprise than I ever possessed, but as a companion. Even if I had
been encouraged to go alone I would have lacked the courage to do
so. This admission must seem strange to the young women of today.

It would have been far more commonplace in the twenties, when young ladies led, or were expected to live, more sheltered lives. My father, who was mainly now living with his sister, my aunt Clara, was proud of my achievements and very nobly put no obstacle in my way. Everything was soon arranged and we sailed for New York on the 30th August, 1924 on S.S. Baltic of the White Star line.

The night before we sailed, with some surprise, I confessed

> 'Perhaps I ought to have some emotion to record but
> I am too tired. Oh how sleepy I am. That and the fear
> that my money won't last out are my only predominant
> emotions. So much for the spirit of adventure.'

It was fortunate that I had not pitched my immediate expectations too high. It was three days before I made any further entries in my diary. Then it was to explain

> 'I suppose I ought to have kept my diary religiously,
> but the melancholy fact is that from Sunday dinner
> until today I have been sick and had no more kick in
> me than a half dead flea. We sailed from Liverpool at
> 3.00 on Saturday having said goodbye by everyone.
> Daddy was splendid; very good and brave and cheerful.
> Then we anchored off New Brighton until nine. So I
> enjoyed my dinner. We had two funny Englishmen at
> our table. One I thought by his accent was a Yankee,
> the other came from Yorkshire. Both were fortyish
> and married. Most of the passengers are in parties
> and it is too crowded to mix much beyond our table
> companions and the people whose chairs are near ours
> on the deck. One is occupied by a Miss Wentworth
> from Boston, (Well connected she would have us
> know) but pleasant with all. On our other side is a
> Mrs Walsh. She fusses a lot over a strong, silent (and

242

slightly sick) husband. Apparently she thought I was going to Vassar as a student. Both the men at our table were very nice to us.'

I had not yet grasped the fact that my mother was an attractive woman of forty four and on later voyages I discovered that the normal roles were reversed. I had to keep the men away when they pressed their attentions on her. All they wished me to do was to go away and find a young man of my own and leave the field open to them.

'The Yorkshireman is a kind hearted, ugly dear, the other a moody cuss, who, to hear him talk knows half the film stars in the USA. The Baltic is a pleasant ship in which to sail, very steady and all the attentions very affable. It is very pleasant to be travelling first (particularly when you are sick). There is no doubt about that. But money wise for us henceforth it is Cabin Class on smaller boats. Not second class if I can help it.

Life on the ocean wave is rather boring. Most of the joys are mythical ones invented by landlubbers. One sits in a chair most of the day, reading, sleeping a lot eating a lot and being sick a little or a lot according to the weather. I shall be glad to land and so will mother. The first day was nice. We coasted off Ireland and anchored off Queenstown. It is a lovely harbour and coast and the sun was shining brightly. It was there that I had the splendid sight of a full rigged ship with all her sails set.' Even in the twenties there were not many of them going about their lawful occasions on the high seas. 'Once we had left coastal waters sea sickness struck. It was certainly not auto suggestion. I was very used to messing about in boats with my father and had never been sick.'

Re-reading my comments on the voyage I am struck by the lack of modern amenities even in the First Class when we approached the American coast

'For the first time for three nights the cabin was cool. Coming through the Gulf Stream (it should be called the Gulf Steam) the heat was terrible.'

Also, there seems to have been very little of the organized entertainment that is so much a feature of popular cruises today apart from a fancy dress dance and at that I did not think there were more than 25 couples.

My first entry into the United States was not without its hazards. In the twenties, after the convulsions of the war masses of Europeans were looking to America to provide them with new opportunities and a new life and the States were threatened by a mass emigration. Theory, or rather sentiment and practice were once again in conflict. It was one thing to say send us your poor, etc. when too many of the Europeans took them at their word. Americans were alarmed at the threat that this flood might submerge their own culture. It had to be moderated and a system of quotas was introduced for people whose intention was to settle permanently, though visitors were exempt from such restrictions. The American consul was himself uncertain as to which category I fell in. I had no intention of staying permanently in the States but I was coming to work there. In the end he gave me the necessary papers and his blessing. The latter I was certainly going to need as I discovered when we prepared to dock in New York. We anchored at 7.30 and the medical officers concerned with quarantine regulations and the immigration authorities came on board. The medical inspection was a farce; our landing cards were automatically clipped and as far as they were concerned we were free to go ashore but I wrote indignantly

'the immigration man was a nasty bully. He knew

nothing about universities and made a fuss. I felt pretty sick when he held over my case for consideration. Then Miss Neil, a sweet old lady who lived at Walton, Boston, Mass., found a Professor Webster from Harvard (he had married the daughter of Emmerson's daughter) who tackled the immigration officer. Once he found we had his authority behind us he positively fawned and stamped my card. It had been perfectly beastly. I was still too upset when we moved up the river to study the Statute of Liberty but it did not strike me as being particularly beautiful or inspiring in spite of an American girl standing beside me who kept repeating "Isn't it Wonderful". I was more inclined to agree with the ironic comment that "It was pointing towards the only true land of liberty, England".'

It was not an auspicious beginning to what was to prove to be one of the happiest and most rewarding experiences of my life. At Vassar I was given a welcome and an encouragement that would never have been mine had my adult academic career started in England. I was immediately happy; Americans are incredibly kind to the stranger within their gates. It did not take long for me to feel at home both in the country and at Vassar in spite of so much that contrasted with England, Cambridge and Girton. A new chapter in my life had opened and I looked forward eagerly to whatever lay ahead. America had given me my chance and I shall always be grateful.

CHAPTER NINE: THE VASSAR DIARY

When I first re-read the diary that I had kept at Vassar, which had lain unopened for some fifty years, I could hardly believe that it had been written by the same person as had penned my Cambridge outpourings. These had been almost entirely subjective in their approach. I was the centre round which everything revolved. Pages were devoted to the chronicling of my emotions, the torments of friendships tinged by jealousy, of introspection when I took out and examined my feelings, casting myself for my failure to achieve the moral standards, pathetically naïve with hindsight, of which I believed every right minded person would approve. Yet under this tumult of adolescent emotion and idealism I was glad to discover that I had retained a solid foundation of commonsense. Both were set in the framework of the life of the college and the wider background of Cambridge and in recording both in the twenties I have found some difficulty in disentangling the realities of that life from the private struggle that I had in trying to adjust myself to them. My task as an interpreter of my Girton years has been to disentangle the things which people today would find interesting from the inner sanctum whose secrets remain my own. My Vassar diary is quite different. It is basically objective. I am no longer concentrating on myself as a bundle of feelings: my theme is Vassar and the American world in which I found myself.

Both fascinated me, Vassar as an academic, America as a historian. Much of the Cambridge scene I took take for granted: only certain aspects, in particular the interaction of being a Girton student not a member of the university and the part that this played in my social life. In America everything was unfamiliar and I was conscious that to concentrate on Vassar without giving the American background that had created it and out of which it had grown was only to get half the richness of the opportunity that spending a year in the States gave me. So my mother and I seized every chance to explore this new country that our limited vacations and finances gave us. As a result, my diary abounds in descriptions of the places most associated with America's historical past. Today modern transport has taken hordes of English tourists across the Atlantic, but in the twenties that was not so. I had never been outside England and Scotland and even my mother had been no further afield than France. The joys of the explorer were ours. What we thought, and saw is worth recording for another reason. The America of the twenties is very different from the United States today, and to record a world that has gone has a fascination of its own as well as being of some historical value, and to preserve it uncontaminated by hindsight, or even from the America that I knew when I spent a year at Wellesley in the sixties, I have quoted more extensively from my diary than I felt was necessary in describing the Cambridge scene.

Though my previous information about America was patchy, and often far from accurate it was by no means negligible. It was haphazard and acquired by accident not design: I had never even thought of visiting that country, certainly not of working there. The first, and most vivid impressions that I accumulated came from my liking for historical fiction. My taste was catholic and included

American authors. I found Fennimor Cooper's *Last of the Mohicans* tough going but the novels of Winston Churchill (the American author not the British Prime Minister) readable, and exciting books like *The Crossing* brought the expansion of the frontier alive to me and I was fascinated by a large volume on the grimy manoeuvres of city bosses. Alas I can no longer remember its title but I have a feeling that the main character was called Jethro Bass. But my favourite authoress was Mary Johnson. I loved both her early romantic stories and her sad tragic novels dealing with the Civil War between North and South. It was a theme on which she was well qualified to write; General Johnson had been one of the southern commanders. Little did I ever dream that one day I should meet her and share the hospitality of her house. The new fangled cinema I have described its fascination for me, added its own quota of information on cowboys and Indians. They were not the Indians of Fennimor Cooper and I did not enjoy them or believe in them over much. I doubt if the romances that figured Mary Pickford, *The Worlds Sweetheart* furthered my understanding of the America scene in the first decades of the twentieth century, and the same could be said of the antics of Harold Lloyd, but Griffiths *Birth of a Nation* was the most impressive film I ever saw. As against fiction and the cinema I received a more factual account of American history from lessons at school. It is easy to forget that in the seventeenth and eighteenth centuries English and American history had not gone its separate ways. The Pilgrim fathers and the Boston Tea Party figure in the classrooms of both.

Two of my courses at Cambridge provided me with a solid factual base: the eighteenth century Whigs were deeply involved in the War of Independence but for any one visiting America, or attempting to understand its politics the study of comparative constitution, part of the course on Political Science was invaluable. I came to America understanding the role of the President, and that of the Vice President, the latter rather unkindly impressed on my memory by a quip on the part of my lecturer that 'a woman had two sons one went to sea, the other became Vice President and neither were ever heard of again' an unfair, inaccurate but illuminating witticism. I had written essays on Congress, on the function of the Supreme Court as the final guardian of the constitution, on the distinction between Federal Powers and those of the States. In short when intelligent people discussed politics I held the key to their conversation. I might be able to discuss American politics but I was soon to discover that the bond of a common language was not as fool proof as I had thought: to them a pavement was a sidewalk and other examples were soon to follow, in many ways we were to discover, when we disembarked on the 8th September, that we were indeed in a New World. One voyage was over another about to begin, our personal discovery of America.

Landing in New York is in itself an experience and how we should have fared had we to do so alone heaven knows what difficulties would have engulfed us? From that at least we were spared. Mother's nephew, Willie Edge, had arranged with the firm's representative to meet us at the docks and see us safely installed in the hotel where he had reserved a room for us. Accordingly Mr McMahon collected our luggage, saw us through customs and drove us to our hotel near Washington Square. I was puzzled as to why he had chosen that area. It may have been that Willie had warned him that we would have to operate on a tight budget and a hotel there would be less expense or perhaps less impersonal. It was not the New York of our expectations and we were not favourably impressed.

> 'It's a funny sort of a place in a rather Bohemian
> quarter' I wrote. 'If we had not had so many traps I
> believe we should have fled. But we decided to stay.
> I don't think it will prove so bad really. The food is
> dull (perhaps the Baltic spoilt us) but we have a nice
> bedroom and are near the fire escape.'

Next day I decided that the hotel improved on further acquaintance and that its position was not inconvenient, but already

I was beginning to discover that American habits and English ones when it came to food were not the same.

> 'We do have the funniest food. For dinner we had melon, mutton broth, duck with vegetables, salad, ice cream and tea' going on to add "They serve cake instead of pudding and when you ask for fancy cakes with your tea in a shop they don't know what you mean.'

This first instance of our differing culinary tastes was the fruit of our exploration the previous afternoon when we had set out from Washington Square to discover Fifth Avenues excitements. Someone must have told us to take tea at Schafts which we found very expensive and where, to our astonishment they served iced water when they brought the tea. If my memory serves me correctly the tea was their delicious Orange Peaks? Even today they still don't serve iced water with either tea or coffee in England, though if you are sufficiently firm minded at dinner a waiter will produce it, but it is significant that the American taste in food has travelled back across the Atlantic. In the nineteen-eighties no one would be surprised to be given melon as a starter, followed by soup, duck, salad and ice cream. There are times when I could wish they had not exported fast food and hamburgers to flood not only the European but the British market!

That same afternoon we had our first experience of public transport. Having done some shopping at Woolworth's and rested our weary bones in the public library we boarded a bus back to Washington Square. Immediately we found ourselves in difficulties. Mother handed the conductor two nickels, having no idea of the fare. He gave her a dime back and said he wanted another. Mother was utterly confused, just as American visitors would have been by our pounds, shillings and pence, not to forget that long forgotten half crown and crown. Then handing out a handful of silver she told him 'Take what you want. I don't understand your money.' He took

251

another dime and then to our surprise instead of giving us a ticket, he put both coins into what I described as 'a little dime slot thing that looked like a small colt revolver.' We were learning; the process of settling in had begun.

The next two days were devoted to sightseeing, the first by bus and the second by car as the guests of the McMahons, who were hospitably determined to show us the glories of their city. Having crammed so much in two days is to expect too much, we were both suffering from what could be described as urban indigestion. Our own exploration was more modest. Our bus took us up Fifth Avenue, which, once we had passed the Library, where the day before we had taken refuge from the rain, I described as a very fine street with public buildings. Then we passed 'a big park with natural rocks and vegetation inside and backing on to it were big hotels and houses.' Could it be Central Park, I wondered? It reminded me of Park Lane, while Riverside Drive I thought was the equivalent of the Embankment in London. Not everything I saw met with my approval. What, from the names of the streets I presumed was the Jewish quarter, I condemned as 'very messy' and I applied the same adjective to Broadway. My verdict on New York as a whole was that 'it is a tiring place'.

When the McMahons called for us next morning and took us on a whirlwind tour I realized that the day before 'we ain't seen nothing'. They must have been determined that such a reproach could never be levelled against them. My knowledge of the topography of New York was patchy and much of it must have been imparted to me by our American acquaintances on the Baltic, so I never discovered whether the aquarium was one of the sights not to be missed but we flew through it, with no time to study the beautiful or strange fish that it housed, so that it made very little impression on me. Our next port of call was the famous Woolworth Building, which I found both impressive and rather frightening. When we had first been deposited at Washington Square I had found the buildings in the vicinity

252

disappointing; they did not seem particularly high. These in this part of New York impressed me.

> 'They were simply tremendous, with the road which was rather narrow, winding like a river of light between them.'

I was equally impressed by their magnificent entrance halls which, adorned with gilt and marble, seemed more like palaces then places of business. Even more strange were the rows of lifts I was destined to commit myself to one of them in the Woolworth Building and confessed to feeling

> 'a bit funny when we started to shoot up to the 54th floor where we changed into a smaller lift for the final ascent to the Tower.'

Today a bird's eye view of a great city is a commonplace event to a generation that takes a plane as automatically as we took a train then, but to our unsophisticated eyes it was wonderful to not only see New York but the rivers, the Jersey coast and Long Island beyond, with the Hudson winding into the distance. The streamers looked like toys, the motors hardly an inch long.

I wonder does the vista from the Woolworth Tower still have the same magic for the present visitor? I doubt it. Having come to earth in more senses than one we were taken to lunch at what must have been the haunt of businessmen. I ate swordfish, my first encounter with that species, but felt embarrassed at the expense I was causing my host. Eating out in America to one accustomed to the modest standard of the London Plane Tree, or even the few restaurants frequented by my family, was a new experience and I found it hard to accustom myself to American prices.

After lunch our whirlwind tour continued. The pace was too fast for me to get more than a few fleeting impressions and a few notions about the American way of life when what I saw seemed to English eyes an odd way of doing things. That was certainly my reaction to Central Park and in particular to Central Drive with its lovely quota of splendid apartment houses, which I discovered is the American term for flats. This was very confusing to anyone accustomed to thinking of apartments providing very modest accommodation. Even more odd was the information that very rich people were content with an apartment of five rooms or so, for which in the best locations they paid enormous rents. And to increase my impression of a topsy turvey way of life, even the wealthy usually had only a single domestic. Even our modest establishment at home ran to a cook and a housemaid, though both were village girls trained by my mother and in their first posts, while the houses of our wealthy families who lived in the magnificent mansions in Park Lane and Mayfair had a domestic hierarchy that stretched from the lordly butler to the scullery maid.

Later we had a chance to see how the prosperous as opposed to the wealthy lived when our odyssey ended with a visit to the McMahon's own house. It was somewhat a little out of New York at Orange and, I supposed, was the equivalent of a well to do English residential suburb. We were surprised to find

> 'the majority of houses, even the big ones, were made
> of wood. They stand back from the road, each in its
> own garden but without any fences; the grass runs
> down to the pavement. There were lots of trees and
> open spaces and the whole effect was charming but
> how, I wondered, did they prevent their children and
> dogs from being run over? In America a man's home
> cannot be his castle, a private place.'

The inside of the McMahon's house seemed to emphasise this lack of privacy. I described it as

> 'very nice but un-English. They have no doors but only

openings about twice as wide to their living rooms, so that the vista is clear right through the hall, dining and living room. In winter they have curtains over the gap where the door isn't.'

Here again, though only with hindsight, could I have realized this, the Americans were innovators in designing open plan houses. Another variation from English family life that I observed on that impression-packed day, was the prevalence of

'eating out, especially when entertaining guests. We had our dinner at the Golf Club as they had no maid. It's a charming place with a lounge, dance room, big dining room. I think people feed out much more in America than in England. Every town is full of lavish eating places. The meal over, "my son Jim" took us back in a Subway, as they call a Tube. They are worse than ours and so stuffy.'

So ended our first acquaintance with New York. Next day we left for Poughkeepsie and my new life. London I had taken very much for granted and much of it had remained unexplored. Geographically my knowledge was limited to the West End, with its theatres, to the British Museum and the LSE. New York, because so much had to be crammed into so few days, I could view as a whole and not in segments, it distilled the essence both of the American way of life and also of its historical background and present problems. In London there were great differences between the poverty of much of the East End and the wealth of the inhabitants of Park Lane but essentially we were one people. Our immigrants had been absorbed more completely because they had not arrived in droves. In New York there was no such sense of unity. The Jewish quarter was clearly marked off, but even more so was Harlem which in contemporary usage I described as 'the negro part', writing 'the change was startling. Suddenly all the people in the streets became coloured as if it were a different city altogether.'

But perhaps one of the most significant facts, like Sherlock's dog that did not bark, was my failure to mention the modern pictures of a city where violence was endemic. The subway was stuffy, not dangerous. No one suggested that two ladies should not go out after dark alone. In New York, as in London there was no shortage of crime but it had not become a public nuisance or a public danger. It was a city to which in the year that, lay ahead I returned with pleasure and affection. Like London I came to take it for granted as I came to take the American way of life. Vassar was to provide another facet, as open a contrast to Girton and Cambridge as New York had proved to London. I was indeed discovering the New World. An exciting, stimulating year lay ahead.

I did not go to Vassar immediately. For my first night at Poughkeepsie I stayed with my mother at the Nelson House hotel where she intended to live when I had moved into the collage. I approved of the hotel which I thought more comfortable than its New York specimen, even describing it as almost English. The town of Poughkeepsie I viewed less favourably at my first viewing, considering it an awful hole with an irregular messy street of third rate shops. Later I discovered that behind Main Street there were pleasant residential areas. In the evening Miss Thompson, the Dean of the College, came to welcome us. I thought her a funny woman, odd to look at but very kind. It was a most informal occasion, or so I thought it then, and furnished yet another example of the American way of life. Miss Thompson insisted on taking me into Smith's across the road and giving me an ice cream soda. Not so I am sure would P.K. Leveson have welcomed a new member of the staff at Girton. Nor could I see her sitting on a high stool at the counter. I should certainly have felt too self-conscious to perch there alone. American drug stores, as they were called then, were a far cry from the gentility of Mathews with its little iced cakes in Cambridge. Nevertheless, strange though the venue was, our conversation was in essence business-like. I was to take charge of three sections of freshmen, each twenty in number, and to lecture to them three times a week. That meant nine hours, though only three hours of new work to be prepared each week. In addition if I wanted to avail myself of the opportunity to learn some American history I would be welcome to attend the lectures of my colleagues. In conclusion I decided that

'Everyone promises to be most kind and I really think things will be well. They know I am green and don't seem to mind. I think I am going to start work under ideal conditions.'

Americans have a wonderful way of welcoming the stranger within their gates and of making one feel something rather special, so building up self-confidence. I could so easily have been deflated and frightened and in retrospect my gratitude to Vassar is great.

Next day Miss Thompson asked us both to have lunch with her at Vassar. Like Girton it stood in its own grounds, surrounded by lawns and trees. But there the comparison ended. Vassar was a sprawling complex, a campus in the American sense of the word. Like Girton it had its own chapel and library but everything was on a grand scale. The small library that I had packed in one of my trunks was utterly superfluous. It was almost as if I had inherited the private use of a public library. The whole complex was a self-contained community. Anything that a student required was to be found on the campus. There were reception rooms for entertaining guests or for social occasions. There was a post office, a telegraph office, stationery shop and even a grocery as well as various halls of residence, known rather misleadingly as dormitories. It did not take me long to decide that once I got started I should like Vassar very much. My approval was soon extended to my new colleagues. At lunch I met Miss Ellery, 'even weirder and older than Dean Thompson'. Odd she may have looked but no one could have been more helpful or more kind and I soon grew very fond of her. As there were eight members of the faculty in the History department and as there had been no changes for years I was obviously going to be the baby of the department and as such they spoilt me.

Even so I was in for an unpleasant shock when I moved into residence on the 16th September. As a member of the faculty I had expected to be installed in a well furnished, comfortable room or a small suite of study and bedchamber, which even freshers at Girton were allotted. So great was my dismayed surprise when Miss Ellery took me over to my new quarters and I found them to contain only an unmade bed, a dressing table and a bookshelf. Even Miss Ellery gave a gasp of dismay and, going back into the passage, acquired a chair, which was hardly a solution to our problem. In my account of what followed I resorted to schoolgirl slang, praising her for being awfully decent. She had obviously forgotten that my room would be so sparsely furnished and handed me over to a girl of about my own age, Anita Marburg. She too was a new instructor in the English department, but as an old Vassar graduate she knew the ropes. Unlike Girton, Vassar students were expected to furnish their own rooms. This responsibility had been crystallized into a routine. When a student went on she deposited her unwanted furniture in a depository from which the new student could buy whatever they wanted or could afford. The price that was asked was whatever the market would bear.

The daughters of wealthy parents might not be tempted to patronize it at all and after four years wear and tear they still represented good value. On the other hand furniture handed down through several generations of students were both cheap and battered. Anita took me in hand, saying that I must inspect the stock now before the hordes of new students arrived. Here is the list of my purchases with their prices. In addition to what was strictly necessary I would have to buy things like cushions, curtains, crockery.

all the little luxuries that made a room a pleasant place to live. Under Anita's guidance I bought the necessities and with my mother's help the luxuries in the Poughkeepsie shops. From the college I bought a chair for four dollars, a table for two, a desk and a couch, both for six dollars each. A desk chair and a waste paper basket, both cost only 50 cents each and a screen for four dollars. I was surprised to have bought so much for the money; my basics had only come to 26 dollars. In consequence I began to feel more cheerful, telling myself that when I had bought some curtains, crockery and a percolator it would be both comfortable and attractive. Meanwhile there was one more hurdle between me and a good night's sleep. The bed had not been made up, and Miss Ellery, who had come to see that I was settled in, and I had to go round and round campus looking for sheets. Next afternoon my mother and I went shopping in Poughkeepsie and came back with some orange and blue cretonne, a green rug and a tea set. As a result I declared myself quite broke and had to borrow from the family exchequer until I got my first salary cheque, consoling myself that 'it will look rather well'. Two days later, when the curtains had come and my mother had covered my chair with the cretonne we had bought and made a curtain to cover my bookcase and I had varnished my furniture, I gave my new quarters my final accolade:

'It looked very nice.'

I was getting settled in in other ways as I began to meet the other members of my department. There was no question of my sitting on a drug store stool when I first met Miss Salmon, who I think, was the senior member of the department. On her I paid a formal call. In some ways a formidable figure, I found her nevertheless to be

> 'quite a nice old thing when you get her alone, though I could not get a word in edgewise. She gave me two books written by the staff and when I protested said she had a hundred copies of each as she had bought up the remainders. I came away with the impression

that within our department it would be a case of live
and let live and that I should be allowed to plan my
work very much as I chose.'

Meanwhile, Anita Marburg was a great support and help and
I was delighted when she propped me. As far as I know this was
more spontaneous in American academic society than the more
formal routine of the Girton 'prop'. It was she who introduced me
to the President, Henry MacCraken. Here again the same friendly
informality prevailed, he took us over to his house as a matter of
course and I lost my heart to him, writing

'He is perfectly delightful and so like an older, darker
Pryor-Wandesforth that I could flirt with him. Their
house is charming too.'

No wonder that I came to the verdict that

'I believe I am going to love this place. Nowhere else
in my academic career can I remember after only
six days being so at home and looking forward with
confidence to the workload that lay ahead.'

Had I had more time in which to worry and to plan I might
have viewed the future with less equanimity but the hurly-burly of
furnishing my room and getting to know my colleagues left mercifully
little time for self doubt. Indeed I recorded ruefully.

'My difficulty here won't be loneliness but the difficulty
of finding a few minutes in which to work.'

The new term opened officially with Convocation and I had not
even decided on my choice of the basic text book for my course.
Indeed it was only at lunch that Miss Barbour, one of the younger
members of the department, had given me a couple of books that
she thought would be suitable. I was slightly surprised to find any

260

textbook basic reading: I could not envisage either Eileen Power or Emma G thinking one necessary. When I had jumped at the opportunity of coming to Vassar rather than Wycombe Abbey in a vague way I had visualized it as being another Girton set on American soil. I could not have been more mistaken. Vassar, like Girton, was a totally female residential community, it had been created by people who were passionately interested in providing the female of the species with the opportunity of an academic education and in this they had been successful. But there the similarities between them stopped. What I was to discover was that both countries, though pursuing the same goal, played a very different game. It is possible but dangerous to generalize except to say that educational standards and practices in both were rooted in the national culture and that by the twenties these had diverged, the English based on class distinctions and the American, with its ideological commitment to the equality of all Americans, more influenced by the pocket. Admittedly this is a gross oversimplification suggested by my unverified assumption that pre-academic education was less class-ridden than the English system. Had Board schools provided elementary education for the workers, the new secondary schools, of which the Preston Park School was a shining example, and the more modest private school catering for the middle and professional classes, and the public schools like Eton and Wycombe Abbey for the gentry and the wealthy. My impression was that in the States though there were private schools, the High school drew its pupils from a wider social spread.

It was only at the level of higher education that divergence became marked, where once again simplifying, the academic world seemed to run along parallel lines. The majority of students attended the State Universities, the privileged minority of brain and wealth went to the private colleges of the so-called Ivy League, of which Vassar was a leading member. Hence the contrast between Girton and Vassar. Both were self-governing communities in so far as their internal life was concerned but Vassar was in essence a self-contained university. It decided its own courses and conferred its own degrees. Girton was enmeshed in a university that refused to accept it as a member. Girton studied courses designed for men, its examinations were set by men and corrected by men. Not until 1922 were they rewarded by being allowed to put BA after their name, and even then the word titular bore witness to the women's inferior status. Yet between the two colleges it was a question of the swings and the roundabouts. Vassar students, when in residence, lived in a female world. Girton students, denied academic equality, on the social level could share in the rich traditions of Cambridge and what we could not share we could observe. Had I been a Vassar student I should have grown into a blue stocking, instead of being punted by white flannelled young men on the Cam or waltzing to Sole Mio once a week. The main social life of Vassar students lay elsewhere, at home or in New York, only sixty miles away, but while they were in residence they lived in a female world where inevitably the pattern was different. It was, however, a more comfortable world in that Girton had to run the college on a very modest budget. Vassar was wealthy though not all its students could be so described. There were scholarships for the clever girl and the American tradition of working one's way through college made it possible, having got a place, for the daughter of parents of moderate means to go there. But the majority came from wealthy families and after graduation as alumni they were loyal and generous to the college. There was money for expansion, for new buildings, for excellent libraries. Vassar students did not have to rely on the Seeley Library for their books. Nor did they have to eat cold curried tripe. I still remember with nostalgia the Vassar Sunday lunch with its enormous slabs of delicious ice cream smothered in maple syrup and chopped walnuts. For me it made every Sunday a very special day! Even New York stores acknowledged that Vassar students were worth wooing. At intervals, I cannot remember how long these were, they would hire a hotel room and send down a fashion display calculated to tempt the young. Such a gesture to tempt the young of Girton would have been unthinkable. Most of us rarely got past looking longingly into the windows of Joshua Taylor's and if we had money to spend it was more likely to be spent on books.

Degree courses and the relations between students and dons, or in American phraseology members of the faculty, were not the familiar ones of Girton. There was much less formality, and I should have said much less pressure on Vassar students than we had undergone, though no Vassar student would have agreed with me. They too lived under stress though this was more short-lived than the crises of my student days, because the framework of the degree course was structured on very different lines. We had two examinations, Part I and Part II of the Tripos, that determined our standing throughout our subsequent academic life. Normally Part I was taken after two years and Part II at the end of the third year. The work of three years had to be crammed into two three-day periods at the end of May. It was of no consequence to the examiners that a student might have a headache, or a period, which in those modest days we called 'our visitor', or be a bad examinee. However outstanding our performance in essays over three years, or in our college terminals, only those three days counted. The American pattern was kinder. The AB (even those familiar letters were reversed in the States) involved four years study, as a freshman, a sophomore, a junior and a senior. The first year seemed to me to be of sixth-form quality, not comparable with my first year's courses in Cambridge. Of the others I could not speak personally. The courses spread over four years, allowed a greater diversity of subjects studied than in English universities. You did not read Honours in only one subject at a time though you could 'major' in a particular field, i.e. select a majority of courses in that field, but the remaining ones could include some very odd stable companions. These were sometimes the expression of a genuine interest but could be a canny selection of easy options. In each year the grade that was awarded at the end depended more on lengthy essays that had been handed in than on any test of comprehension of the whole course tested by a written examination at the end. Memory was not unduly strained: what had been quickly absorbed could be equally quickly forgotten. At Vassar I was dealing only with first-year students and these views are coloured by my experience much later when I was at Wellesley, another Ivy League college, in the sixties. There I found repeatedly that a student who could present an admirable minor thesis on a particular aspect worthy of a first class grade, in a more general paper at the end of the course might quite well slip from an A to a B or even B-. Cambridge and Vassar used a different yard stick in measuring achievement and who can say which is the better? Today English schools use continuous assessment as well as the burden of a final examination, Heaven help the teacher faced with a flood of mediocrity if parents or pupils can see their private reports! I had never taught in England, never spoken in public except in debates or the LSE Research group. Tomorrow I would have to face my first class. Two days before I had written,

'If I like the teaching I am just going to love the life.'

The acid test was about to begin.

The new academic year opened with the formal ceremony of Convocation for which I could find no Girton parallel. Girton was not given to ceremonial occasions and there was no dramatic dedication to the opportunities that lay ahead. I did not find the proceedings either particularly impressive or interesting. We all trooped in, taking our places on the platform, and the President addressed the assembled college. The Dean and the President then made what I described as

'moral speeches to the assembled students, an activity
that I could not imagine dear Kitts indulging.'

What gave the occasion importance in my eyes is that we all wore our gowns and I considered that

'I looked rather nice and my rabbit skin, (a reference to
the Cambridge gown and hood) was much admired. It
was the only skin there.'

As only on formal academic occasions I had the opportunity of wearing my white furred skinned hood, the insignia of a Cambridge BA, my vanity was excusable After the speeches we all trooped out again and classes began. I had hardly had time to be nervous and my ordeal was short. Convocation had taken up most of the morning, so that I had only a twenty minute period with my first class. Afterwards I wrote

> 'I hope I did not make too great a fool of myself.
> Anyway I did not dry up or gasp or pant for breath.
> On the whole it wasn't so bad and I think I'll like it
> later on. I had to work hard that night though in order
> to get my next lecture ready and it will mean working
> at pressure for a bit I fear.'

But at least I had my mother to support and cheer me. In the afternoon she came up to college bringing me fudge and cake and peaches to cheer me up or celebrate, whatever seemed most appropriate. I was always conscious that life might be full and exciting for me but that, stuck as she was in Poughkeepsie with no friends of her own, life must have been dull and I worried about her.

I was, however, finding my feet. Next day I had periods with all my three sections, whom I described as 'very nice', and I was relieved to find that I was not unduly nervous when facing them. It did, however, mean the hard work that I had foreseen and my diary became full of such comments as 'I am very sleepy now' or 'I am too tired to write'. I needed to be well prepared for I soon discovered that American students often crossed the barrier between the lecturer and themselves that existed at Cambridge. Though in a Cambridge tutorial it was expected that a student would discuss an essay with the supervisor to ask a question in a formal lecture was unheard of. Behind that barrier one could ignore whatever inconvenient aspects that might give away one's own ignorance or muddled thinking. Next day, when routine classes began in earnest, I began to sense something of this, to me, novel approach. I met two of my three groups for the

265

first time and made another discovery. To both I had expected to give the same lecture but that was not what happened. I found that, like baking two similar cakes, the ingredients might be the same and the method of mixing identical but what spelt success or failure was the temperature of the oven. Audience response differed and so did the lecture. The first group responded, they had as I wrote 'my heart'. The second I felt were more critical. I described them as 'sticky', though the fault was possibly mine. It is not easy to give the same lecture twice in one morning. This would have been even more of a problem if I had been faced by bent heads and scribbling pens; to continue the analogy, an oven whose temperature remained constant. The Vassar students were not autonomous and were not afraid to ask a question or raise a point. In this more intimate atmosphere I relaxed with surprising speed. As a consequence even next day

> 'I had collected so much material for my lecture on the Rise of Christianity, and I got so thrilled by all those ancient dogmas that I just talked and talked and did not finish. Hastily I told them to get ahead with their reading and I would continue next day. Accordingly I asked them 'Where did you go to?' meaning how far ahead had they read? I was surprised to be told 'To the religious shelves' and they looked puzzled when I laughed. My colloquial English had stumped them.

The discussion that followed showed that I must not expect historical perspective from a nation whose history only started in the mid-seventeenth century. The course I had been imported to take was to trace in outline European history from the end of the Roman Empire to the emergence of the modern world and the subject I had been discussing was the small influence that the early Christian Church could exercise when it was only a persecuted minority. To my bewilderment one member of the class launched out into an account of how the Jews were persecuted by the Huguenots, or vice versa, it really did not matter much. While I was struggling to explain that the early Christians and the Huguenots were not synonymous another student broke in with the statement 'Christ was not born then'. Whether she meant that the early church preceded the birth of Christ or that He was preceded by the Huguenots, I could only guess. But certainly this fog of confusion did not make the task of teaching medieval European history an easy one. I could only hope that I might fare better with the barbarians, the next subject to be tackled. Sadly I wrote,

> 'I do hope that something is going into these girls'
> heads. As a result of my having set them a couple of
> written questions I decided that it wasn't. So in the
> next class I pranced from my desk to the map and
> back again, expending much energy over the wretched
> barbarians. It was all very depressing from an academic
> point of view.'

From the personal angle the situation was much more encouraging. As individuals the students were charming, friendly people, apparently quite unconscious that members of the Faculty were superior people and to be treated as such. Even after I had graduated, in all my dealings with Eileen Power and Gladys Jones something of that ancient awe remained. American students felt no need for it. Even on the first day of term a couple of seniors, who had been in Cambridge the previous term, called to see me so late that I was half undressed and had my hair down. Definitely they were no respecters of privacy! Within the first week a fresher, Faith Waterman, call late one evening and stayed over an hour when I wanted to go to sleep. Departing she pressed a small box of toffees remarking,

> '"In future just remember that my name is Faith" I felt
> like remarking that mine was Charity.'

When after a long afternoon walk with my mother and Wanda Freaken from the English Department with whom we were becoming increasingly friendly, I came back to my dormitory, 'Davidson', to find a party of some kind in full swing, but I was too tired, as I described it

> 'to put my nose in. Out of politeness two sweet
> children brought me up some ice cream and candy as
> the spoils of the party.'

To me at the advanced age of twenty five they seemed very young, hence the title 'children', but my verdict on going to bed was

> 'I like students: they are awfully nice.'

I felt that I must do something in return and as I was too hard up to do much lavish entertaining I revived the old Girton ritual of jug, starting with some of the members of my groups who lived in my dormitory. The jug was a success, I thought.

> 'There were four of them and they all talked fourteen
> to the dozen. Mercifully, they went at ten.'

It seemed as good a way of getting to know them as any and I resolved to give another jug next week. But happy as I was with my young flock there were times when I looked back nostalgically to my own salad days and on one occasion, as a reaction to a play given by the juniors, I once again took refuge in verse. Here it is. I was not, I think, as old as I felt myself to me.

> *Life is growing stale and grey,*
>
> *Youth and laughter flee away,*
>
> *Every dog must have its day,*
>
> *Mine alas is over.*

Once I joined in laughter free,

Now it comes no more to me,

College days are over.

Once my life was gay and sprightly,

Dancing through the small hours lightly,

I would love at least twice nightly!

Flirting days are over.

Now I must a stern don be,

Asking freshers into tea,

Petticoats alone I see,

Giddy days are over.

But oh for Cambridge once again,

King's and Caius and Jesus Lane,

And the haunting sound of a dance refrain,

Alas that those days are over.

Though I felt deprived by the lack of young men in my life and confessed that 'I would like a nice man to flirt with' in my petticoat world my social life flourished. The President's reception was the first of many college occasions. Like most parties it was a squash and babble of noise but gleefully I recorded that

> 'I have invitations out or things fixed up for Friday,
> Saturday, Sunday and Monday.'

Americans I soon concluded were great givers of parties and invitations from both my colleagues and students to dinner or lunch were frequent. What pleased me was that their sense of hospitality was beginning to he extended to my mother which helped to break the monotony of her semi-isolation. In my free time we began to explore the countryside, Poughkeepsie might not have much to offer but the ferry across the Hudson opened up a world of great beauty, I had never been out of England until I came to America, so the Thames was the largest river I had ever known. So it is not surprising that I lost my heart to the Hudson, with its sweep of water and its background of hills. To me still it is the most beautiful river I have even known and loved: far, far in my eyes superior to the vaunted beauty of the Rhine. I have never been back nor do I wish to lest I find it fringed with hotels and its loveliness invaded by the demon of progress. I prefer to remember it as when my mother and I took the ferry and set out together with Wanda Freaken to find Lake Mohawk, Through the trees were glimpses of wide country and the jagged line of the Catskill beyond. The trees were just beginning to turn. Already the sumac was a glowing red and the leaves of the maples were golden and pink. There was however a fly in the ointment, or rather two. The first was a monstrous hotel that towered above the lake and the second was that my mother demanded a cup of tea, which the hotel refused to serve until four, so we had to make do with cups of cold water. Then when she tried to buy some cigarettes they only had cigars. So we departed in high dudgeon. Before we reached the ferry we were weary and more than grateful when a car stopped

270

and offered us a lift. This was a pleasant custom that had not yet, I think, spread to England. There to own a car was to be a privileged person and privileges are not to be shared with passers by. Later in the term we set out to explore the Catskill, a complicated expedition that involved the ferry and a bus to Woodstock, a lovely ride. But the summer was nearly over, the leaves though still beautiful, were falling fast and, the visitors having departed, it was with difficulty that we at last found a hotel still open where we could eat. However at The Twin Gables of Woodstock we got an excellent lunch for a dollar. Once again we were lucky enough to be given a lift for part of the way of our trek back to the ferry.

Not all our expeditions were devoted to exploring the beauties of the Hudson and its mountains. New York was easily accessible by train and we decided to go up to see *The Farmer's Wife*, which the Birmingham Repertory Company had put on in New York. I imagine that Cyril had managed to provide is with free seats, as I do not think our finances would have stood the strain of New York theatre tickets. I had seen the play many times when I had been in London and to see it again was an exercise in nostalgia. Like most such exercises it was not a success. Disgustedly I reported

> 'They had made it into a farce and all the character
> was gone. I feel that I ought to get compensation
> for busted illusions. Nothing made me feel so much
> a stranger in a strange land. The house was full and
> people seemed to enjoy it. But oh for Keith Johnson
> and Cederic Hardwicke.'

However being a stranger in a strange land had its compensations. Though I was only a humble instructor when visiting eminent persons came to Vassar, if they were English on some occasions I was invited by the Principal to meet them, as when the poet De La Mare came to lecture. Of course my conversation with him personally was brief, 'mere crumbs' I described it. But my love of food was at least gratified for as well as

271

'the crumbs of conversation I got a very good dinner, duck and ice cream and melon etc.'

De La Mare I described as

'rather dark, blue chinned and he has a charming smile. I thought him much more charming as a guest of honour at dinner than as a lecturer. His is an intimate charm. People in the hall were rather restless, partly because they could not hear him, and partly because he read his lecture, which is never so arresting.'

Still for me it was an interesting evening. Indeed, my life in every way had been interesting. It had also been exhausting. There had been the constant pressure of preparation of the remorseless routine of new lectures to give, of the strain of getting them over to my students, of entertaining and being entertained, of expeditions and of the need not to leave my mother too much on her own. So I was looking forward thankfully to what I had been led to think of as the great American festival of Thanksgiving. At least it meant a break and a short vacation. Not that we regarded this as a rest. Instead we planned to seize the opportunity to extend our acquaintance with the United States and what could be more suitable to a budding historian like myself than to spend it in Boston? Vassar even in so short a time had become not an alarming adventure but a fact of life, I was ready for 'fresh woods and pastures new' when on the four o'clock train, after my last class, we departed for Boston and my first impression of New England.

CHAPTER TEN: VASSAR IN CONTEXT

In England, as a student, I had found myself leading two different lives: in Cambridge academic and in Old Hutton as a member of a family. Between the two there was a great gulf fixed. The pattern of my days was different, the environment was different, even the inhabitants of my two worlds were different and there was very little overlap between them. Only occasionally did my Mother come to Cambridge or a special college friend come to stay with us during the vacation. At Vassar this dichotomy vanished; term and vacation became a seamless robe, one as important as another. I was immersed in the American story of which Vassar was only one part, a microcosm of a sprawling nation that stretched from sea to sea and the more I could comprehend the whole, its traditions and aspirations the more and more I could hope to understand my own small fragment, the colleagues with whom I worked, the students whom I taught and this knowledge I could only acquire in my vacations.

Until the late eighteenth century Britain and America had shared, admittedly under an increasing strain, a common heritage. Lexington,

Concord and Bunkers Hill were as much part of our history as of theirs. As a historian to spend Thanksgiving in Boston, where the past and present were inextricably linked seemed both right and fitting. The New Englanders were indeed new Englanders. They were as unwilling as their countrymen at home to submit to what they thought was injustice or exploitation. It was there that the first fires of this new nation were kindled and kept alive until the conflagration spread to Virginia and New York. Had the crisis been more skilfully handled would the United States have been the most powerful of all the members of the Commonwealth? Few Americans would answer 'Yes' to that question. But to the historian it remains interesting if unlikely speculation. So I was agog to see the places where so great a break with the past, and potent for the future, took place. What had been names were about to become realities; I was to experience History, not at first hand, at second hand. Much would have to be crammed into my Thanksgiving brief break. English and American colleges and universities planned their academic year differently. English vacations were longer, American ones less generous at Easter and Christmas and Thanksgiving was accorded a mere four days.

After a journey in a crowded train, half of Vassar seemed to be going to Boston, and after a good night's sleep in a comfortable hotel, we were ready to explore Boston. Dutifully we concentrated on the major sights that linked the city's colonial past with the bustling present. To catalogue or describe them would be meaningless and boring. To Americans the so called 'Freedom Trail' is well known. To the average English tourist, unless historically inclined, of little significance. Judging by the average brochure advertising American tours concentrate mainly on seeing modern America, on Disneyland and its like and on the beaches of Florida. Those energetic people who commit themselves to absorbing the American scene in a fortnight rarely spend more than a night in Boston. Only to the discerning few do New England's towns and ports and historical memories appeal or the glories of the Fall hold spellbound. Whether my own impressions, gathered in that hectic three days are naïve or penetrating I can no

274

longer judge. Nearly forty years later, when I spent a year at Wellesley, Boston became familiar territory, a town where I took its historic past in my stride and bought the sherry that, Wellesley being so according to local option a 'dry town' was not allowed to sell or where, like all good citizens I searched for bargains at Flicman's Bargain Basement or soaked myself in the special exhibitions sponsored by its favourite region in the States. So my memories blend and mingle. From them I have tried to disentangle my more immediate impressions I seem to have been a little superior and amused. We wondered round the Common and found our way to Chestnut Street

'where the old houses are supposed to be. They are eighteenth century. It's rather pathetic the way the Americans treasure and call old things we should never notice. As a historical city Boston was rather a wash out. Most of the interesting places are merely marked with a tablet saying "on this site etc" but the buildings have gone. Boston was disappointing too in a more personal way. My mother could never break her habit of demanding a cup of tea when in need of refreshment and we could not find a tea shop. Presumably all supplies have been disposed of in the historic Boston Tea Party of revolutionary memory so she had to have ice cream soda with a long spoon instead. As I observed "You need one to sup with the devil".

'Having at last found a tea shop, refreshed and invigorated, we made our way to the old Burial Ground where several of the signatories of the Declaration of Independence, together with notable people from Boston's past are buried, including a character called Paul Revere, though why he deserved this honour I am yet to discover. Like so much of the city's colonial past the old is encircled by the new. The quiet graveyard is surrounded by buildings almost tall enough to count as skyscrapers while the tombstones have the quiet dignity of an English country churchyard. Incongruous as the comparison may be it reminded me of that at Dent, where "God's Acre" is surrounded by a girdle of cottages, the living and the dead in close proximity.'

Forty years later, when I was at Wellesley I came to the old Burial Ground again with a more personal interest. An ancestor of my sister-in-law is buried there[1] and I came to seek out his grave. Opposite it stands the King's Church, the oldest Anglican church in America, but now a Unitarian place of worship.

'Boston' I observed 'is dotted with churches showing their influence in the past and all proudly stating the date of their foundation, mostly seventeenth century.'

That ended our sightseeing for the day, which ended I was happy to note with a good dinner. Next day we planned to go further afield to visit the battlefields of Lexington and Concord, the beginning of the end of British rule in New England.

For this we took a bus to these battle fields, a grandiose name for what in military terms were little more than skirmishes. Irreverently I described the sacred turf as

'simply sprinkled with tablets where anyone died or fired a shot or where the British were driven back.'

But I was impressed by the statue of a Minuteman, portrayed as young, intense and eager. From Lexington we went on the Concord, following what I now was informed was the route of Paul Revere's famous ride to alert the Minutemen that the British were on their way. Rather unkindly I noted that the famous bridge which the English regulars failed to cross, being forced to retreat, was not the original

276   [1]Judge Samuel Sewall (of Salem witchhunt fame)

but a replica in cement. Once again however I was impressed by the statue of the Minuteman guarding the ex battleground. This was not personalisation of ardent youth but of the backbone of the popular resistance. He was portrayed as a farmer in the prime of life

'with an intense face and active frame, his musket in his hand and his powder horn behind him, his coat flung over the tail of his plough, now abandoned. Nearby the lonely grave of the first two British soldiers to fall. We drove back a different way through a countryside rich in the past dwellings of famous literary people. We were shown the shabby looking frame house, with its two gigantic trees standing guard over it where Louisa Alcott wrote Little Women, the house inhabited by Emmerson and not far away the one in which Hawthorne had resided.'

Our last day we devoted to the remaining sights of Boston and Cambridge. Because of John Harvard's connection with Emmanuel and with my memories of charming Americans who had enlivened my first May Week, I was anxious to see Harvard. It was a wet dismal morning and I was not impressed. I described it as

'a cluster of red brick buildings round a campus, or yard as they call it, not so large or beautiful as Vassar. There was little atmosphere or charm or character about it and only the oldest hall looked a little like Emmanuel with a vestibule on top. The buildings were all divided amongst the various departments, the school of this and that and the other and there were some dormitories in the Yard.'

I was equally unimpressed with Radclyffe, the women's college. I thought it looked quite small and a little dingy. Coming back to Boston we collected yet another historic battlefield Bunker's Hill which was in fact Breed's Hill. The historians unfortunately got it wrong; so Bunker's Hill it is likely to remain. Unlike the Minutemen at Lexington and Concord even the monument that commemorates the battle is dull and unmemorable. Our next port of call, literally, was the Navy Yard where we went over the old frigate, the Constitution, built in 1790. It was my first experience of an eighteenth century man of war and I wondered, as anyone going over these old ships must wonder, how on earth they managed to stow away her compliment of 460 men and, about which there can be no doubt that in battle the gun deck must have been hell. Having passed the house where Solomon Levi's shop once stood in the Italian quarter, which I thought was reminiscent of Soho but with narrower streets, we relaxed and had lunch in the down town area.

In the afternoon we continued our hectic sightseeing and clocked up Old South Meeting House and the State House red brick with white facings and still adorned with the Lion and the Unicorn. We even found time to spend half an hour in the Museum of Fine Arts where I was fascinated by the El Grecos. Having crammed our minds full with the memory of inanimate objects we finished the day with a privileged peep into the living world of Henry James. We had been given an introduction to an old Vassar student who had graduated in 1874, a Miss Cushing and on returning to our hotel found an invitation to drink tea with her. I use that old fashioned term deliberately, that afternoon. She was indeed a period piece. She lived in a grand mid Victorian house, complete with marble fireplaces and characteristic furniture. Her family had lived in Boston since 1707 and she had many links with the past. She still spoke of the Southerners in the Civil War as 'the Rebels', she spoke without trace of an American accent and was proud of her English blood.

Later in New York we went to see a play, *The Best People* which annoyed me. I thought it was intended as a skit on the English with their airs of social superiority. It was only later that I realised it was directed against that section of Boston society that our hostess so vividly represented. I was glad of this peep behind the scenes. It completed my first impressions of Boston with its jumble of the past and present and gave reality to what previously had existed only on the pages of my history books.

We had left on the 26th and returned on the 30th. On the 14th of September I had seen Vassar for the first time. Now I could write

> 'Home again. My roomed looked very pleasant when I went into it and my bulbs are sprouting nicely.'

It was easy to slip back into what had now become a steady routine. My feelings about my students continued to be mixed. Academically I could not decide to what extent I was failing or succeeding in my role as their lecturer and tutor. Was I expecting too high a standard, the exacting Girton level of performance, or were American freshmen the product of a different system of education, and facing a different pattern of examinations, not expected to achieve what I expected of them. There were times when I felt utterly disillusioned writing

> 'I don't believe they know anything. They seem so muddled. I must do something with them.'

After a morning spent correcting their papers I moaned

> 'I have decided that M.J. Butcher is the only intelligent person in section 8.'

Part of my difficulty was due to the fact that my contact with them was on two levels, the academic and the social. If Girton standards were more rigorous academically, social ones were much less. I did not have an automatic vague aura of authority to act as a barrier between me and my students. The same day that I was bemoaning their unsatisfactory papers I had been invited out to dinner by a couple of them. I think it was their social expertise that baffled me. When for instance I asked Faith Waterman to come to see me and warned her that I feared she might fail the course

> 'she turned it into a pleasant social interview and
> offered to give me some apples!'

However before the end of term I did have a very reassuring conversation with Miss Ellery who said

> 'half jokingly, she hoped I would not fix up any
> contract for next year without consulting her, the
> department was being organised again etc. and they
> really wanted a well known permanent person but
> anyhow I felt very cheered as she would not have said
> that if she hadn't thought I was justifying myself.'

In other ways the remainder of the term continued to provide new excitements and experiences. Already the first snow had fallen and the time for exploring the countryside was over. In compensation was an unexpected opportunity to explore another side of New York. *The Farmer's Wife* was having a great success on Broadway and Cyril was coming over to cast a managerial eye over the American production. He sailed from Southampton on *SS Olympia* on the 26th November, the day we had left for Boston. He wanted us to join him for a couple of weekends in New York. We went up in a mad rush on the Friday after my last class and installed ourselves in the only hotel that we knew, the one in Washington Square where we had stayed when first we landed and which now seemed shabbier than ever. We were about to be introduced to a very different New York. When I had heard that Cyril was coming to America I had hoped that he was flush as I was decidedly broke. He was. He was staying at the Ritz. I described it as

> 'a very elaborate place with lots of green and gold and
> flunkies and lights in the flowers at the table when we
> had dinner.'

My experience of hotels had been confined to the unexciting Thackeray in Great Russell Street, now long defunct, and I was much impressed at this display of luxury. Next day he took us to lunch at the Fruit and Vine and in the evening we again dined at the Ritz where he was also entertaining two women he had met on the voyage out. He had travelled first class and his guests were a new breed of Americans. Miss Gillies was charming, white haired and beautifully dressed. She was also wealthy. After dinner we went to the theatre and saw a piece *Pigs*, which means nothing to me now though I thought the leading actress, also nameless, extraordinarily funny. More in keeping with our usual pattern of living next day, before we left New York we found 'a nice new tea shop called the Peg Woffington at 50 St East'. Then we returned for another uneventful week so empty of anything worth recording that my diary remained blank for the entire week until we returned again for our second weekend with Cyril.

This time we had abandoned our dismal quarters in Washington Square for the Hotel Seymour. Cyril had made our reservations and we found ourselves installed in the unknown luxury of a sitting room bedroom and bathroom all en suite. My first reaction was one not of pleasure but dismay. I feared it might be well beyond our pockets, as similar hotels in London would certainly have been. In America apparently private facilities were already within the means of the prosperous as opposed to the wealthy and I was most relieved to find that the charge would only be eight dollars a night. Once again we dined at the Ritz, then went to see Abbie's *Irish Rose* and next day returned to Vassar for the rest of the term which was less than a fortnight away. The problem that had faced us was where most enjoyably should we spend the Christmas vacation. It was our dear Principal who came up with the answer, another example of the unremitting kindness that Vassar showed to an insignificant young English Instructor. He suggested that we went to Hot Springs in West Virginia where General Johnson's two daughters were managing to hang on to the old family estate after the financial collapse that followed the Civil War in which he had played an important part.

What made the idea particularly attractive to me was that one of these daughters was the novelist Mary Johnson, whose novels had been part of my schoolgirl reading. In order to see still another historic city, and also to spare us too long a journey that meant overnight travel we decided to stop en route at Philadelphia. The previous night we spent at the Seymour; already we were beginning to take for granted comfort we had never expected in England. The Philadelphia hotel, with its ornate decor of gold and green and with gilt chairs in the dining room put a strain on our budget. In addition it was large and impersonal and though the food was excellent it was so expensive that 'we were never able to choose the nicest things.' Philadelphia too at first sight was disappointing.

Fortunately help was at hand to reverse this impression. We took Blue Line Tour of the city that I enjoyed. What pleased me most was the old Independence Hall where the famous declaration was signed. It has a quiet eighteenth-century dignity. In front is Independence Square, half-flagged and half-well kept grass and flanking the Hall either side were the Congress Building and that of the Supreme Court. I found it easy to imagine the bewigged gentlemen with their swords pacing to and fro on the Square and discussing the latest enormity perpetrated by England. It was the very essence of the United States to be. The other building that gave me pleasure was, in some sense, the reverse of the coin, Mount Pleasant, the home of Benedict Arnold, who later defected to England. When he lived there it was still in the country though now it has been overtaken by the growing city and part of Fremont park. Even so it remains a dignified and self possessed house, the relic of an age long past. The other relics of the past that we saw were the house where Betty Ross sewed the first stars and stripes, and earlier still the small house where William Penn had lived. It too was brick built but very small, almost like a toy, and a silent testimony to the poverty of the early colonists when bricks were a luxury. My final verdict was that

'Philadelphia must have been charming in colonial days with its small quaint houses in Chestnut Street ranged round the old brick, white painted Independence Hall and with the houses of the gentry dotted over the countryside. There is very little of it left now, though it is easier to construct now in memory than Boston. But as a town I prefer Boston; it has a more friendly air.'

Next day we left for Hot Springs and to delve still further into the American past.

To go from Philadelphia to Warm Springs was to travel from the historic past to the living past. The Johnson's house that overlooked the valley below, stood some 6,000 feet above it, a tranquil scene dotted with trees and interested by many small streams. I loved it. The house itself was old and rambling and utterly charming, comfortable and overflowing with bookcases and books everywhere. Outside its garden and carefully trimmed box hedges added to the general air of stability. It was a house and a setting whose roots went deep into the past. The historian's role is to make a link between former days and the present. To interpolate one to the other and the task is not as easy or as simple as at first sight appears. A past constructed from its inanimate remains that includes every kind of documentation, and what remains in the more tangible shape of buildings or the evidence of the countryside can at best produce a fallible picture. To step into that past and feel its reality for the historian is a valuable experience. Imagination is turned into reality and this experience my Christmas at Warm Springs gave me. When the visit was over, writing in the swaying train that was to take me back to Vassar, 'I shall love America if only for Virginia.' Everyone was so nice all the time we were there and I hated to say goodbye. The remoteness of Warm Springs was apparent as soon as we had left the train when we first arrived. It was already dark and the drive was so long and so lonely that I began to wonder if the driver were a bandit and we were being taken to an unknown destination. Then the lights of the house appeared and the two Miss Johnsons came out to greet us and take us into the friendly warmth within. I pronounced them

> 'dears, Miss Mary a little more compact and well put
> together and we have lost our hearts to them.'

In atmosphere the world in which they lived was the world of Southern gentlewomen before the Civil War. Their hospitality was so genuine that we seemed a gathering of friends. Breakfast next morning was a further example of Southern ways in that we were faced with waffles and maple syrup and eggs all on the same plate and hot bread and heaven knows what. In the afternoon, as a courtesy to my Mother even tea was produced. The company, whether at meals or in the living room or in Miss Mary's private sanctum, with its blazing fire and multitudinous book cases, where we were sometimes invited, was stimulating and eminently civilized. The people that I remembered best were a Mr Benedict, an older man who professed himself to be an admirer of mine and two spinsters, a Miss Jenny Eliot and a Miss Mary Street. The former kept a school at Richmond. I described her as

> 'old and she wears a green dress, her hair is almost
> white, her skin rather parchmenty and her lids fall over
> her eyes in a funny triangular slit. She is terribly pro
> English and appears to regard me as an authority on
> education. Miss Street is big and country looking with
> glasses, rather wind blown greyish hair and a brusque
> manner.'

Rather belying her matter of fact appearance she was fascinated by some kind of unorthodox religion, tinged I think with Theosophy. Anyhow she informed me that I had a rose coloured aura.

Christmas Day was a day of enchantment. I declared that

'It was the nicest I have ever spent since the childish glamour went from it.'

It started with the giving of presents at breakfast and, though almost a stranger I was not left out. Miss Eloise gave me a box of delicious candies in a pink tin tied up with a splendid ribbon that I could keep and I had another box 'from a new admirer' who I was sure was Mr Benedict. Then Mother and I together with Miss Eliot and Miss Street walked down to the little chapel below, a simple wooden structure, its interior turned into golden light by the sunshine that streamed through the windows. I thought I had never seen the valley look more beautiful than it did as we walked back that morning. But the highlight of Christmas Day came in the afternoon when the tradition of the good plantation owner, which I am sure the Johnsons had in those pre civil war days been. In the hall there stood a gaily decorated Christmas Tree erected not for our pleasure but to make the focus of a party given to the coloured people who worked on the estate. I recorded the scene in detail. Here is the picture that remained with me when I remember my Virginian Christmas.

'There must have been about 30 people from a tiny little girl of about three or four with her hair in two tight pigtails that stuck out on either side of her face to older girls of fifteen or sixteen. There were all colours and types from the real Negro with fuzzy hair to a girl who was no more than dusky whose hair was mid brown. First they all marched round the tree and then sat down while Santa Claus (Mr John Johnson) distributed the presents. Everyone got something and some of them were very handsome sleighs and trucks and things. All the older people got presents too. Then the children recited their little pieces, all gabbled in their soft southern voices so I couldn't hear a thing. Some of them were as solemn as judges, others beamed all over their faces but the littlest little girl never even smiled. Then some of the older sang their old spirituals, *Roll Jordon Roll* and *Swing Low Sweet Chariot* and some I did not know

Hand me down a silver trumpet Gabriel,

Hand me down a silver trumpet Lord.

Hand it down, knock it down,

Any way you get it down,

Hand me down a silver trumpet Lord.

There was another sung by a mother and her three daughters that struck a less religious, if more practical note.

Ain't it a shame to steal on Sunday,

Ain't it a shame

When you've got Monday, Tuesday Wednesday, Thursday, Friday, Saturday too.

Ain't it a shame.

This concluded the more organized part of the proceedings and the grown ups left while the children devoured ice cream. We in our turn trooped into the dining room for our Christmas dinner.'

This was the one part of the day that I criticized. The turkey was as it should be but the plum pudding did not taste like an English one, but there were no three penny pieces in it, or thimbles or any surprises and there were no mince pies. Still it had been a wonderful Christmas and at dinner I had worn my new golden coloured dress.

Warm Springs was a small and scattered community, the fashionable Hot Springs Spa whereas the nearby Hot Springs was, or perhaps it might be more accurate to say had been, a fashionable Spa and next morning we walked over with Miss Eliot to explore it. The main feature was the hotel, built to create an illusion of glamour, with white walls and soft coloured carpets and hanging to soothe those coming to take the treatment. As well as treatment rooms and bath it had lounges and a ballroom and shops. But at this time of the year it was empty. It was a great contrast to the primitive bath house in Warm Springs. It was a domed wooden building, very primitive both in structure and design, while to describe its provision of facilities for dressing and undressing as adequate would be grossly flattering. Nevertheless it had a certain charm and for me some practical advantages. The pool was circular, the water only came up to my chin and there was a rope stretched across the centre. In short it was a bath in which I could have no fear of drowning. It had two other attractions. The water was pleasantly warm; it was also buoyant so that even I could swim in it without sinking after the first three strokes, though even here I must confess to being put to shame by a small eel of a child, hardly more than a baby, who swam around with utter delight and abandon. Not to be outdone I swam across three times. Outside the bathers were forced to face a chilly world. Shortly after Christmas the first snow had fallen. All the trees were outlined in ice, turning the valley into a fairy world but my most vivid memory is of the overflow from the bath house, still steaming as it escaped between its frozen banks. By New Year's Day the snow lay thick enough to reduce the party to the level of rollicking school children. Mr Benedict and I started things off by a little feeble snowballing. Then someone produced a sledge and the fun began. To begin with I lay at the bottom of the logged contraption and as I had not the slightest idea of how to steer we always ended up in a snow drift or fell off at a corner with us all shrieking like two year olds. In the afternoon Mr Benedict lay underneath with me on top of him and Miss Derby on top of me. It was not a success. We were all too helpless with laughter that we kept rolling off. But it was great fun, though after my sedate and sedentary life I was so stiff and exhausted that by 8.30 I retired to bed.

Before the snow came and made exploring impossible I got another glimpse into the past, a past even older than my memorable Christmas Day peep into the pre Civil War Plantation traditional celebration. We had gone for what our companions called 'a stroll' down the yellow dirt road and along a trail that wound through the hills until we came to another valley, so remote in its appearance and way of life that it was, like a fly in amber, imprisoned in the seventeenth century.

'Here and there were quaint, unpainted and sometimes ramshackle houses. Near them a few cows, their bells gangling, were grazing, and some hens clucking. Once we passed a man with a huge bundle of corn stalks on his shoulders, to be turned into fodder I suppose. He wished us "good evening" though it cannot have been much after four. They go to bed with the sun in that valley; another medieval touch. It is inhabited by a quaint sect of Dunkards who follow the Bible literally and hold the ceremony of washing feet once a year – the Middle Ages again. Their minister too follows his trade and preaches on Sunday. It all seemed another world, not English, not American but a strange breed of its own rooted in a mixture of the New World that attracted the religious descendants of the seventeenth century grafted onto the wilderness where they had sought the right to worship God in their own way.

'I felt Dunkards can be compared to an old vessel stranded on the sands of History, never to be re-floated the fact that following the Christmas junketing Miss Eloise organised a debate for the coloured people on "Is the world better than it used to be" was surely a portent for the future, one in which black and white would be equal citizens. The speakers were very different, a fat jovial man who was a licensed preacher, next a sombre man with a black beard spoke. He was followed by a little man like a frog who spoke more intelligently than some, and lastly a thin man with a drooping moustache and a voice that nearly tore him by its emotion; he tied himself into knots with his vehemence.'

I thought the majority of the speakers resembled children. The facts tumbled out without making a reasoned argument. Yet here and there were sudden flashes of wit and a keen intelligence. Such consistent thread as could be discerned in their arguments was their reliance on isolated biblical texts as the ultimate authority, a distinctly medieval way of arguing. My final comment was that

'Mr Walter who presided and Mr Parker who gave the verdict both acted with complete and absolute courtesy and ease. But I could have kicked Mr Brewer and one or two of the others who treated the performance rather as a show of cute animals. I do think it says something that they can debate at all and they are so like kids, so pleased with themselves. The minister clapped when his side won. They stopped singing in the middle of *Sweet Chariot* to hear the verdict. I ought to have said that they started off with a hymn and sang between each speaker, which was rather a quaint but pleasing custom.'

It was the first time that I had seen the descendants of slaves treated with equality. Hitherto, in the States I had regarded them as men and women born to serve their white employers and my condescending comments were as out of touch with the future as the offensive attitude of Mr Brewer and his like that I had condemned. They were however pretty typical of even the majority of people in the twenties. The days of Martin Luther King lay far ahead and the debate was an episode no more than I found interesting but not significant.

By the 4th January the party began to break up and there was a general exodus, the Seiglimands, the Derbyshires and Mr Benedict. He travelled with us to New York and was most helpful in looking after our comfort. He gave us dinner, got the beds in our sleeper made up and called us next morning at 7.30 so that we could get our breakfast before the crowds emerged. I was sad to leave Miss Eloise and Miss Mary, who gave me a signed photograph and the friends we had made with whom we exchanged addresses and spoke of future meetings. Mr Benedict really seemed quite upset.

> 'Mr Benedict' I reported 'looked very glum, said he
> hoped he'd see us again as having met "two such
> attractive ladies" he did not want to lose sight of
> them.'

My mother thought he was fishing for an invitation to visit Vassar but, characteristically I never realised this. Yet I had come to like Mr Benedict in spite of what I described as

> 'his funny looks. He had dark eyes, dark hair going
> grey and combed over the bald spots, goggles, and
> brown toothbrush moustache, a mouth that looked as
> if it were going to break into tears, a red complexion
> and a double chin. I should think he was 38 or 39 but
> his expression was very benign and he was good to
> children and his conversation could be sensible. I think
> he had a nice mind.'

Obviously he was no Adonis. On re-reading this description sixty years later I feel that it reveals more about me and my judgements and aspirations than it did abut Mr Benedict. I did at least consider sending him one of my doggerel verses that registered the fact that the time for play was over and that the claims of work had once more to be met.

'I must confess to feeling glum

When the last goodbyes were done

And we had turned our back on fun

"Honest to Goodness" I did.

I love not work, no more do you

If what you confess is true

And we must still pretend we done

"Honest to Goodness" we must.

Business men don't play with snow

Instructors must sedately go

Responsibility brings much woe

"Honest to Goodness" it does.'

This Christmas interlude had not only been pleasurable it had been profitable in that it had widened my knowledge and understanding of America and its people. With Virginia I had already had a historical sympathy, born of Mary Johnson's novels long before I was privileged to count her as a friend. Now the South with its tradition and its 'darkies' had become a reality to me, though a reality with the shadows omitted, if indeed that can be counted as reality. The fight to free the ex-slave members of the community from the restrictions and assumptions of the past lay in the future; my own comments on the black speakers, likening them to children is proof of that. The other bonus that accrued from my stay at Warm Springs was that it enabled me to meet another section of American society. Hitherto my friends had been confined to the academic world of Vassar. The party at Warm Springs was composed of a mixed group, all of them civilised and people of culture or Miss Mary and Miss Eloise would not have entertained them, even as paying guests, but drawn from the business world or from the prosperous, but not wealthy middle class. They were the counterpart to our circle at Old Hutton, the older generation whose sons had adorned my first May Week and whose daughters I was attempting to educate at Vassar.

When we got to New York snow was piled high on either side of the streets and it took us ages to get from the Pennsylvania to The Grand Central Station. It felt odd to be back and sad for Mother and me to resume our semi-separate lives after so lovely a holiday. Next morning I slept until 11.30 and then went down to Poughkeepsie to stock up my private store of provisions. After Virginia it seemed an alien place. Then it was back to the old routine. Classes started next morning so I spent the evening reading up for the Hundred Years War.

Next day I reported that

'Nothing much happened. Classes went alright I think.
One thing I have plenty of energy after my holiday'

so I settled down to get ahead with my reading. Keeping one lecture in advance of a class does dictate an academic living from hand to mouth but at least there is never time to grow stale. The next day, the 8th January I found more interesting. James Baldwin, the eminent constitutional historian, whose great work on The King's Council I had done my best to mark, learn and inwardly digest for my constitutional paper in Part I, was to spend the term as a guest lecturer at Vassar, and I was thrilled to think that he was actually to be a colleague. In the morning he waylaid me before my class to find out if I had told them about the lecture that Herbert Hall was to give that day. He too was a distinguished medievalist on a lecture tour in the States. I approved of him 'Slow, sleepy voice, his almost white pointed beard, that had been sandy, and a pleasant manner'. He was lecturing on the demesne farm in fourteenth and fifteenth century England and I congratulated myself with the comfortable thought that my students would at least know enough about medieval agriculture to understand him. This was satisfactory but what I really loved was going back to the Baldwins afterwards. As I confessed that I was

> 'still young enough to enjoy going behind the scenes
> for a time and meeting the leading lights. It's fun being
> a don even though I have to take Miss Ellery's next
> semester. I knew that she approved my work because
> towards the end of last term half jokingly she had told
> me she hoped I would not fix up any contract for next
> year without consulting her. The department was being
> organized etc. and they really wanted a permanent
> person but –.'

That she trusted me take her class was certainly encouraging which was pleasant but in what I described as

> 'the nicest way that there would be no place for me
> in the department next year. They wanted one person
> to do ancient and required another to do American,
> neither of which I could do. Of course I was only
> engaged for a year but after what Miss Ellery had

said herself earlier I think she felt a bit bad. I don't believe things went in the department meeting quite as expected. She told me that my work was quite acceptable but just there was no place. I did not mind anyhow as I should not have stayed.'

Indeed we were already making preparations for our return and were hesitating between the Mount Royal which sailed from Quebec on the 19th June and docked at Liverpool and the Melita sailing from Montreal to Southampton on the 17th. On one thing we were determined and that was to include the Niagara Falls, and see something of Canada and the St Lawrence as it seemed unlikely that we should ever have another opportunity. Finally we settled for the Melita and made our reservations.

After the Christmas vacation I found it much easier to settle down and get into my stride. This was fortunate as my responsibilities were increasing. For the first time in my life I was setting exam papers and not sitting them. This was both a thrill and also a worry in that scrupulous fairness is important and this is hard to achieve. Candidates are a mixed bunch and the examination to fix their class or grade is supposed to separate the sheep from the goats. One must be fair to the sheep, good hard working students who, at a superficial level have covered the course and who can write a straightforward factual answer. But the question that provides for them must also give an opportunity for the goats to show their intellectual ingenuity, to demonstrate that they understand as well as know and can bring their own interpretation to the question. To achieve this is not easy but it is an academic problem. The men who set the Tripos papers were impersonal in that they had no contact with the students who would have to answer it. But at Vassar, where the examination was an internal affair that was not so. The students who would sit my paper knew me and I knew them. Most of the subjects that must make the foundation of any paper I set we had either discussed in class or in conference. It was rather like two chess players who know each other's

294

game. And it is impossible not to have favourites, to see potential in one that should be given its chance and the temptation to provide it must always be resisted. Nor was it only a question of the individual. If you have taught a class you have a pretty good idea of the paper that will suit its particular aptitude and interests. Set one kind of paper and the results will be good. Set another and they won't. At this, my first trial run, I do not think I realised how tricky the course could be. All I wanted was not to disgrace myself in the eyes of my colleague. So great was my relief when at the departmental meeting my papers were approved a few minor alterations and when, next day, another of my colleagues, Miss Brown, told me how good she thought my paper was.

All the same there was something that I could not quite place in that departmental meeting. I had a feeling that

> 'there were wheels within wheels. Either there had
> been a fight about me and Miss Ellery had wanted me
> back or I've put my foot in it but there was a certain
> feeling that I can't quite grasp. How I would love to
> pull my people through without a 'plough[1]'.'

It was the first time I had got into contact with departmental politics and sensed the bitterness that they could engender. In the running of a department American and English practices differed. In England in the twenties there was only one head of a department, THE PROFESSOR, and he was only one remove from God if he aspired to assume that role. In America only the humble Instructor was denied the professorial title. There were associate professors and assistant professors and full professors and I think the headship of the department rotated even then at Vassar, as it certainly did when next I was in America in the sixties. Today the practice has spread to England. With the creation of personal chairs there is no longer a quasi deity in charge, as throughout my own academic career when on the whole a benevolent despotism prevailed. I think my supposition

[1] Cambridge slang for a failure

that there was strain in the department was correct, for a couple of days later Miss Ellery went out of her way to tell me

> 'how she wished I could stay on and that I fitted into the department and the work better than anyone else they had ever had who was not an alumna. I wish I felt I really had deserved it but I do know I have not done badly for a beginner. At least my examination results had not disgraced me. About half of them got a C, which is a respectable but not an impressive mark, 19 got Bs, which meant good steady, intelligent work, and only 10 sank to the lowest pass mark, a D. But what pleased me most was that two of my group got As, equivalent to a First Class. Polly Butcher, who in my first term I had decided was the only one of her group who had any intelligence, was one of them and the other Anna Jane Philips. Because I thought that she had potential and a keen interest in History, or was it a G.P. on me, I got Miss Ellery to read her paper and she agreed it was worth an A. and that Anna Jane was worth keeping an eye on.'

I cannot remember whether it was before or after getting an A. that she flabbergasted me by her reaction to a suggestion of mine that she should have consulted the Encyclopedia Britannica when she wanted information not available in her text book. Two days later she informed me that she had bought an Encyclopedia Britannica! Anna Jane came from Pittsburgh and apparently money was no obstacle but how American her lavish gesture was I am afraid she was one of my favourites and I was glad that she had done so well. But I was perhaps ever happier that Lucille Johnson had pulled off a B. because she used to be a rather shaky C. and I flattered myself that at least I had done a good job there: 'There is more joy in heaven etc.'.

It was pleasant too to be asked to meet distinguished English

296

historians when they came to lecture at Vassar. When Seton Watson came Miss Barbour asked me to tea to meet him. Then after the lecture there was a departmental dinner, so I had a pretty good dose of Seton Watson. Alas I was not impressed either by his appearance or his lecture. I summed him up as follows

> 'He is big, wears badly made tweeds and boots, glasses and has a short brown moustache, but has rather a pleasant way of talking. He might be interesting in a small group but he was no good as a lion as he refused to roar, the only lion like thing about him being devoted to his dinner rather than conversation.'

I had however to concede that his analysis of the situation in the old Austrian Empire after the carve up at the end of the War was interesting when, as I said 'he got down to it'. I voted the evening as a whole dull, but I had at least done my best to improve the not so shining hour by sitting next to Mr Baldwin and doing my best to be charming. By now I had decided that he fell into the category of being 'a nice thing' but what gave me the greatest pleasure that evening was that Prizzy came over to speak, whom I regarded without qualification as 'a dear' and even cherished the hope that, because he was so nice to us he might even visit us when next he came to England. Much more enjoyable was the lecture given by one Mr Leicester B. Holland, who would be joining the faculty here next year, on St Denys as the cradle of Gothic architecture. He was a complete contrast to Seton Watson and regaled us with amusing and delightful stories to form the legends of the past. Once again there was a reception afterwards but that I condemned as dull.

Meanwhile winter had set in. By the 11th January it was so bitterly cold that I realized how accurately the phrase 'iron cold' represented my feelings. To be as cold as that was a new experience, as also it was to live in a world that seemed perpetually white. On the 20th I awoke to snow so persistent that it almost amounted to a blizzard, a grey veil of tiny flakes that stretched across the sky while underneath it was incredibly soft and white. On the 24th there occurred an event that, while it had no place in the academic calendar, was, as far as my mother and I were concerned, a unique experience. At the time I do not think I realised quite how privileged I was to see a total eclipse of the sun in perfect conditions. Even so it made a great impression as I hope this extract from my diary will show

> 'It was a clear cold morning – oh so cold with the thermometer below 7 – ugh! Mother got over about 8.15 and we went to the New England Building to watch from a window as the moon nibbled into the sun. Then when it was three quarters over and the light was getting queer we went to the top of Taylor Tower. It got all queer and odd. Then the moon slipped over and outburst the corona, a beautiful thing like a veil of light draped round its dark body. To the right were three stars while the sky behind the hills was a weird, unearthly pink. So it stayed for a minute, then the edge of the moon seemed to waiver and crack and outburst the rim of the sun, blotting out with its light the corona, the pink of the sky and the reluctant stars. It was over and the rest of the day seemed a little flat.'

Looking back I seem to remember a lack of warnings given to the onlookers. We were provided with squares of smoked glass and told not to look directly at the sun except through them. Meanwhile it continued to snow and for a few days my mind as well as my body froze. This was because at the beginning of February there had been a shuffle of classes and I was now to have Miss Thompson's students, or at least one section of them, which gave me 91 instead of 68 with whom to cope. When I first met them I confessed to feeling

> 'a little frozen and at a loss how to go on. I expect I'll get into them in a few days. Anyhow I am forward in my work.'

Already I was becoming conscious of my ability to hold a class's attention and my panic reaction was over. To some extent my ego had been boosted when Miss Ellery, my academic fairy godmother, told me that Mr Baldwin had commended my papers very highly and that it was unusual for him to praise anything. All the same I was ready for a little relaxation and a break in the monotony of college life so we decided to go up to New York on a shopping spree. As our intention was to buy material for summer dresses and as the snow lay a foot deep outside my window I called it an act of faith. Moreover, at my mother's instigation we were to meet Mr Benedict for tea. So at least for one day I was prepared to put college and my responsibilities behind me and become young again.

CHAPTER ELEVEN: REFLECTIONS ON AMERICA (AND THE WAY AHEAD).

Whether it was a pride in authorship or a liking for Mr Benedict that made me send a specimen of my doggerel to him I cannot now recollect. It brought back a response in kind which privately I considered inferior to my own effusion. Here is a specimen to back up my effusion

'Oh fondly on the past I dwell

And oft recall those bumptious moments

When hilly flopping down the hill (pardon the USA slang)

I missed the snowy bumps.'

Though hardly up to Poet Laureate standards I felt it merited some reward hence the meeting in New York for tea. It confirmed my opinion that 'he's a funny man but a dear.' I came away feeling rather sad at the thought that we should probably not meet again. Our visit to New York in February enriched my knowledge of American society. Miss Gillies, Cyril's sea voyage acquaintance asked us to stay with her for a week and had promised to take us to the opera. It was my old favourite Carmen, so I felt in a position to criticize the production. I approve of *Don Jose* and *Marcella* but was disparaging about *Carmen* and the *Toreador*. Nor did I find the celebrated Opera House very impressive as our seats were in the second tier box and I found it difficult to get a clear view of the stage. The evening at the opera turned out to be the least interesting part of our time with Miss Gillies. If at Vassar I lived in an enclosed academic world I had various opportunities to widen my understanding of the American way of life. Staying with Miss Gillies was a fascinating glimpse into the lifestyle of the wealthy New Yorker. As a budding historian I thought myself privileged to see something of the world into which normally I never expected to penetrate. I am not too sure that my comments are not a betrayal of hospitality for she was a kind and thoughtful hostess, even to the extent to making sure that we had iced water in our bedroom at night. Yet the impression I got was one of emptiness.

> 'Her conversation was determinedly highbrow and her
> sentiments elevated as she was living up to a picture
> of what she thought her position required. Yet there
> were lapses into commonsense that hinted at a sensible
> woman behind the facade. It is as if she can never free
> herself from her wealth and her important friends.
> Her conversation is peppered with Sir Somebody this
> and Lady That. Yet I think she tries not to be a snob.
> I think we might like her much better when we know
> her better. In the afternoon she had asked some 14
> people into tea to meet us. Most of them were women,
> and apart from a young married couple whom I liked, I
> found them dull.'

One of them would talk moral platitudes. Sometimes I think that passes for worthwhile talk over here. She certainly did us proud in the way of social contacts.

Another of her friends asked us to dinner. Mrs Chandler, our evening hostess occupies a charming apartment in 23ʳᵈ street. In atmosphere it was a complete contrast to Miss Gillies' more formal apartment. There was a log fire and sofas and books and soft lights. There was nothing brittle, no desire to impress and no worthwhile talk, just civilised conversation and a pleasant meal. On Sunday morning we were taken to hear Dr Fowstick the fashionable preacher of the day, hold forth at the Presbyterian Church. He was a man who invariably filled it, though his sermon was a direct contradiction to the materialism that I assumed, perhaps unfairly, dominated his audience. His theme was that one must give to the Lord not merely worldly goods but something that involved personal effort. He had the gift of touching an emotional nerve and my response was a decision once I was back in England

'to try to give one evening a week to the W.E.A. It's the only social work that I can do but I could do that.'

Alas the impulse vanished as the memory of his eloquence faded from my mind.

However in the immediate future I was to be given yet another example of the failure of material possessions to bring contentment. We went to lunch with another friend of Miss Gillies, a Mrs Rodgers, who had a house on Park Avenue. I was impressed by the fact that it was equipped with a lift and that Mrs Rodgers employed a butler. Both luxuries she was more than able to gratify as she was a millionairess. The house I described as

'It's a beautiful house in a soft, subdued sort of a way but there was no joy in it. I sort of liked her. She was easy to talk to but Miss G. says she cares for her money above all else. One room downstairs was decorated

with pale green panels and gilt taken from a room of
Marie Antoinette and the furniture was gilt and green
and brocade from the house of the Polignacs. There
was a big green harpsichord and all the statuary in
the room was museum worthy. It was a polite, remote
room, haunted by the memory of powder, paint and
patch of silks and satins and swords and at us, in our
modern garb, it levelled a gentle reproach.'

My final comment on a world with wealth and without the
tempering influence of tradition and responsibility was that

'they live in a different world and between us is a great
gulf fixed which they can hardly cross even if they
wanted to and I'm glad I'm on my side. I guess real
happiness lies in having a congenial job and being able
to earn enough for one's reasonable pleasures.' After
which assessment came the work-a-day postscript 'I
must go to sleep: I have an 8.30 class tomorrow.'

Looking back over the years I have found nothing to make me
change my opinion on the advantages of being a round peg in a
round hole, even if both are of modest size but perhaps, lest such
a judgement appear limited and smug, I should also add the dictum
that 'Though wealth cannot buy happiness it can make you unhappy
in comfort' though even there work can still be a better antidote.

Apart from an occasional shopping spree in New York for
summer clothes or to buy presents as the time for our departure
grew nearer the rest of the term provided little in the way of new
experiences or excitements. As I observed on 23rd February 'It's
difficult to write when every day is pretty much the same' but just
to prove that one should never generalize five days later Vassar had
a very minor earthquake, indeed it was so slight that I did not realise
it was a quake until it was all over. Perhaps my ignorance was due to

the fact that my mother and I were in the lift when it happened and the swaying sensation as if the walls were closing in on one and then relaxing and steadying I put down to the motion of the lift. As we emerged a couple of students rushed onto the landing asking us if we had heard or felt anything. We laughed, saying it must have been the noise of the lift or our feet, when they were joined by two more agitated people, wanting to know what we thought of it. In retrospect I can reconstruct the odd motion but how far this is memory and how far imagination I should not like to say. But if it appeared in the local paper next day I was determined to cut it out and boast of my American earthquake at home. This uneventful term ended on the 28th March when college closed for a brief Easter vacation. Anxious to see as much of America as we could within the geographical limits of our purse and our time, we intended to spend it in Washington and in Richmond where we looked forward to seeing Mary Street, who lived there, once again.

Our time in America was coming to its end; in a little over two months we should be leaving Vassar with its friends and its memories. A couple of days before leaving for Washington I had a letter from Joan in which she enclosed an extract from Philip Gibbs, whose novels by now only older readers will remember, summing up his impression of America. The time was coming when I too, consciously or unconsciously, would try to sort out my impressions and, as a check list, I copied out the extract

*'I regard the people of the U.S.A. as the greatest menace of the world. They are emotional without intelligence. They are a collection of races without being a nation. They mistake abstract idealism for practical morality. They have a tremendous vitality and efficiency and strength undirected by any historical tradition or any conscious purpose except the pursuit of wealth. They are verbally sentimental and professional advocates of liberty but at heart they are intolerant of free thought and action. They scorn the rights of the individual, they have a blind worship of the State and they wish to lay down the laws to the world with a self righteousness that to me is repulsive.'

* PLEASE NOTE: This is the opinion of Philip Gibbs, NOT Dorothy, although she does make her comments further on pages 306 and 307 in contradiction. ED

It is a swingeing and bitter indictment. A cruel mixture of accurate observation and black prejudice and it provided the backdrop to my visit to Washington.

Washington was not as other cities. Like Topsey they had grown unplanned through force of circumstance and human need. Of these I had visited, Boston and Philadelphia were rooted in the English colonial past. The founders of New York were not English but Dutch and geography and economics had turned it into the melting pot for the immigrant hordes that swarmed there. It had energy, vitality, efficiency all devoted to the pursuit of wealth but it had a spirit, an identity and if wealth brought luxury it fostered that broad band of interests known as 'culture' in its libraries and art galleries and to me it was a city in which I felt at home. It was an adjunct to my Vassar world where I went for a day's shopping. Washington was unique. It had been planned as the centre of the newly born independent United States. It was the embodiment of the American dream, a city worthy to give substance to it. As we did all the things that sightseers do unconsciously I was trying to assess how far Washington helped me to understand the America that had created it. With its tree lined vistas and public buildings set in well tended lawns I conceded that it was a beautiful city, attractive and beautiful

> 'but I wonder if it would twine round your heart
> as London does? Anyway it is too young to have
> much soul. It was too like an exhibition, even its very
> beauties emphasised that, the tree lined street, the
> flowering shrubs and the white buildings moulded by
> formal architecture, gave the same impression of a
> planned beauty.'

Parts I thought unfortunate. The approach to the Capitol from the station was a wasteland of vacant plots, unplanned buildings, and cafeterias. The outside of the Capitol, with its dome, floodlit at night, was impressive but my comment on the inside was

'it was gaudy and pretentious. It looks as if they had
tried hard not to be English and had achieved a Roman
Italic Gallic nightmare.'

There were many pictures of historical subjects (all to the greater
glory of America) that seemed to me crude and dull and in places
the walls were frescoed that made them look like a mixture of a
Moorish mosque a la movies and the outside of a musical box of a
roundabout. In the case of the White House too, though I admired
the simple dignity of its exterior I was critical of the famous East
Room which irreverently I said reminded me of the Ballroom of the
Palace at Blackpool. Finally I decided

'that to be perfect at all Washington must be all
perfect, which it wasn't and for its blemishes it hasn't
the excuse of history.'

Two things however, and possibly three, I found as near perfect
as anything made by human hands and designed by human hearts
and minds could be. These were the Lincoln Memorial, the cemetery
at Arlington and, in a minor way, George Washington's old home
Mount Vernon. The Memorial facing a formal oblong lake and built
in marble a gigantic statue of Lincoln, with his deep seer's eyes and
a sense of uncouth power, created for me the atmosphere of an
ancient Greek Temple. It called up the power of the graven image
and the priests of long ago. Here was the soul of America committed
to serve humanity at whatever the cost[1].

The cemetery at Arlington carried the same message. Here in
series ranks of simple headstones were buried those men who had
died in the service of their country and whose bodies could be laid
to rest in its soil. The great memorial amphitheatre framed in dark
Cyprus trees was an utterly satisfying miracle in white and green.
Summing up these two great monuments to the dead I wrote

---

[1] cf. Phillip Gibbs' quote on p305.

'When the Americans do a simple thing they do it with dignity and well but more elaborate things tend to be gaudy. But one should never despair of a nation that could build and love the Lincoln Memorial and Arlington. That I believe is Washington's answer to Philip Gibbs who wrote the truth but not the whole truth when he analysed the United States so clinically.'[1]

The third building to give me a less exalted pleasure was the visit we paid to George Washington's old home, Mount Vernon. Sentimentally it gave me pleasure to be back again in what I affectionately called 'The Old Dominion'. The house itself was charming, an old Virginian mansion, a three storied white house, red roofed and set amid lawns and trim box hedges, It stands high, overlooking the slow moving wide waters of the Potomac. I described it as soul satisfying and peaceful. To me it was a place where happy gentlefolk had lived and nothing less American (in the modern sense of the word) can be imagined than Mount Vernon. The English serenity of its atmosphere made me realise how deeply Washington must have felt his break with the past. I wonder what he would think of the U.S.A. today or whether he would regret it? After visiting the simple church where he used to worship I was driven to declare that 'I never knew a country where its past was so out of joint with its present'. I was soon to dip very happily into that past when we arrived at Richmond late on the afternoon of the 2nd April with the daylight just fading. I loved Virginia and to be back felt like coming home. Our hotel, the Jefferson, had resolutely refused to move out of the Victorian era. The hall is very lofty, at least two stories. It has massive marble pillars festooned with iron grapes and the dining room was adorned with red velvet curtains draped in Victorian fashion. One could imagine stocks, and cut away coats and crinolines better than anything else against such a background. How has it managed to survive. Even the music they played fitted the scene. But then Virginia itself is a survival.

[1] cf. Phillip Gibbs' quote on p305.

Next day Mary Street called for us at eleven and then followed what I called 'a perfectly lovely day'. We drove out to Westover, that almost legendary mansion on the Banks of the James river. The sky was a brilliant blue, making the young green of the trees and lawns even more intense and the old red brick more mellow. It was Virginia's past transfixed in time and because its owners were people of wealth it boasted a tended graciousness that helped to imprint it on our memory. From there we went on to another old house, Shirley, that was built in 1664 and which belonged to Mary's friends the Carews.

Like so many Virginian families the Carews had been all but ruined by the Civil War and now only two old, old sisters remained. Then another of the old colonial families would be lost to history. Once it had been an outpost of defence against the attacks of marauding Indians. It drew from me once again the cry

'I love Virginia and I wish they had won the War
though that is wrong I suppose, seeing that in some
sense slavery was an issue. But they suffered so terribly,
sons, slaves, money all gone and then the years of
bitter humiliation that followed. In many ways they are
the finest stock in America. They would have built up
a different place. Virginia is only just recovering now.
Lincoln's speech that perhaps it was God's will that the
Civil War should go on until all the money piled up by
slave labour was destroyed and all the blood drawn by
the lash was atoned for by the blood spilt by the sword
was literally true of Virginia, whatever it might be for
the North.

'Next day, when Mary came to show us the sights of
Richmond and we came to the house of the Lord
Chief Justice, John Marshall, I began to wonder,
but without much conviction, if I too might claim
a connection with Virginia's past. This was when I

discovered that in 1783 he had married a Mary Willis
Ambler, the daughter of the Treasurer of Virginia and
I was struck by the coincidence that my father's name
was John Willis Marshall. It would have been fun could
we have proved that he married one of our Willis
crowd, apparently they are a bit of a mystery.'

Our next visit was to the White House of the Confederacy where
all the previous relics of Virginia's heroes still speak of the valour and
heartbreak of those war torn years. There was Stonewall Jackson's
coat still sprinkled with the blood of his last wound and J.F.B. Stuarts
rakish hat, full of bullet holes. He was only 21 when he too died.

'It was a temple to a useless sacrifice. They had such
fine faces, almost all of them, and they were so young,
almost all of them and all the agony of the South
shown in plaited straw hats, in wooden soles because
leather was scarce, in old battered grey Confederate
coats riddled with bullets, in homespun grey dresses, in
all the little makeshifts of a stricken country.'

Later, in the sixties when I was lecturing at Wellesley I came to
love New England but in the twenties my loyalty was to Virginia.
America I thought would have been a finer place if it had won.

This jaunt to Washington and Richmond was our last break before
we were due to leave Vassar on the 9th June. I was sad to say goodbye
to dear Mary Street, with her silver rimmed spectacles and ungainly
body made for tweeds. She was such a genuine person and had been
such a kind and stimulating companion. But already my thoughts
were concentrating on the future when I had returned to England.
Vassar had fallen into my lap but this was not likely to happen again
and my prospects were not promising. The academic world was still
a man's world and university posts for women, as women, were few;
only residential tutorships in women's colleges could be regarded

as a female preserve. Only in comparatively few universities had the masculine monopoly been successfully challenged, notably in London and at the LSE. My qualifications were good. Not only had I a Cambridge First but I was about to become one of the early batch of Ph.Ds. I had my viva to face when I returned to England but EEP had told me that it was a mere formality and she even went so far as to speak of being able to find a publisher for it after some reshaping. So already I had started to put in for any likely opening. I was moderately hopeful that I might be considered for a part time post at St Hugh's where I should have to concentrate on medieval history. One great advantage of my Vassar experience was that I had been forced to cover the whole field of European History, but by no stretch of imagination could I claim to be a medievalist as Oxford considered the term. Still it was worth a try. Moreover, though I did have the backing of Eileen Power and Miss Jones, I was marooned in America and not available for interview. So when I got back to Poughkeepsie I was not unduly surprised to find that the St Hugh job was filled and that I was prospectless once again, other attempts having been also abortive.

I do not seem to have been unduly depressed. Spring, which had shown its tentative face in Washington, with its early parade of blossom had arrived with an un-English speed and flourish. The snow had gone and the ice caked earth was free. A sight that I shall never forget was to see the great chunks of ice, almost floes in their massiveness, break up as the thaw released the Hudson from its winter immobility. It was as if a giant hand was suddenly tossing them to and fro as the force of the water took control. Also my summer clothes were a success. I had bought a new grey coat at Altman's a la Princess of Wales and a new grey ribbon hat. It cost 12 dollars 50 and I confessed to being nearly beggared, but I had not been able to resist it; it was so sweet. Moreover I was happy in my work and was beginning to indulge in the euphoria of personal success. Miss Ellery had always been encouraging but now I was getting confirmation from the grass roots. Via my grape vine it was reported to me that

> 'a freshman had said how sorry she was that she had
> put off taking History until next year because Miss
> Marshall would not be here then and she was such a
> good teacher!'

Ah well. One is soon forgotten but it's nice to hear that someone said it. Actually it would have been difficult for me not to know that I was popular with my students. By the time I had settled into the American way of life I was very conscious of the wide differences that separated a Cambridge College and one of the American Ivy League and one of the first of these differences was my relations with my students which had an informality that I had never felt, and indeed never did feel, towards my Girton tutors. I am not sure how much these were influenced by the age factor. Eileen Power was eleven years my senior and Gwladys Jones twenty. The gap between me and my average student was eight or nine years; not I should have thought enough to make a difference in EEP's case. Nor do I seem to remember quite the same lack of formality marking the attitude of my students towards my older colleagues, but that was more a generation gap than an academic one. Frankly I had more at a personal level in common with some of my students than with my older colleagues. They were increasingly my friends as my year at Vassar drew closer to its end.

The manifestation of this took different forms. One that I remember with pleasure was my twenty-fifth birthday. Everything contributed to what I described as

> 'a lovely birthday'. The weather was perfect, 'hot
> enough for cotton dresses and everything smelt of
> spring and the grass is getting green again until I went
> quoting all the time "Bliss was it then to be alive but to
> be young was very heaven." '

- as if I had not already reached the age of twenty-five. I told

312

Anna Jane as I was coming out that it was my birthday as I was feeling conversational and the class had gone well. Mother had organised a small party for me to which I had invited some of my younger friends like Wanda Freaken and Anita Marburg, suddenly I was presented with a huge box of flowers from Anna Jane Philips, 'tulips, wallflowers, daffodils, narcissi and sweet peas. I felt like a movie star'. It was only that morning that I had told her as my last class broke up that it was my birthday and on her way to the station she must have ordered them. I was very touched. There was however, like most things, a less comfortable side to this semi intimate relationship. When a student fell by the wayside and had to be told that she was in danger of failing to make the grade, I found her stricken face devastating and I agonised over poor results.

Here again my Cambridge background made it difficult for me always to be fair. When I had taken my first classes at Vassar I had been depressed by what I, by Cambridge standards, thought their poor performance, fearing that my own might have been to blame. That was before I had realised that the wide differences that separated Girton and Vassar were due to a fundamental difference of outlook. The Cambridge Tripos aimed at high achievement in one or two subjects and lectures and tutoring were focused on this. Everything else that made Cambridge what it was, from the cultural pleasures of the Union or the Marlowe society, the athletic enjoyment of the rugger field or the Cam, tea parties, river picnics, *Vingt en Un* were there to be enjoyed or spurned as a matter of individual choice. Women were forced to aim at excellence. They were only admitted to Girton and Newnham to read Honours. But in the twenties, when apart from scholarships students had to be financed by their families, competition for places was less keen and many managed to pass degrees or, if they read Honours, were undeterred by the fear of getting a Third. American objectives were different. Vassar and its Ivy League set out to give their students an all round education. It was an education for citizenship not scholarship.

Students who aspired to an academic career went on to take a higher degree that, like the Ph.D entailed research. The nearest equivalent to the classification of the Tripos was the five Beta Cappa and even this aimed at all round excellence. Once when Miss Brown, a colleague of mine in the History department, was bewailing the fact that however excellent a girl might be in one subject she could never be capped, another colleague made the crushing remark that 'whoever was not an all rounder was sloppy minded!' My private comment was 'In that case heaven help me: I never excelled in anything but History.' Not only were the aims different, the structure of attainment was different. In Cambridge it was only attainment in the final race that counted. Everything depended on three of our days in May when we sat Part I or Part II. However brilliant the performance in Time Papers in essays made no difference. The full burden of a year's or two years' work had to be unpacked and displayed in a three hour paper or it had no official recognition. To Americans, and indeed to many people, this fixation of examinations as the only deciding factor, would have seemed unfair. American achievement was judged partly on examination and partly on an assessment during the term. Admirable in theory, in practice this put a double load of responsibility on the faculty, namely how to judge written work handed in during the term or contributions made in class. Like Francis Reyburn, it would be possible to write a brilliant, first class essay on Mary Queen of Scots and to know nothing of her son James the First. In other words her knowledge of History could be but a thing of threads and patches. It is not surprising that at times I agonised over my assessments wondering had the mark I had given been fair.

As the academic year moved into its final stages college routine was disrupted by annual events and ceremonies. Americans, I soon discovered, took their traditions with solemnity, possibly because they were so recent. Certainly they loved 'an occasion'. The first to occur was Founders Day in honour of Mathew Vassar. In the morning a singing contest took place, the four years being competitors. Each year wrote and sang an original composition. The best of the four

314

songs was handed down to subsequent years. It was a very un-Girtonian affair

> 'All the girls were dressed in white and each class
> filed into its position on the steps displaying its own
> banner. The seniors wore their gowns and looked very
> composed, the freshmen like a flock of sheep, willing
> and anxious to do what was asked of them but a little
> uncomprehendingly. The sophomores sang with much
> vim. I liked the juniors best but the judges awarded the
> prize to the seniors. We then went in to get our coats,
> being frozen, and went to hear Prezzy make a speech
> about old Mathews from the steps of his house. After
> lunch there was a friendly student baseball match
> and in the evening a performance of Treasure Island
> which was very good. Half the audience were dressed
> as pirates. The next event was the Third Hall play. We
> were frightened that it might rain but it cleared up and
> was warm in the evening. The show started at nine and
> all the chairs were ranged on the steps of the open
> air theatre. The stage was quite dark until lights were
> thrown on it and then it looked lovely with its circle
> of grass and the dark trees beyond. There was a good
> deal of singing, to which the frogs made their own
> contributions and the staging, dresses and grouping
> was most effective.'

By the 23rd May, the day of my last classes, I commented that

> 'The place is full of ceremonies now. The last week
> seems calculated to put the seniors under the greatest
> possible emotional strain before the examinations
> as far as I can see, what with handing down golden
> spades and senior songs and Rocky Steps and last
> songs in chapel etc. They all wore caps and gowns for

the last class today. I am so tired I could sleep for a week.'

With June we were suddenly struck by the heat of summer. We had gone to New York for the day to do some last minute shopping and when we left Poughkeepsie the heat was bearable. But in the pitiless glare of 42nd street I thought Mother would collapse. It seemed to eat you. We ate nothing but salads and crawled back utterly exhausted. It was the first but not the last time that I had to face that terrific New York heat; it is something one never forgets. Next day I was supervising while my students wrote their final history papers. When I had set my Part II examination it had been hot but that heat was bearable when compared with the devastating heat of Poughkeepsie in the summer. My heart bled for the candidates. Goodness knows I thought

> 'how these poor children will fare. It is too hot to think
> coherently and every time you put your hand on the
> paper it sticks. They look so different, hot and with
> their hair scraped back behind their ears.'

I did so hope that my lot would do well. Meanwhile the heat continues to pursue us by night as well as by day. Sleep was almost impossible, though I had pulled my bed under the window and wore only the thinnest of nightgowns. It was a relief to know that term was nearly over. To correct my exam papers was a nightmare until finally I went into the basement of the Library where it was cooler. Considering the conditions in which they had been written the results were what I described as fair to middling. But at least they were done and now only the final end of the year ceremonies remained. Then we would leave for Canada and be homeward bound. The baccalaureate service for the seniors was a gloomy affair. It took place in the chapel

> 'with all the seniors looking like dying ducks in their

black gowns, processing between rows of people. If it had been their own funeral it could not have been slower.'

Next day was the great day of the academic year, Commencement. Luckily it was cooler as I had to wear my rabbit skin for so formal an occasion. The faculty, having been marshalled, walked in line to the chapel, preceded by the seniors, and went to our places in the choir stalls. Then the President gave the address. The theme he chose was Leisure and Study as the two pillars of a liberal education and I think he intended to give a warning that organised leisure, to which American students were prone, and individual leisure were not the same thing. I was not too certain if I understood the implications of what he was saying or whether I read into them my own thoughts, but my reaction was to realise that what made both Oxford and Cambridge what they were was just this combination of Study and the chance to live one's own life. The life of the university was open to all its students, well anyway with some modifications for women in Cambridge, but the students as a body were not organised when out to enjoy themselves. The Pavement Club had been a spontaneous rag, college songs an informal get together, I cannot imagine each year marching in to partake of either. Americans loved occasions; I think Prizzy was telling them not to mistake the wood for the trees.

The speech over the students went up to receive their diplomas. It was very dull and not a bit impressive and I was rather disappointed. Having got out of my rabbit skin and gown we then assembled for the Trustees Lunch which took place in Main. It was a good lunch, which was some compensation but I decided that

> 'we paid for it by listening to three dull speeches,
> sandwiched between delightful interludes by Prezzy.'

Then I slipped away, it was a quiet farewell to Vassar, and joined my mother to catch the 8.16 train to New York, where we got the train for Canada. By now we had become accustomed to spending a night on the train and having changed at Buffalo, where we had breakfast, and having crossed the long bridge that connected the States with Canada, we had our first view of Niagara Falls.

Our American year was over. It had been for me a most enjoyable year, and for my mother, like the curate's egg, good in parts. She had enjoyed our vacation trips and our visits to New York, and she had become very friendly with some of my younger colleagues, particularly Wanda Freaken, soon to become Mrs Neff. We had watched the budding romance and the Neffs continued to be our friends when we returned to England where they in turn visited us. To me the experience had been most valuable. It had given me self confidence, not to say a swollen head, and in a friendly atmosphere I had learned the elements of my craft. I knew how to plan a lecture, correct an essay and handle students. Only later did I realise how valuable this propagating year had been. I was not by nature self confident and had I been faced with unresponsive students, or indifferent colleagues, or, even worse unruly pupils I might never have blossomed at all.

Dear Vassar. I owe you much. I had come to America with the memory of my first May Week, of Mr Martin, my partner at the Girton Ball, and of Sherry and Lathrop who had paddled Elspeth and me lazily up to Granchester in the sunlight and brought us back as the shadows had begun to fall, and for their sake I had been prepared to like their country. And yet, in spite of my initial feeling for America and all the kindness that I had met there, I left almost without regret. This surprised me. I had made such good friends, whom I should never see again, favourite students, whose work I had seen grow, of whom I was fond and of whom I still think with affection. Francis Reyburn and Polly Butcher and Anna Jane Philips. If my reminiscences should ever fall into their hands, though they too will be old ladies now, it would give me much pleasure to hear from them. And yet, ungrateful as it seemed, we both left with a sense of relief at getting away from something alien. Nationality and kinship is a strange emotion that goes very deep and bypasses both approval and disapproval. I remembered that when I threatened to wear a Union Jack pinned onto my sleeve for Empire Day I was told

'If you do you must wear an American flag too or you will be suspected by the Loyalty League'. 'No I won't' said I 'Or if I do I'll wear it with a bar sinister.'

Alas they did not even see the joke. More than once when it came to Anglo-American History I found I had to tread carefully. I was lucky not to be lynched when once in class a student asked me 'What do the English think about the War of 1812?' and I looked at her blankly. My mind being full of Napoleon and the retreat from Moscow I had completely forgotten that owing to a little misunderstanding we had drifted into hostilities with the United States and had burnt down the White House. So when I asked, in all innocence 'What War?' I realised that between us was a great gulf fixed.

Canada was different, we shared a King. In Toronto, when we went on a conducted tour round the Parliament house our little guide was magnificently Canadian. He treated the party, who were mostly American, with 'a you can't beat that in your rotten old States air' and the way in which he said 'Gentlemen remove your hats' when we went into the Chamber. There was only one fly in the ointment; it made my blood boil to be taken as a Yankee.

My last American memory was of the old river boat that leaving Toronto took us past the Islands and through the rapids of the St Lawrence, in itself a link with the past and worth recalling. We shall not look upon their like again. On the other hand our reaction to the power and magnificence of the Falls is shared by what now must amount to millions of tourists and is therefore irrelevant. Briefly we returned for the last time to American soil, to board our steamer at Lewis. It was a final goodbye when we boarded *S.S. Caragyer* for the first stage of our journey home. I described her as a darling ship, clean and ship-shape and once again we experienced that sense of belonging at being under the British flag once more. After the strain of the last weeks, culminating in our concentrated last minute sightseeing it was bliss just to sit on the deck at leisure at last while slowly the land faded away across the vastness of Lake Ontario. Next day, after a stop over of some three hours in Toronto, we seemed to be sailing over a softly jewelled sea of amethyst and amber as the sun disappeared into the shadow of night. Next day we threaded our peaceful path through the Thousand Islands that dotted the St Lawrence. Then peace and dignity vanished. We had to leave our 'darling boat' for a beastly little tug called the *Rapid's Prince* that was crowded with an American men's fraternity, a side of American social life that hitherto I had been spared. They horrified me and with venom I described them as

> 'horrid materialistic brutes who roared comic songs at one another in the over crowded dining saloon – ugh! Women unrelieved may be pretty dull but men in groups are loathsome, unless they are Varsity men and have learnt to shield that side from the public view.'

The boat was small and men swarmed everywhere, playing poker with huge piles of bills around them in the cabin. There was no room to walk on deck and we had to have lunch at 11.30. Historically maybe this disgust and discomfort was a small price to pay for an experience now denied to posterity that of shooting the rapids in a river boat. It was something to remember. For some time the water had been uneasy, with round smooth centres and funny little soft dimples surrounded by whirls. Then suddenly we saw a line of white breakers tumbling over each other like a sea. As the ship struck them I could feel her tremble as the water seemed to seize her hull and twist it towards the shore. We dipped and quivered but steam being stronger than water got safely through. That hazard surmounted, we sailed past an Iroquois Indian Reservation where I was disappointed to see that its inhabitants, though fishing from their traditional canoes, were wearing European dress. 'The age of standardisation' I moaned. The more formidable Larachine Rapids were still to come and we were in some danger of missing them. Having been fasting since our early lunch Mother suddenly discovered that it was possible to get a cup of tea in the saloon below. Declaring that 'a cup of tea was worth all the rapids in the world' she devoured a cheese sandwich, but luckily, like Drake, it proved possible to have her tea and see the rapids too. It would have been a shame to have missed such

> 'wicked looking things, white capped with a deep
> treacherous sucking movement that showed for a
> moment deep hidden brown fanged rocks that seemed
> almost under the ship itself.'

Then the moment of danger was over and soon we disembarked at Montreal where we transferred to *S.S. Sagneny* sailing through the night towards Quebec. The ship was spacious and uncluttered and peace returned as we strolled the decks, had dinner and went to our cabin. The American venture was over. When we docked at French speaking Quebec Europe reclaimed us. Here the Atlantic had culturally disappeared over night. After a few wonderful days, staying at the Chateau Fontenac in luxury and soaking up the atmosphere of Quebec, we sailed on *The Melita* for home. There in our cabin, like a gracious memory that blotted out that of the 'Materialist brutes' of the Rapid's Prince, I found flowers with love from Anna Jane and I was touched by this last farewell. At least I was not yet forgotten. I wonder if, as I remember her, she still has some lingering thoughts of me?

When I returned to England the second chapter of my academic life had been completed. What the third would contain I had no idea. I had returned without prospects and without a job at a time when these were hard to find. Also, though EEP had been reassuring I still had to face my viva before I could become Dr Marshall. All that I had was my Cambridge First and a year's experience as a junior lecturer and, because I had not got back until the end of June, and so had not been available for interview, the best posts in prestigious schools like Wycombe Abbey, where I might have found a permanent niche in 1924, had been filled. What I felt was my best asset was the fact that Miss Jones, who had given me a wonderful testimonial was doing her best to get me placed. My diary is imprecise, there are vague illusions to Alexandra College and others that indicate the possibility of an appointment for one term in Dublin, whether that and Alexandra college were the same or two different probabilities my memory is too hazy for me to be sure. In any case it is immaterial; I went to neither. Fate again had an expected card to play, though I was inclined to rate it no higher than the knave, not even of hearts or diamonds, maybe of Clubs, the most undramatised of the four. But at least my appointment had the suddenness of surprise.

Because I was pretty desperate and did not want to be a financial burden on my mother I had applied for various teaching posts, one of which was for a History teacher at the Reigate County School for Girls and, rather to my surprise, on the 9th July I had received a letter from the headmistress asking me to let her have more information. While not expecting to be offered the vacancy nevertheless I was full of uncertainty as to whether I should accept it if I were, or whether I would wait and hope that one of the other possibilities materialised. I rather favoured the idea of Dublin but my Irish History was very sketchy and the syllabus laid great emphasis on this. My mother was more in favour of Reigate. Things moved rapidly. On Saturday, while I was alone in the house, I heard the phone ring and went to answer it. It was a wire phoned through to save the telegram boy cycling over five miles to deliver it. Starkly I received the message 'Offer you the History post at Reigate' followed the request for an immediate reply. There was no time to think and almost automatically I wired my acceptance and then had cold feet, hoping I had done the right thing. At least I had landed a job and on further consideration decided that I was lucky to have got one so near London. At least I could hope to renew my connection with LSE and in particular with Smellie. It was at least reassuring that a few days later I got what I described as a nice letter from the Head, Miss Jean Aitkin, though the fly in the ointment was that my term would start on the 10th September and that meant leaving Old Hutton on the 8th. It was certainly a new world and I was not looking forward to it. My school days at Preston seemed a very long time ago and my class room memories were dim. But, assuming that all schools were like the Preston Park and all headmistresses were the same calibre as Stoney, both of which assumptions were very wide of the mark, I thought I could manage. Though after Vassar I was not enthusiastic.

The more immediate milestone was to get my viva safely over, so that I could use my new title to impress my world. It was to take place in Cambridge and I had arranged to stay at Girton. To return was to see my American year in perspective and my reactions are, I think, worth quoting

> 'There is something very sane about Girton, no Vassar
> hysteria. There was a welcome of course but one
> would have to be a very big whale to disturb that pond.
> This is the place from which so many clever women
> had come that not to have done something would have
> been an exceptional matter for wonder rather than to
> have achieved something in life. One sinks into one's
> right position after America, even if one misses the
> fun a bit.'

At least I had the gratification of both EEP and Miss Jones admiring my American clothes. During my stay at Girton I revived a very old link indeed with my own school days. When I used to travel from Thornton station to Preston I was joined by a member of the junior school Ellen Parkinson, five years my junior. Each day we walked that dreary mile through Preston's streets in the morning and back again at night. She had become very much my satellite, as children do, and in 1923 had come up to Girton to read Geography.

In 1926 she was in her last year and we had a long gossipy tea together. Later she went to work in Canada and married a Professor at Toronto, so I lost touch with her. I also had a visit from Margaret James, who like Ellen had come up in 1923 and whose college career had closely resembled my own. She held the Cairns scholarship from 1924-5 and the Old Girtonian from 1925-6 and intended to present herself for a Ph.D in London. I was not over pleased to have another Girton Ph.D treading on my heels and wrote

> 'It's going to be terribly common and some of us will
> have to clear out for there won't be enough posts in
> England to go round.'

My prophecy was to be fulfilled, though not in the immediate future. Today Ph.Ds are almost two a penny and the academic world is flooded with thesis written only too often because a Ph.D is now almost a *sine qua non* for university posts. But at least I belonged to an early edition; my viva posed no problem and in 1926 I became Dr Dorothy Marshall. Then in 1984, to my intense pleasure, the University of Lancaster made me one of their H.N.D.Litt. a distinction I had never expected, which meant that in the academic world I had arrived.

But in 1926 a Ph.D was still something special. Had it not been, and had Miss Aitkin not thought it would look well on a prospectus, I should never had been appointed, for I was indeed, as far as teaching was concerned, a pig in a poke and a reluctant pig at that! It would be a complete break with my academic past. On my last brief visit to Girton I had written nostalgically

> 'If one has any love for learning at all the life of a
> Girton student is most pleasant; just to have the day
> all one's own, a decent room and at the end a hot
> bath and cocoa. I hope I am like the Girton type for
> they are so delightful, such a relief after Vassar, and I

want to drink it all in. They are so unaffected in their friendliness and healthy and well turned out in a quiet way and so restful in their minds and conversation. I am awfully glad I came back, if only to get a grip on myself again and realise what are the things that really count.'

My reference to Vassar is, on the face of it, base ingratitude. I had been happy there and it had given me much for which to be thankful. But coming back to Girton with its tradition of understatement must have been in sharp contrast to the more vivid way of life that characterised Vassar, where on the surface everything was sweetness and light and a desire to please that papered over cracks, so that I had come back with the feeling that I was a very special person. Certainly I was going to need to take a grip on myself in the immediate future. Today no Headmistress would appoint a woman utterly without training or experience to take charge of a subject throughout her school. Miss Aitkin had been bewitched by that Ph.D and I was thrown in at the deep end without the slightest idea of how to swim. At the end of my first term the verdict was

'Though I don't exactly loathe it I don't like it or do it very well. I hope to get out before too long.'

My trouble was that though I was a born teacher in the making I was not a born disciplinarian and Miss Aitkin was not Miss Stoneman. Had the school been under her iron control I should have had no difficulties but Miss Aitkin, never quite succeeded in imposing herself on the school. In her presence the pupils were respectful but in her absence discipline was lax. As a consequence the upper Fourth made my life a misery for the first term. Actually they were a nice bunch of children but at first I hadn't a clue as to how to control them and the little wretches knew it. What made my life even tolerable was that I taught English, Religious Knowledge and History to the Upper Seconds and from the beginning we liked one another.

Religious knowledge, a subject I had never been taught to teach, I turned into concentrating on St Paul's journeys with the religion left out, so that they made a lively travelogue. For Medieval History I discoursed on the latest views on King John and explained the writs of Henry II which they took in their stride. The Lower Third, which seemed to be composed of the dregs of the school, reduced me more than once to tears and I could do nothing with them. But my victory over the Upper Fourth I consider the moral highlight of my teaching career. Occasionally they would listen and behave but generally they played me up until at last I took a leaf out of my own History mistress at the Park, and decided that I would take no notice of their behaviour but, whether they listened or not, would continue with whatever I wanted to say. Oddly it worked. If I took no notice of them there was no point in their taking none of me, so they began to listen and be interested. Moreover I began to establish some personal relationships. At that time the contemporary hobby was autograph albums and I was duly asked to write in these. My talent for doggerel came in useful, writing in one, if I can remember it correctly

'Oh Phyllis of the Fourth Form

What can I say to you?

Though you say you like your History,

Then how explain the mystery,

Of all the hum and chatter,

If I should for any matter,

Take my eye off you?'

My triumph was that in my second year that once unruly crowd, now promoted to the Fifth Form, became my form, Miss Aitkin telling me that I was one of the few teachers who could control them.

326

So I became a successful teacher but it was an exhausting business to hold the attention of lively school girls, whatever their age, and I could never relax while Miss Burchell, who became my junior history mistress in my second term, had only to say 'Quiet girls' and the little brutes were silent. Later she became the redoubtable Head of Camden High where she did a magnificent job. For the most part we had a pleasant staff and I suppose I was not unhappy once I got on top of my early incompetence but the horizon of my life during term was very limited and I knew that school mistressing was not for me. So dull I found my life at Reigate County School at the end of my first year, that I declared myself ready to flirt with the curate! Could life be less exciting? I was trapped until once again fate played an unexpected card, though I must admit that I had done my best to shuffle the pack.

CHAPTER TWELVE: WITWATERSRAND AND SOUTH AFRICA.

This is the chapter that was lost, the loss of which so disheartened my aunt, Dr. Dorothy Marshall, that she never completed her memoirs. Indeed it was not until after she had died and after all her papers had been lodged at Girton College Cambridge, that the archivist, Miss Kate Perry, found them. Even now there are gaps which I will point out as we proceed through this chapter.

It is sad that this is the chapter so badly damaged, as it is the highlight of her academic experiences in the twenties, which so influenced the rest of her life. It was also the time when she learned about the evils of racism. I don't think she ever forgot the hurt she caused a gentle kind and considerate Jewish family who had befriended her. This unworldly 26-year-old, with her mother in tow, was venturing into the unknown academic world of South Africa at a time when the affects of the Boer War were still keenly felt. The hurt was caused by a gaffe and loose language. Even in today's enlightenment such gaffes occur, and I only hope we learn our lessons as well.

From the advantage of the 21ˢᵗ century, we can look back in this chapter to see how racism, anti-Semitism, and apartheid grew. We can witness the growth of fascism. Hitler, Mussolini, and the incidents leading to the imprisonment of Nelson Mandela, and the horrors caused by apartheid. In this we are privileged and the insights such as described here help us to do this.

ED

Of my three experiences of academic life in the twenties my year at the university of the Witwatersrand is the most difficult to analyse and describe. Like Caesar's Gaul the South African scene, or at least my impression of it, is divided into three parts. The difficulty is to combine them so as to produce a well-balanced and authentic picture. Within the frame has to be fitted three main subjects, the South African background, a society divided by racial tensions, and my day to day life in the university. In the composition of the picture the country itself may be said to provide the background, the society of which I was both an observer and a part, the middle distance, and my life in the academic world, a rather uninteresting foreground. My difficulty is to portray the relations between these three and at the same time to fit together the detail that illuminates the whole. Since the background determines the light and shade that determines the subject as a whole it seems sensible to begin with the African scene as I first observed it when we landed from the *Caernarvan Castle* on the 18ᵗʰ July 1926. Though it attracts more attention today than when I visited it, it is not a country to which the British short stay tourists flock in their hundreds as of late they have gone to America. The British who come to South Africa are people who come for a purpose, to stay with members of their family now settled there or to engage in business concerns or as politicians and journalists coming to comment and observe. Tourists find the prospect of a safari in Kenya, observing wildlife more tempting venues. Most Britons tend to form their views on South Africa if they have any views at all via the media and the picture they produce deals only with the more dramatic aspects of its troubled society. As Oscar Wilde observed 'The truth is rarely pure and never simple.'

330

We docked about 6 am and unlike our arrival at New York, both Customs and Immigration people were friendly and polite, so soon we were sightseeing, as until the *Caernarvan Castle* left port we were allowed to use her as a hotel. Here are my first impressions. Cape Town itself I described as

> 'a little shabby and dingy and nondescript in the
> shopping part the location at the foot of the mountain
> is lovely with the bay like a silver and opal carpet
> spread out before it. The sun was very bright and as
> we walked up the avenue, with Table Mountain in
> front of us and the white buildings set in the trees, the
> whole effect was so brilliant and soft and warm that
> one could hardly realise it existed. Along the shore the
> water was a soft blue, except where the waves broke
> in a quivering line of jade and opal, and dissolved
> in spray like the soft smile of some Eastern beauty
> hidden behind her veil of lace.'

Already the magic of the sunshine, of which later I was to get so tired of, longing for the coming of the rains, so that I wrote,

> 'One can hardly describe the effect of the sun here.
> It makes one feel that South Africa is going to be
> worthwhile after all.'

Next day we entrained for the long journey to Johannesburg. Our carriage was shabby but comfortable; my mother was depressed at the idea of a 39-hour journey, but cheered up when she found she could be served with tea. Later we had a very good dinner and I recorded happily that the wine was only 1s/6d (9p) for a half bottle. Once again the beauty of South Africa delighted us as the train journey through

> 'long stretches of bush and scrub with arum lilies
> growing wild and masses of vivid green low growing

331

bushes. Behind the mountains, very bare and serrated, soared cleanly into the sky and the sun pervaded everywhere with its brightness. Here and there were white farm houses and cultivated fields, but the Kaffir huts were little better than cattle shelters and always an eyesore.'

It was my first comment on their existence; they were sordid blot on a beautiful landscape. Next morning we saw a very different Africa, an Africa cruel and stark, as we travelled through the drought stricken Karoo. It was unspeakably desolate. There had been no rain for two years and the land I described as having been scorched into aridity.

'The hills were gaunt bony structures like the ribs of a half starved world breaking through the skin of dry brown earth. There was nothing green, except some shrubs still were tinged with a paint greenish grey, but most of them are shrivelled up. Sometimes huge boulders and stones lie scattered about, as if the gods had played at destruction and suddenly, growing weary, had gone away. Just here and there were a few patches still green where settlements had grown up around water holes. It's a heart breaking sight, and makes one pray for rain even though no-one one knows is involved.'

Had I had the gift of foresight I should have known that my brother, now farming in Rhodesia, was himself a victim of a drought that destroyed his budding attempt to carve out a farm for himself. That was in the future. Now we were looking forward to his being on the station to greet us as he had travelled down to Jo'bugh to spend a few days there and see us settled in.

For the first few days until we could find more permanent quarters,

332

we stayed at the Langham Hotel. From the first I was not impressed with Johannesburg. It was crude old makeshift and half finished, or so it seemed to me. Even the station suggested improvisation with its galvanised roofing. The general impression was messy, and the shops I considered only so-so. I concluded:

'I don't think there will be anything to do here.'

When we finally moved to a guest-house near the university I had another shock. Parkville, our highly respectable suburb, like Girton in my first year, had no modern sanitation. Indeed Raymond Lodge was worse. The earth privies were outside and I was never quite reconciled to them! Each night a long line of bullock carts with their red lamps swinging could be seen making their stately progress to remove the night soil.

The terrain made draining difficult and Johannesburg for all its wealth had not got round to supplying the necessary facilities everywhere. It still bore the marks of a mining mushroom town. Forty years ago with the opening up of the Witwatersrand, and after the opening up proclamation for gold mining, and the mad gold rush, that what had once been almost barren and sparsely populated veldt became a mass of thriving activity. Coal also was discovered near at hand, with which to supply the necessary fuel, and the prospectors and investors flocked in, avid to make their fortunes. Everything had to be improvised at once, housing for the influx of people, transport to feed them and to carry away their precious gold. That was in 1886. It was no wonder that in 1926 the railway station was still roofed by corrugated iron. It was a miracle that the community it served had been so swiftly created.

Since my only reason for being in Johannesburg was supplied by the university, it seemed logical to block in my foreground, at least in outline, leaving that detail to be added later. My new professor, William MacMillan, called to take me to the university. Later I grew fond of him and nicknamed him to myself 'Pinky' because of his reddish hair, but at first I found him pleasant but almost nervous in manner with none of that warmth that had greeted my arrival at Vassar. There would be no red carpet here for an, English visiting lecturer from England. Indeed I almost got the impression that since I was here he hoped that I would cause him no trouble. Looking back I am sure I wronged him: he was nervous and uncertain how to treat me. My first impressions of the university were that

> 'the main building is nice but it's all new, yet crude and unfinished.'

I had a nasty shock when I discovered how meagre the resources of the library were which I judged to be not much more than a sixth of the Stanley Library in size at Girton. Once again there was to be no repetition of Vassar.

When I had gone to America I had taken with me almost a cabin trunk full of books, only to be greeted by a magnificent library where the difficulty was choice, not scarcity. When I came to the Witwatersrand I was determined not to be caught in that trap again. I wasn't! This time I had no private supplies on which to fall back. Luckily I had brought some of my old Cambridge notes to cover the subjects on which I had expected to lecture and these, combined with such standards as the library possessed, had to suffice. At least I had a study of my own a room at the top of the building. This as soon as possible mother and I set about making habitable in a civilised way. We bought pretty green curtains for the window and the wherewithal to do a little modest entertaining.

> 'We bought some delightful odd cups, a yellow one, a black one and a mixed one for 2s/6d (25p), plates to match and a big one and a teapot. I shall be so elegant.'

That at least was Girton and Vassar over again and so equipped I was ready to face my new world.

For me the Witwatersrand was a new experience in that before I had lived over the shop; I had been in residence. Now my room had become merely my office and the lecture rooms my workplace. Here I arrived at stated hours to do a stated job and that done I could go home. It made a most enormous difference. I now lived two lives, my professional life and my personal life and the overlap could be as generous or as limited as I chose. At Girton and at Vassar I had been part of a community, at the Witwatersrand I was part of an institution. The effect on my relations with my colleagues and my students was to limit both, but particularly those with my students. This is apparent as I turn over the pages of my diary. For the most part they remained a row of faces though tutorials in my room were slightly more human. There, as I began to feel more at home sometimes I produced my elegant china and biscuits adorned the large plate. Over the years I became more and more convinced that tea and biscuits were great looseners of tongues. As lecturers became human so did one's fellow students. But in Jo'burg though coachings and tutorials became less formal it is significant that, unlike the diaries that I kept at Vassar, in my South African ones there is rarely the mention of an individual student's name. There are no Mary Jane Phillips no Francais Reyburns. With my colleagues my 'cup of tea' routine was more humanising, particularly with MacMillian and later, when John Hicks came out to fill an emergency vacancy. Both increasingly dropped in, stayed for an elevens and a chat. It was time wasting but pleasant and I began to feel less of an outsider.

On the 28th July I gave my first lecture. My reaction was

> 'It's rather an inhuman job but I found my voice all
> right, though I nearly got through too soon and when
> I talked about sovereignty I could feel that they felt
> quite blank.'

I had a more varied schedule with which to cope at the Witwatersrand than had faced me at Vassar, where I dealt only with

European History. Here during my first term my main course was constitutional, so once again it was a matter of keeping one step ahead of the class. One advantage of the Cambridge History syllabus was that it left us with a wide, if rather outline, picture. Specialisation was expected to take place later but at least we knew where the pieces fitted and what authorities to read to fill up the outlines. Hence my involvement with sovereignty. My second class that day, a small group of four, was less of a strain in that I was on familiar ground, eighteenth century European. My impression was that

> 'two of them will be nice and jolly the other two grimly earnest. One man, Noble by name, complained that one could get so few details about Joseph II, which having discovered the extent of the university library I could well understand but felt like telling him that he ought to be grateful. Still I think I shall manage quite nicely.'

Next day I reported

> 'I am correcting some of MacMillian's papers. Of course they are only half way through their first year but they are pretty bad. The Vassar standard was better. I am glad I have not taught them, still mine may be no better.'

Having completed their exam papers I decided that only two were really good. Unlike Cambridge and Vassar I was committed to taking evening classes specially provided for students who could not attend during the day. They at least were eager to learn and I felt more at ease with them though still apprehensive at the prospect of having to drag my day time group through the mysteries of sovereignty. However by the beginning of August I was generally more cheerful writing

> 'I am finding my lectures easier, perhaps because I am on more concrete ground now, the Farm Acts.

MacMillian after leaving me alone for most of the week was quite chatty today and Leifelt asked me to go to a dramatic society. If I can arrange about getting home it will be rather fun. On the whole I am settling down better but I felt very empty at first. Among my new colleagues is a Miss DuPlessis from the Philosophy Department.'

By now we were also installed in our temporary Johannesburg home. This was Raymond Lodge, a pleasant guest-house conveniently situated both for the university and near a tram that ran into the centre of the town and was our lifeline. A Mrs Sinclair kept the Lodge, which was approached by a long garden that sloped down to the road. I suppose that someone from the university must have recommended it to us. It was clean, reasonably comfortable and inexpensive. We paid ten guineas (£10.50) a month, for which we got a double bedroom, plain but well cooked food and rather restricted public rooms, a dining room, a lounge and the inevitable and invaluable stoep or roofed balcony that fronted the house. The company ranged from the middle aged to the youthful. They were a pleasant enough group. Two of the youngest members were a good looking youth called Hutchinson, popularly known as Hutch, and a chap called Malan. William liked the latter but remarked that 'Hutch made him feel sorry for Owen Nares', the matinee idol of the theatre going world. During the months to come his various romantic attachments provided me with a continued saga but at least he was intelligent, and he and Malan between them did something to redeem the Philistine atmosphere of Raymond Lodge. It also provided me with a window on the average attitude of the average Jo'burger towards the society of which he was a part At least mother was not lonely, as often she had been at Vassar because here we shared a common background. but she was most dreadfully bored.

I was correct in the assumption that both intellectually and culturally this would be a dull place in which to spend a year. Such public entertainment as was available we patronised which in practice meant regular visits to the cinema and to the theatre when anything worth seeing was on. We even on occasions went to the Cabaret at the Carlton, but that was when William was with us at Raymond Lodge. Our chief refuge from an evening spent at Raymond Lodge was the cinema, which varied from the sometimes good to the frankly awful – as witness this entry;

> 'We went to the world's worst picture tonight. It was called *A Window in Piccadilly*. Sickidilly would have been more appropriate.'

However there were many good movies for the film industry was flourishing and the best as well as the worst films came to Jo'burg. One evening when I had not really wanted to turn out to see *The Eagle of the Sea* as I was tired, but poor mother was so bored that I went and was rewarded by a really good blood and thunder. I quite lost my heart to Riccardo Cortez as the pirate Jean Lafitte. Another star who redeemed an otherwise poor film was Ronald Coleman, always a favourite of mine. There were some great films too like *The 49th Parallel* that I would have been sorry to have missed. The theatre also put on some good shows. For instance I much approved the production of *Trilby* but the star event was a visit of Sybil Thorndyke in *The Lie*. Condescendingly I remarked she really is fine and I rather like Lewis Casson.

The university also made a spasmodic contribution to the drama. Soon after our arrival

> 'we went to *The Clouds* by the university dramatic society. The scenery was quite good and so was music, while the lead was excellent, could not have been better, but the rest did not compare favourably with Cambridge.'

Throughout the year there were other performances, not all of them full length plays. On one evening the menu was for four short plays;

> 'Two were by Susan Gasfelt which were very smart.
> Wynne was very winish but quite good and so to my
> surprise was W.G. Murray.'

It is perhaps symptomatic of the little impression most of the people I met at the Witwatersrand made on me but in some connection I described Wynne as 'an engaging youth' which rather suggests that he was a student. Later he asked us to a performance of *The Madras House* given by the dramatic circle.

> 'They put up a jolly good show in spite of the
> difficulties and Wynne was really quite good. That is
> where his heart lies. He's really quite decent looking.'

There must have been college societies of a more intellectual kind. We certainly went to a meeting of the Philosophy Society but that was because Professor Haaroff was speaking and by now both my mother and I were on friendly terms with them. It was a relief to get away from both Raymond Lodge and the university when they asked us, which increasingly happened to tea. It was through my friendship with Theo that I got some insight into the African point of view. No one could have been nicer or kinder or more honest a person and he remained a significant piece in my efforts to sort out the jigsaw of the problems of a divided society. To be fair to the intellectual side of the university there were the usual crop of invited distinguished speakers. On one occasion I heard Smuts himself lecture on Evolution and Holism but alas it was one of those evenings when I was tired and great man though he was he made little impression on me.

One side effect of the lack of both mental stimulation and of a wide choice of books from which to choose was in desperation I started to tackle the Russian novelists my criticism of which reflected naïvety of my literary appreciation. My reaction to Dostoevsky after having read *The Brothers Kamanazov* was that the author would have been more aptly called 'Dot-and-of-fsky because he won't stick to the point. One gets to an interesting climax and then suddenly is confronted by 50 pages on the existence of God.' I fared better with Tolstoy having taken *War and Peace* with me to read while on my Christmas vacation at the Cape chosen because it seemed to be the fattest book in the library shelves and that it would last longer.

After reading Helen Waddel's *Holoise and Ablard* I came to the conclusion that

> 'on the whole I do not think grand love affairs are
> worthwhile. For a little feverish ecstasy one gets
> nothing but trouble ever after.'

After two such disclosures of my standard of literary criticism how fortunate it was that I read History and not English at Girton! Not all my criticism reactions were so personal. After reading *The Mummer's Wife* I wrote

> 'There is no doubt that Moore is sordid but he does
> write well and certainly gets the effects he wants.'

Perhaps among my strictures on the Witwatersrand and Jo'burg I ought to be grateful that for the first time in my life I had the time to read widely and to be able to digest what I read.

My frantic search for leisure reading heralded the end of term and the beginning of the long Christmas vacation. This we had decided to spend not in Cape Town itself but in the neighbouring small sea resort of Fishock. As there was no friendly Prinny to organise our holiday; we were determined to get away from Johannesburg and the Rand. We had liked the little we had seen of Cape Town and its environment when we had landed. Fishock, unlike Muzenburg was a small place of sea and sandy beach, more to our taste and pocket while being in easy reach of Cape Town. We took up our quarters in what I described as being

340

'quite a nice hotel though the other guests do not seem very thrilling, but there is a big lounge and stoep.'

On the 4th January, after we had settled in I decided,

> 'I really think we are going to like Fishock. It has a long bay, almost horseshoe shaped to itself, which gives it a snug air of privacy between the towering hills. The slopes of the mountain run on both sides On the lower slopes the houses perch, white and gleaming and covered with brilliant creepers or surrounded by gaudy rock gardens. The atmosphere and setting reminds me a little of Como, or anyhow of Italy. It's all so much more peaceful and secure than Jo'burg. This evening we went down for a walk, and it was new life to feel the space of sea and mountains and solitude to move in.'

Fishock had other merits in my eyes. It was perfect for bathing and to my joy, being no swimmer despite the efforts of my Girton friends, the sea 'kept my legs up in a most satisfactory way.' We explored the vicinity, going one day to Simons Town, then still a British naval base and, out of curiosity to Muzenburg, which I hated I found it 'cheap and flashy and boarding-housey with the spirit of Jo'burg transported to the sea'.

During our stay at Fishock we contrived to see much of the Cape with its lovely scenery as well as exploring Cape Town itself. The pages of my diary are full of the magnificence of the one and the charm of the other which has given me much pleasure to re-read. But our finances for such delights were limited as we were husbanding them so that we could also visit the Wilderness, renowned for its beauty and then sail up the coast as far as Durban. So there were many days when walking as far as Kalk Bay or bathing had to suffice and I was apt to moan

'I wish there were a little more to do here. I am
inclined to get too restless just hanging about though it
is very lovely. But I can't just bathe and read and sleep.'

On the 6th February we said goodbye to Fishock and to Cape
Town and, alas, to my brother William who had been with us and
was now waiting for a passage to Australia. A prolonged drought
had scorched his farm and killed his cattle, so that there was nothing
left of his gallant effort to own his own farm. As we should not
be returning to England until later in 1928 he decided to see what
Australia had to offer but his intention was to return to England and
look for a farm there, now that the threat of lung trouble was no
more. Looking back with hindsight I am thankful for that early, heart
breaking disaster. Otherwise he would have settled in South Africa or
in Rhodesia. his farm had been in an enclave between the two race
dominated countries. Yet who can tell? He might still have been alive
had he not volunteered for the RAF and been shot down as an air
gunner. But at least between his returning to England and his death
stretched many happy years.

As it is certainly not my intention to write a travel book I shall
not attempt to describe the beauty of the Wilderness, nor our voyage
after we had boarded the *Durham Castle* for Durban. In the end we did
not disembark there, deciding to suffer the discomfort of re-coaling
there and so stretch our finances to go on to Lorenzo Marques and
then catch a train back to Jo'burg and work.

For me the voyage, short as it was, was another milestone in
my own voyage through life On our first day on board one of the
passengers, I called him Holly an abbreviation of his name, started
to attach himself to me. He asked to play deck tennis and, having
survived my efforts, we danced together and later strolled round the
darkened deck at night. This became our routine and I purred into
my diary

'It's nice having a man of one's own on board. You need it.'

A sentiment which I feel most young women would echo. The moon that turns the glittering wake into silver, the starlight darkened sky and the steady throb of the engine, even without an attendant swain is pure magic. Ours was more than a flirtation, certainly on his part but hardly a love affair, though had it been longer, who knows? Certainly not I. When at Lorenzo Marques we said goodbye in the moonlit garden of the hotel where mother and I spent our last night, Holly kissed me. It was the kind of kiss I had never met before, a lover's kiss. Then, because he was no philanderer, abruptly he took me back to my mother waiting in the lounge. That was the end of Holly, though I wrote to him while I was in South Africa. But for me it was the beginning of my own comprehension that sex and my airy-fairy dreams of Pryor were different things. A man, an attractive man, an older man had found me desirable and my self-esteem began to blossom. Dear Holly, I owe you much.

We returned to Jo'burg as children return to school; our holiday was over The night before my first lecture I wrote 'I hate starting but I expect it will be alright.' The following entry was more cheerful, comforting myself with the fact that,

> 'it really was not so bad on the whole. I had cold feet but did not feel quite so much of a dithering idiot as when I began. At least I believe in the value of the subject that I teach.'

A few nights later I summed up the situation by writing

> 'if teachers of History took their work seriously it would wear us out but it might do something. I must try to get over the fact that History is about living men and women and not a string of happenings scribbled in a note book.' Then I exploded, 'Those

343

beastly exams! How can I manage to inspire students who only think in terms of examination papers and who judge their attainments by their marks? I must struggle to give them of my best and not put things off through laziness, for my sake as much as theirs. After all half my life may be over. I must justify the remainder. I have done little yet except perhaps Reigate.'

I was thinking too that youth and decent looks will go soon and my brain will remain.

'It is my one resource and I must not let it wither away.'

I had reached the mature age of 28; no wonder I was worried!

From time to time I monitored my progress reporting as follows:

'My lecture to the first year was quite good but the second year not so good.'

Later in March I congratulated myself that

'I lectured quite well yesterday and today.'

This was partly due to the fact I was beginning to break down barriers at least with my Honours students whom either before or after sessions I entertained to tea and biscuits in my room. Thus with a small group I found an effective way of loosening tongues and weaning them from their note taking. I continued to be rather pleased with myself writing a little later

'I lectured really quite well today. I think with some energy and go.'

In other words I had enjoyed the lecture if no one else had

which in itself was encouraging. My performance was not always so satisfactory. On occasions I found it difficult to organise my material but I was beginning to discover that I had that within me that could tide me over sticky moments as when

> 'my third years tutorial went off better than I expected, or had any right to deserve, as I hardly prepared it.'

Of my larger groups I found the evening class the most responsive. They at least wanted to attend enough to sacrifice an evening's leisure after the day's work had been done and were more adult in their whole attitude. Not only did they listen but also of all my classes made a tangible gesture of appreciation. At the end of term I experienced

> 'a great thrill in that my evening class gave me a lovely brass vase with the university arms on it as a farewell present. I could really have sunk through the floor with surprise. Still it is nice to be appreciated and it was nice and very unexpected of them. I have always treasured it.'

Because I was putting more into my work than I had done during my period of adjustment when everything was unfamiliar and impersonal it became more enjoyable and I more at home. Moreover any strain between MacMillian and me had disappeared to be replaced by an easy friendship with both him and his wife.

At this point in her manuscript there is half a page blank. The reason for this I do not know and can only surmise that either there is some text missing, or that she intended to write an extract from her diary. The flow has not been affected.

ED

Life at Raymond Lodge was equally uninspiring. I was conscious, perhaps over conscious, of the fact that there too my life lacked colour and excitement. It too had its own routine. I did a little dress making when mother and I had seen some material that we liked but once made there was no one in particular who I hoped would admire them. In the evening we might go to a theatre or, more often the movies, but generally we just sat around and talked with our fellow guests. I fell between two stools. I felt myself too old for the younger group, Hutch and Malan, Iris and Margery and too young for the older members. My poor mother was even more bored than I was. So it was a matter of soldiering on. I think I was inclined to exaggerate my sad lot. There were alleviations and life, even at Raymond Lodge, had its pleasurable side.

> 'One evening Margery, Mrs Sinclair's daughter and I
> got tired of the men doing nothing and carried the
> gramophone down the garden. The men emerged later
> and followed us (as secretly we hoped they would) and
> we lay in the moonlight on a rug watching the stars.
> Nothing much happened but it was nice. Margery and
> Malan went to make tea and Hutch and I followed,
> after an interval in which I read Granchester by the
> light of the moon. Then in the lounge we had a long
> conversation about poetry.'

Obviously there were compensations, islands of content amid a sea of boredom. In Johannesburg everyone played tennis and for the first time in my life I made a serious attempt to learn the game. That everyone played tennis was taken for granted and when I had lunch with the MacMillians quite early after my arrival I found to my horror that as well as the MacMillians there were two other people invited for tennis.

> 'I was pretty awful at first. I think I improved, anyway
> on the hard court I was playing better than at home
> and I quite enjoyed it. I do hope I shall be tolerable
> and must get some lessons.'

This I duly did but with no outstanding success. Inevitably there was a court at Raymond Lodge and

> 'Hutch is really worried to find my tennis so bad.
> He taught me a new service which I found I could
> get over with the result that I played Margery today
> at singles and was much better. We had some quite
> decent rallies and my serve did go over.'

Gamely I struggled on and even bought 'a new racquet. It is a pretty one and cost £3.3.0d (£3.15)'. Little did I ever think I would pay that for a racquet! As a month's board and lodging only cost me £10 I am not surprised at my surprise. Alas, even the new racquet failed to turn me into more than a very, very average player, but at Jo'burg to play at all was a must.

Once I got settled in I found colleagues friendly and wives of the married ones hospitable both towards my mother and me. Sometimes I thought the social life of the place revolved round the teapot. In the mornings MacMillian or another colleague would drop in on some vague errand or merely for a chat and a cup of tea, but the main social institution was afternoon tea. I think its popularity was partly due to the climate and to the coming of the rains.

For half the year there is no rain and it is surprising how tired one can grow of constant sunshine Everything is hot and arid and one longs with what can only be described as nervous tension for the coming of the rain. The effect of living at so high an altitude may have something to do with the fractious irritability that both my mother and I felt waiting for the beginning of the rainy season. On the 7th October the first drops fell.

> 'We went out on the stoep to greet it. Somehow it was
> thrilling. Behind was the lighted lounge and a quiet
> house With the sudden patter, patter of the rain and
> the darkness of the stoep. It fell on my arms, through

my red dress and I smelt the wet dust.'

Unlike England or 'the rains in Spain' those in Johannesburg had the convenient habit of falling approximately at the same hour every day. When it fell it lashed down so fierce that it almost drowned the sound of any accompanying thunder. So nobody wanted to be caught out in it. Fortunately that could usually be avoided. Teatime fell within the dry hours and was correspondingly popular. Lunch parties too were popular and tennis could be played with impunity. So in Jo'burg it was not difficult to organise a pleasant social life. Pleasant but circumscribed; one always met the same people and for my mother, who had no work to fill her days, life was indeed boring. When she could stand it no longer we could flee the town and spend a weekend at some convenient country town. Our first expedition was to Kroonstad a small town on the banks of the Vaal.

> 'It's about the size of the Lune at Kirby Lonsdale,
> sluggish and a greeny grey, with willows just coming
> along its banks. Their feathery green against the blue
> of the sky was lovely and the whole place bathed in
> sunshine and deserted was very gentle and peaceful.'

The drive itself had been exciting; some friends had given us a lift, in that we encountered a dust storm. It swirled over the land like a plague obscuring the sun and smothering everything with a greyish white cloud. The car was an old fashioned tourer with curtains and the dust got in everywhere. But afterwards, as so often happened in Africa beauty followed harsh reality. The sunset was almost unearthly in its splendour. The veldt spread out before us like a golden carpet while the sky was an intense cobalt blue, not the ordinary blue of even an African sky but something strange and vibrant. On our return journey over the sun baked veldt the mirage danced down to the blue hills and tree hung Vaal at Parys. It was a heavenly spot and when I got back that evening I wrote

'The love of Africa and of wandering caught me by

the throat and I wondered whether any man, even K.S. was worth marriage and settling down. I love Africa.'

No wonder that the Afrikaners, to whom the Veldt represented a haven against the money loving encroaching English, rebelled against a way of life that was not their own and that white society was a divided society. I think it was a mingling of pride and affection that made Professor Haaroff drive us to Pretoria to meet his aunt, so that we might sense something of the past to which he and his fellow Afrikaners belonged. I described it as

'The public buildings were simple, beautifully placed and in themselves beautiful, particularly Government House. I like the rural Dutch very much. Our host had been secretary to General Botha; they had a great affection also for Smuts. We stood on the balcony of the old Volkray house where Kruger stood etc' Why the etc.? I no longer know. 'The Government schools are very fine.'

Everything in short was a great contrast to the brashness of Jo'burg. So was the old fashioned courtesy of our host and hostess. At lunch mother and I had almost taken up our knives and forks when we were shocked into embarrassed immobility by the delivery of a long grace. Driving back that evening the sunset was almost unearthly in its splendour. The veldt spread out before us like a golden carp while the sky was an intense cobalt blue. The impression that it made on me I have never forgotten. No wonder that the Afrikaner, to whom the veldt was both home and a haven against the money loving encroaching England rebelled against a way of life that was so alien. I could respect and even understand them but the longer I lived in South Africa the more I came to condemn his attitude to the black men who shared his country.

This I think is the major piece of text which is missing. However I think

she had made her point about the Afrikaner attitude. It is sad not to know how someone persuaded her to fly. My aunt was always terrified of flying, even in a modern jet airliner. How someone managed to get her into a flimsy biplane such as a Gypsy Moth, we now will never know. It was quite an achievement and there must have been a considerable attraction! At any rate she seems to have enjoyed the experience.

ED

That night I wrote,

> 'Anyway it was not so bad. One sat strapped in a deep cockpit and off one went. My thought was anyway it's quite a pleasant death if things do go wrong and with that calming thought I hung on to the side. It was not really bad, or even as bad as a lift and one had a rather wonderful sense of pushing against something very strong as one mounted and mounted. The earth seemed very near and yet the trees in the plantations and the animals were like toys. One soon calmed down and I almost took it for granted. It was a calm day and I did not feel sick. They told me to look out for the shadow and for ages I could not see it, and then I saw it below, not looking much bigger than this book, I was surprised it was so small. As we landed a photographer rushed up to take my picture as I leant out of the little Gypsy Moth all smiles. Somewhere there is a photograph to prove it.'[1]

No ceremony marked the end of term, as it was not the end of the academic year so it was only a matter of private farewells, after which we departed as inconspicuously as we had arrived. The following extract, written on my last night in Jo'burg, followed by some doggerel verse reflects my farewell emotions.

> 'Pinky and I had our last tea together. Then I insisted

350   [1] See front cover

on taking his photo in his chair, only he scowled terribly. Then we went downstairs and found a very disgruntled Hicks, who had failed to go down the Crown Mine, so I took him scowling mightily and rather against his will. Then Raines who was the Principal and for whom I had a warm spot hoved into view. So I took him too, giving him a friendly wave of my arm. He posed like a nice big dog and I think Hicks was a little comforted.'

Finally I wrote,

'Our last night. It will be a blessed relief. I think everything is in order now; touch wood. No more boarding house and dark avenues at night.'

I am not a poet and never shall be, but in those far off days I found it easier to express my emotions in verse than in prose and if these that follow have no other merit at least they sum up my feelings after a year in Johannesburg.

'Bare feet patterned in the dust of the town

Cars that rush endlessly up and down

Natives, town bred or fresh from the kraal

And the damming sunshine over it all

Johannesburg.

Houses and gardens that hint at peace

Contrast With a rush that can never cease

And underneath there still holds sway

Morals and manners of the mining day

Johannesburg.

Whisky and sunshine, kisses and dust

Piling of fortunes and breaking of trust

Where women lack virtue and men lack strength

What retribution must come at length?

Johannesburg.

Where natives are huddled in yards of shame

And wealthy businessmen guzzle champagne

Where even the sun no respite gave

Gold thy snare and golden thy grave

Johannesburg.'

So ended the last of my three academic experiences in the twenties. Girton had nurtured me, Vassar had encouraged me and Witwatersrand had hardened me into a professional. Inevitably in ten years I had been turned from a schoolgirl to a woman, knowing the career that I wanted and knowing too that I was capable of holding my own in the academic world. Nevertheless the future was uncertain and for women university posts hard to get. Would luck still hold? I could only hope and pray and trust that my academic godmothers Eileen Power and Gwladys Jones would somehow contrive my future.

CHAPTER THIRTEEN: FAREWELL TO SOUTH AFRICA (RETURN TO LONDON).

When I set about describing my year in South Africa and my impression of that often unhappy country I used the simile of a picture describing Africa as the background, with the University of the Witwatersrand and the town of Johannesburg as the foreground. The middle ground, the complex pattern that together made up the society that inhabited both has yet to be filled in. In it there is more shadow than sunshine, more potential conflict than peace. Today South Africa is news in a way that it was not in the twenties. In the main this is due to the Western World being aware of and shocked by the avowed policy of the South African Government to retain complete domination in the hands of a white minority, denying to the black majority any share in running the country which they also inhabit. Because apartheid is indissolubly linked in British minds we are apt to think of South Africa as a society that is sharply divided into two opposing sections, black and white. That is to simplify a complex situation. It is arguable that South Africa is no more than a unity than the United Kingdom. Just as England, Scotland, Wales and Northern Ireland is each rooted in its own separate histories and traditions, so are the English and the Boers, and the rival tribes that confront them. During the eighteenth century there had been more than enough for everybody. For the Dutch burgers of the Cape and the tribes that occupied the interior there was land to spare. Within the Cape settlement itself, black and white lived amicably together, intermarrying and so producing still another strand in South African society, the Cape Coloured, who, even in the twenties, were not yet victims of racial segregation. This developed first in the new towns that grew with such amazing rapidity after the discovery first of diamonds and then of gold round Kimberley and the Witwatersrand. Labour was needed to work the mines and build the towns and gradually a black proletariat grew up within them. But in the early days of expansion the conflict was not between black and white but between the older Boers and the thrusting wealth creating English influx. The result was the Boer War, and English victory and finally the Act of Union in 1910, which combined in one self governing member of the Empire the four original provinces, the Cape, Natal, the Transvaal and the Orange Free State.

When I came to South Africa in the twenties there was no national policy of apartheid though in the mining areas it had already taken root. Because diversity continued and because I am determined to write only that for which I can give chapter and verse my observations must be confined to the Cape and the Transvaal. Here I think it would be true to say that I was more conscious of the tension between the Afrikaners and the English. The early white settlers were the Dutch who brought with them their architecture, their way of life and their religion. It was not until our stay at Fishock with Cape Town on our doorstep that I realized how Dutch in its origins it was. On one of our explorations we wandered into the old seventeenth and eighteenth century parts of the town and discovered its magic. We started our sightseeing at de Wit's old house on the Strand. Everywhere it spoke of the quiet dignity of harmonious architecture combined with old furniture that harmonized with the white and marble floors and the ubiquitous blue and white tiles. It was as if we had been transported into those Dutch interiors, hitherto seen only in some art gallery. Only the people were absent. Later that evening, writing in my diary I concluded

> 'One can understand why the Dutch cling to their traditions and their race. If more English people would linger in the atmosphere of the past and learn a little more Dutch history both races might get on better. There is something galling in the Englishman's assumption that of course the Dutch are an inferior race. They are "Dutch" in a half contemptuous phrase often used.'

One of my favourite colleagues at the University, Professor Haaroff, stood for everything that was fine in the Afrikaner tradition. I think it must have been a mixture of his liking for us and his pride in his race that inspired him to drive us to Pretoria where his family lived. It was a great contrast to that creation of the gold seeking English, Johannesburg. Though Boer and English considered the African inferior their attitude was not identical. To the Afrikaner, rooted in the Bible they were God ordained hewers of wood and carriers of water. To the average English person they were a necessary supply of cheap labour since no white man, however poor would condescend to manual labour. Only missionaries regarded them as equals in the sight of God, hence Pinky's enlightened views. When I first came to Africa I had no views on a problem that I hardly realized existed. Gradually, as the months went by I began to realize that the Bantu too had possibilities and herein was a problem that would not go away. Even as we journeyed to Johannesburg I commented on the well cultivated farms of the whites contrasted with

> 'the Kaffir huts which were little better than cattle sheds and always an eyesore.'

That the servants at Raymond Lodge were all natives I took very much for granted; Alan, the chief house boy was both capable and pleasant and no doubt thought himself in a lucky position. I saw the other side of the coin when on Sunday Miss Hodgson, the senior woman in the History Department, took me, as one of the tourist attractions, to

> 'the big compound where the mine boys all go before being drafted off to the mines. They were in clothes, curtains and blankets of every hue and sat on the ground eating their meal and beans out of tins with a spoon. They seemed happy but it's a sort of slavery. We went round the hospital too, very clean but plank wooden beds and blankets, no mattresses.'

It was my first critical observation.

Already I had become conscious that the white minority had a sense of unease, even fear, of the black majority that they ruled. The Sinclairs slept in a bungalow in the grounds and when Margery went to bed her mother saw her across the yard and locked her in, not trusting even Alan. Every black person had to carry a pass and their movements were carefully controlled. The mine boys lived in their compounds, black work people not residing on the premises of their employers, had their homes on specific locations. They could not wander at will in town at night but lived under what was in effect though not in name a perpetual curfew. The people at Raymond Lodge thought my mother and I brave, even rash, to walk up from the train and through the long garden without an escort. Certainly I was never allowed to be out after dark without an escort though in London in the twenties it would never have occurred to me that I could be in any kind of danger. But from the first I realized that Johannesburg was different. When Professor Leifeldt asked me to go to a meeting of the university dramatic society my comment was 'if I can arrange about getting home it would be fun.'

Apparently it was arranged. Here is my account of the evening, a rather ungrateful one.

> 'It was not over until 11.20 and a young man drove me
> home. It was not very thrilling even though there was
> a moon. He had horn rimmed spectacles and was tall
> and lanky.'

That precautions were necessary was made dramatically clear when in November an Irene Kantfoord

> 'was murdered by natives just outside the zoo. It has
> made us all feel rotten and mother very jumpy about
> my working at the university now it's half empty.'

The zoo was an area that we knew well, we often went there to walk to get away from bricks and mortar.

It was not until I was in the more relaxed atmosphere of the Cape that my sympathies and understanding of the root of white tension started to change. We had gone, I don't know why, to a lecture 'by Jatabu, or some such name.' Translating sounds into letters was never one of my strong points but having tried to check my assumption I think it was probably D.D.T. Jabavu, an active propagandist for native rights. Here is the extract in full.

> 'He turned out to be a native in a London M.A. hood.
> He was very good with a simple but keen sense of
> humour and showed by his face exactly how he felt all
> the chairman's remarks in a way a white man would
> not. He had a good command of English though his
> enunciation was a little thick. It was a good lecture,
> though the subject Bantu Literature did not lend itself
> as it meant translations that robbed them of their

357

poetry. Still when some of the race can be so good not
only in imitation but in understanding it makes one
think and I do think the Negro has a very real future
especially if wisely guided now.'

My eyes had been opened, or rather my ears had been unblocked.
A few days later I received a moral shock, driving home the callous
indifference of perfectly nice white people towards their black
neighbours, whom they hardly regarded as human. We had been
going to the theatre that evening when someone, rushing past us,
said there had been an accident at the station. We then saw that at
the end of the platform there was an overturned engine and a coach
splintered into matchwood. It looked as if the engine had run into it
and overturned on impact. Then a couple of women hurrying back
told us that they were taking out the injured and that we had better
not go any further. So we turned back. Apparently two people had
actually been killed. When we returned to the hotel the accident was
the main topic of conversation and to a perfectly nice young woman,
a fellow guest with whom we had become casually friendly, I informed
her that two people had actually been killed, she replied, blandly and
quite without any trace of compassion, 'Oh no: only natives.' In my
diary that night I wrote

'It seems to me that this country must have a
reckoning for its attitude towards the natives.'

I returned to Johannesburg intrigued and puzzled by the two
contradictory facts that a black man, in the person of Mr Jabavu was
my academic equal and that a conventional young English speaking
South African was less moved by the death of a couple of natives than
in all probability she would have been had a pet dog been run over.
During my first term at the Witwatersrand my attitude too had been a
conventional acceptance of the place of the Kaffir in society. All that
I knew of them, apart from the servants at Raymond Lodge, whom
I certainly thought of as human beings, was, the sight of raw recruits

358

in the mine compounds draped in blankets and eating out of tins or performing their tribal dances for the amusement of a Sunday crowd. How could I reconcile that picture with Jabavu in his London MA hood and gown? I could not. It was with a heightened curiosity that through the train windows on our journey from Lorenzo Marques I saw, how ever curiously, something of the rural native way of life. Both their living conditions and the people themselves seemed very primitive. When the train stopped at the few isolated stations en route the men would come to sell their skilfully carved wooden animals to the tourists. Them I described as

> 'wearing only aprons but were a fine lot. Some of them seemed to bleach their hair a ginger shade.'

Their air of quiet dignity impressed me in that it did not suggest an inferior race in spite of their scanty attire. When I returned to the university with my interest in the position of the natives now aroused I found that my own professor was one of the small minority who did not share the current view of the native inferiority. Perhaps this was because he came from Scottish missionary stock. Towards the end of my first term he had given me a copy of his first book dealing with the native question, The *Cape Coloured Question* that he published in 1927. I was not then particularly interested so it was not until I returned that I realized his genuine commitment to the belief that the black man could be gradually raised by education to the white man's standard. The gap between the two could be bridged though it would be a slow process. Three years later, after I had left South Africa he published *Complex South Africa* and followed this with two more important books, one in 1949 and the other in 1963.

That I was able to see something of this slow programme of education at first hand was due to an unexplained tragedy. Unlikely though it seemed, Professor Leifeldt had committed suicide by electrocuting himself in the bath. When I first met him I described him as 'a bit of an old stick but pleasant,' and in many ways he had been kind to me. When I first heard this I could hardly believe it. I had seen rather more of him than I might have had not Miss Hodgson and I done some lecturing on economic history for the department of Economics of which he was head. In the second term Miss Hodgson had gone on leave and to hold the fort until a new Professor of Economics could be appointed an S.O.S. was sent to the London School of Economics to send out a temporary replacement. They sent John Hicks, a brilliant young economist. Smellie, who knew him at LSE had written asking me to look him up, which I did and found him

> 'quite a nice youth, middle sized in a grey flannel suit.
> K.S. had told him about me so when I collected him I
> gave him tea. I don't know if I shall see much of him.
> I think it rather depends on him. I think we neither
> jarred nor clicked very perceptibly.'

I was rather surprised therefore when he appeared next morning to ask me about some form or other. Whether he would have retreated when I had given him the required information I don't know but I was not alone. Pinky had come in earlier asking for tea and talked and talked. So Hicks joined the party and

> 'there they were with their pipes puffing and me
> caught between them. K.S. must acknowledge that I
> am being a mother to him but remembering how lost
> I felt unless he had actively taken a dislike to me I
> represented a segment of the known in an unfamiliar
> world. Stepping into a dead man's shoes when both the
> dead man and the shoes were unknown is not an easy
> situation in which to be placed.'

He was not an easy person to get to know. K.S. in a later letter wrote he would write again perhaps when I was busy trying to understand Hicks, who was a deep and subtle young man. By the end of term we had established an easy but never intimate relationship; our private lives remained unexplored. But I grew to have an affection for him and hoped when I returned to England, if I frequented the Common Room at LSE as Smellie's guest, we might meet again.

The fact that he and MacMillian got on so well had for me a very welcome consequence. I had become very aware of the puzzlement of the native section of the divided society of South Africa and was anxious to learn more. Whether Pinky would have taken active steps to enlighten me further I do not know. As a woman he might not have taken me seriously but an intelligent young man who was also an economist was another matter and he too had shown an interest. The upshot was that Pinky took us both to a meeting of the Bantu Joint Council which was a joint organisation, perhaps discussion group would be a better name, composed of liberal whites and professional men of the Bantu race. It was the first time I had met a native on equal social terms and I was very impressed.

> 'It was quite a nice building with a big hall for films and games, some smaller and more comfortable lobbies and upstairs, round a little courtyard, class rooms for various subjects. The students had such pathetic striving faces, and they grasped their pens with such determination. The meeting was interesting. Several natives spoke and never off the point. James the secretary, speaking of the Bolsheviks that if South Africa did not make the blacks a part of South Africa there was no loyalty to restrain him from thinking that the Russians might do more. They were such restrained, sane speakers and so restrained and dignified. I am sure they can't really be kept down and intelligent white cooperation in the early stages is the only hope for the country. Yet they are so politically trapped and patient.'

This first encounter with the small educated black minority made a great impression on me. It is an opinion from which I have never wavered and I am a little proud that I saw so clearly and so soon. At least I could begin to understand that vague background of fear that haunted Johannesburg's lonely places, particularly when the night was dark. Indeed after returning to Johannesburg we had apparently explored the possibility of buying poisoned pistols but

> 'as we would need a licence, we are going to have taxis on dark nights instead'

and this became our practice unless the moon were full. We never had to face the slightest trouble when walking up from the tram but there was something eerie by being overtaken by feet that had padded along soundlessly behind me. I still deep down don't like being alone in lonely places. That is one legacy from my other African experience.

My visit to the Bantu Social Settlement was more than enlightening. It was revolutionary in that it at once resolved my puzzlement over Jabavu and his London M.A. hood and changed my attitude to the race that he represented. The gap between him and the raw natives in a mining compound was enormous but it could be bridged and Pinky and his friends were doing what they could to close it. It was the professor's if not the widow's mite. I did however manage one more visit to the Settlement when Pinky took Hicks and me to a meeting of the Joint Council on the 7th June. I found it intensely interesting, particularly when the new South African flag, whose first unfurling Hicks and I had witnessed, came up for discussion and

> 'the natives spoke pretty freely. One member,
> Tamar, spoke hotly of the conduct of Hertog in not
> consulting the natives on the flag if they were a part of
> South Africa they should have and until they were how
> could they be expected to have any love or respect for

it. Hearing them speak one felt that with all our faults we British at least won their respect and that anyhow the Union Jack meant something to them. One felt too that the speakers were both logical and practical people. To white women they are a danger partly from their standpoint and partly from circumstances but as men there was good stuff in them and South Africa will have to reckon with them sooner or later. They rarely talk hot air and they know what they want. Of course there are exceptions but what some others will do in time. Without MacMillian's introduction I should never have had the opportunity of judging for myself both the potential of the African and the conflict that could lie ahead if it were denied its legitimate expression and some hope for the future.'

I had not then fully realized the quality of Pinky's commitment to this hope, a hope which he saw could best be brought to fruition by the gradual education of the black man until he could attain the white man's standard.

It must have been he who invited Ray Philips, another doughty fighter for the black man, down to lecture at the university. To my disgust it was disgracefully attended, though Hicks was there. Later I met Ray Philips and he took Hicks and me round a couple of mine compounds so that we could see something of the conditions in which the migrant natives who worked them live. They were strictly masculine communities. No women or children were allowed to accompany their men folk. Families had to remain in their native reserves, often too poor to support their population. On my second visit to Durban I recorded that the native reserve in the Valley of the Thousand Hills

'was rather poor land except for grazing. The two compounds that we visited were very different. The

first one we inspected was an independent mine and
the compound was very old fashioned, only doors no
windows to the rooms and horrid kitchens. Ray got
the manager to show us round as he said the place
was too dirty for him to take the risk of showing us
round without permission. The other mine was a great
contrast, an airy compound, some trees and though the
rooms were all cement the beds were all clean and the
walls white washed and the kitchens really modern.'

We then went on to Benoni which I think was a location, namely
areas outside the towns where Africans who had passes were allowed
to live if they were not housed by their employers and the prototypes
of Soweto. I have memories of tin roofs, of dirt streets and a general
grey squalor but this is an impression only. Unfortunately I did not
put into my diary what then I did not realize I might have forgotten
as the years went by. I was chiefly concerned with noting that

'we had lunch at a weird cafe. Afterwards the men
disappeared down a yard. So I had to follow suit. They
got back first but obligingly chattered animatedly when
I emerged. I was introduced to all sorts of blacks and
felt rather a fool.' But I concluded, 'I think Philips is a
fine man.'

That was my last contact with the racial problems of Africa. One
is often asked if History provides any guidance for the future, if it
had lessons to teach. My year in Johannesburg taught me one, it is
that when a pot is boiling and the lid too firmly fixed then sooner or
later the pot will explode. It may be serious and, if the head of steam
is too great, do much damage. It may do more than cause temporary
inconvenience. Not all risings, however just the reasons behind them,
succeed. That too is one of History's lessons. But they happen until
the protest is successful or is smothered in blood and wise rulers
let the steam escape little by little. Parliamentary representations in

England in the eighteenth century was limited, illogical and unfair. The so called Reform Act of 1824 let a little of the steam out by letting some of the middle class in. The safety valve was gradually opened until eighteen-year-olds, male and female can vote for the members of the Commons.

Perhaps the British tend to be smug as many detractors of the now defunct Empire will no doubt feel at my reaction. Just before leaving Johannesburg I went to hear Bruce Mitchell speak on Native Administration in Tanganyika

> 'Apparently we are building up on the tribal system,
> making it almost the best native base, giving them
> responsibilities and educating them both economically
> and politically. There was something very staunch and
> steady about Mitchell like a man who was a man.'

At least our Empire for the most part broke up piecemeal and without a blood bath, or at least one in which we did the slaughtering though the racial problem we left behind may well have been responsible.

In the summer of 1928 and for the second time, I returned to England jobless and without prospects. On the first occasion I had accepted the post of History specialist at Reigate County School without too much dismay. Indeed I thought I was lucky to get a post at such short notice. But after the publication of *The English Poor in the Eighteenth Century* and my year's experience at the Witwatersrand I was determined, so long as the faintest glimmer of hope remained and our finances would stand the strain to accept nothing less than a lectureship. I knew that this would be difficult and might well be impossible. The male historians who had been up with me at Cambridge were job hunting too and in the twenties unless a post involved only women students, a man would automatically be appointed. This was so much a fact of life that looking back I cannot even remember resenting it. In these circumstances a sound financial base was vital. Opportunities were few and, like a cat watching a mouse hole, I had to be ready to pounce but also to wait. Without this a First was no guarantee of success. My friend from the Fourth Form at Preston had so impressed her department at Liverpool that one of her professors was anxious that she should take a temporary junior lectureship which unexpectedly became vacant. The snag was that it was temporary and there was not much prospect of its being made permanent. Ethel's parents were getting old and without private means and my friend felt that she dare not risk being a financial burden on her family, so she turned the offer down and went to Luton as the History specialist there. It was ironic that the Liverpool lectureship became permanent in an unexpected way. The woman who was appointed in Ethel's place married the professor in question and so was comfortably provided for for life. Ethel was very attractive as well as clever, there had been a distinct rapprochement between her and her favourite professor; had she been able to watch her mouse hole, I have very little doubt that the mouse would have emerged and that one pounce would have sufficed. Her history was demonstration enough that, like King in the parable, it was necessary to assess the cost of a campaign before embarking on it.

Certainly Old Hutton could never provide a base for operation. It was necessary to be where things happened and in my case that was London. I already had contacts at more than one level at the School of Economics. Among the academic hierarchy I could count on my dear Eileen Power, who was becoming a power in the land, no pun intended, and most probably on Dr Knowles. Among the juniors there was Smellie and his friends, Mrs Anstey, Ginsberg and that group with whom while working on my Ph.D and subsequently at Reigate, I had an easy friendship. At intervals during the last four years Smellie and I had been seeing a fair amount of each other, even to the extent of his sometimes spending a day with me at Reigate. It was an odd relationship, trembling sometimes on the brink of sentimentality but never quite landing on the other side. While I was in South Africa we had written to one another spasmodically and at Christmas he had even sent me a copy of *The Bridge of San Louis Ray*. This had given me much pleasure, both because of the book itself and even more because of its donor. My own feelings were complicated and mixed. From the days of my first lectures at Cambridge I had been conscious of him and in my thoughts at least he had a place in my life. The puzzle was what that place might be. My views of life were romantic yet of men I was distrustful, though whether this sprang from my own desire to attract them and my uncertainty as to my ability. Sexually I was still only half awakened and Smellie was not the man to awaken it. Looking back I think he may have needed more encouragement than I could provide. One thing is certain. While I was in South Africa, Kingsley Smellie was much in my thoughts. Did I love him or didn't I. Would I marry him if he asked me? Did I want him to ask me? What were his feelings towards me? In the barren desert of Johannesburg such thoughts were apt to absorb me and slide over into my diary. When I came back the problem had solved itself. Kingsley was engaged, officially or unofficially, to another young woman. I don't know whether I was relieved or hurt but heroic but the absurd fact remained that we seemed to see as much of each other as we had in the past.

This was partly because we both of us spent a good deal of time in the Round Room of the British Museum. In October my Mother had rented a furnished flat in Beaufort Gardens, near Harrods. It was a top floor flat in an old house and had no lift but it was comfortable and, with a few additions of our own, charming. The ostensible reason for my requiring a base in London was that I decided to occupy myself by doing research, a highly respectable reason in the academic world for my presence in their midst. After my book had been published EEP had stressed the fact that many people had written one book and then had never been heard of again. One must go on writing and for this reason it was necessary. I had been mulling over my choice of a subject for some time. During my work on the eighteenth century poor I had discovered a number of stray references

367

to domestic servants that seemed interesting and in Johannesburg had stumbled across a published diary of an eighteenth century footman which I found absorbing. So I decided to make domestic service in the eighteenth century my subject. As far as I knew nobody had yet tackled it and there was a good deal of scattered material to be found in plays and novels and social comment as well as in long forgotten or printed diaries. In that century, as in pre war twentieth century England, servants were a perennial subject of conversation. Meanwhile to secure my legitimate presence at LSE I decided to enrol as an occasional student. As usual I confessed to

> 'nervousness but no one ate me and I made my
> arrangements.'

The course for which I had enrolled was a series of lectures by Hugh Dalton, now recognized as a leading economist and I had thought that a little knowledge of Economics might not come amiss. Also twice I had heard him speak at the Union when he was a budding politician and was interested to judge him as an academic. My verdict was that 'he has perfected his technique which is good of a kind but very cheap.' I had intended to look up both Smellie and EEP but ran out of time. I thought it wiser to wait until I could make a more casual seeming approach to EEP but I had less inhibitions about phoning Smellie who I reported

> 'sounded quite pleased and we talked for a long time.
> He isn't at the School on Fridays as he keeps it free for
> the British Museum so I said I'd look him up there.'

This I duly did and my vanity was gratified and my feelings soothed by his suggestion that we lunch together at the Plane Tree. It seemed no effort to either of us to slip into our old easy friendship and to lunch together at the Plane Tree became part of the pattern of those days when we both were working in the Reading Room.

Smellie provided me with a very useful link with LSE particularly when I went to meetings of societies that met in the evenings. Then it was pleasant to be able to join him and his friends, who were becoming my friends. He proved a good friend in other ways but perhaps most particularly in re-establishing my connection with the Laskis. While I was working on my thesis he had taken me along to the Laskis' open Sunday teas and once while I was in Johannesburg I had been delighted to get a letter from Mrs Laski. So I was anxious to renew the connection but a little diffident in setting about it. While I hesitated K.S. acted and far from being grateful I was distinctly put out writing

> 'All on his own he had arranged for me to go to tea
> at Laski's on Sunday. It makes me look both a fool
> and his property. Also I don't know if my frock will
> be ready. I sent a polite note to Mrs Laski but did not
> mention Smellie.'

The visit was a success. The frock did arrive in time and with some vanity I claimed that I looked very nice in my new clothes. Certainly I enjoyed the afternoon. It was a large conversation, to revive an ancient name and I wondered

> 'how could they get 40 people into that tiny room.
> Professor Laski asked me about my work some time.
> They were both very nice and I like them very much.
> The atmosphere was so friendly and Mrs Laski is a
> lady. After all I do owe a good bit to Smellie.'

Laski was as good as his word. About a fortnight later, at the end of October, I went to see him and we had a long and very helpful talk. My impression of him is that he was a man who put all of himself into what he was doing whether it was politics or helping the younger generation. It is a tribute to his memory that I recorded our talk that afternoon.

'He was direct, to the point and nice. He suggested
W.E.A. work and that I wrote to Mrs Wootton.
Professor Gregory came in and wrote me a card of
introduction to her. Also if I wanted stray guineas to
Garner (? I cannot always read my own handwriting)
at the L.C.C. He offered to help me write a letter of
application if any jobs turned up and if I would do
an article on the Domestic Servants he would put it
in Economica (the LSE Journal) in February, which
was very useful. Also he advised me to go and see
Sir William Beveridge with the idea that if he took a
fancy to me he might do something. But anyhow he
was cheering and said I should certainly get something
sooner or later without going abroad (in desperation I
had thought of going to Canada).

Encouraged by Laski's optimism, at my mother's suggestion I
wrote to her nephew, Willie Edge, asking his advice as to how best
to approach Sir William Beveridge. As fellow Liberals, Willie was MP
for Bosworth the two men were friendly if not close friends. The
response came more quickly than I had anticipated.

'Indeed I nearly died of shock when I got a note from
Beveridge's private secretary saying that Sir William
would see me on Tuesday. I had never expected Willie
to act so quickly I feel very nervous but hope I shall
make a good impression. Anyway if Sir William is a
snob it is better to be well introduced. Mrs Wootton
says there is no W.E.A. work going but I may go and
see her on Wednesday so I am really trying to set
things in motion an do, do, do hope I'll get a job.'

The interview rather dashed any hopes I might have cherished.
Rather sadly I wrote

'I don't think the interview with Beveridge was very
fruitful. He was very pleasant but not to the point
of making vacancies that don't exist. He suggested
that I sent him a written statement of my academic
qualifications and I shall add my book but I don't feel
there is much doing there. Of course he may think me
over more favourably. I think, I just think he might.
I don't think he is very impressionable and I do wish
Willie had not sent my letter on to him as I know I said
I want to get hold of Beveridge. Anyway I must hope
for the best.'

It was not quite the end of my hopes. mother and I went to have
lunch with Willie at the Russell Hotel, his *pied à terre* in London when
the commons were sitting.

'He was very sweet and said he would do what he
could. There were some other politicians there:
Sylvester, who is L.G.'s private secretary. He had just
come back from the U.S.A. where he says they produce
everything by mass production except children and
those they produce by accident.'

Having recorded this *bon mot* I continued

'I had quite a nice letter from Beveridge he says he has
heard my book highly praised and that after he has
read it he might possibly like to see me again. Anyway
it was a nice letter and he sounded willing to do what
he could. Willie knows Sidney Webb quite well and will
talk to him. So I think I shall be able to count on his
reference for the next job which I apply for.'

In the matter of Sidney Webb, Willie's intentions had already been
forestalled by Smellie who some days previously, when he saw S.W.
in the Reading Room had bullied me into going up and speaking
to him. So the great man already knew my face and later gave me

the gratification of knowing that he had taken my *English Poor in the Eighteenth Century* seriously. One day, when I was quietly at work at my seat, he came up especially to tell me how much he regretted that he had not been able to make more use of it in his volume on *The Old Poor Law* but the proofs were so advanced that he had only been able to refer to it in a footnote. This was fame enough and I glowed with pride. His approbation however seemed to have no effect on my chances of a job. I was obviously peeved when I heard that Peggy James had been appointed to Holloway when I was in South Africa. That was the luck of the game and for me the loss of an opportunity to get a lectureship in one of the few colleges for women. Her qualifications were precisely the same as mine. She had held the Cairns in 1924/25, the Old Girtonian the following year and had then proceeded to a Ph.D., though hers was a London degree. So her good luck was rather bitter to me. Once again I wrote

> 'Surely I'll get something in October. I must, I must,
> I don't think our finances will stand my being idle
> another year. I'll try some articles too and my play'.

My love of the theatre was as strong as ever and in London I was well placed to indulge it: if I could write a book surely I could write a play. Moreover I thought I might make use of my connection with Cyril Phillips and the Birmingham Rep to break into the charmed circle. Clearly as a student of eighteenth century political life had convinced me of the adage that it is not what you know but whom you know that puts the young careerist on the first step of the ladder of preferment. Nothing came of it though I don't think that my attempt at a light comedy was too bad. The plot revolved round an impecunious young graduate who had taken a post as a chauffeur, assuming an accent intended to suit the part, who won the heart of his employer's daughter, to the dismay of her parents. In itself it bears witness to the social morals of the twenties. Neither did my efforts to get an article accepted. The one I sent to *The Spectator* came back, though I was partly consoled by the fact that it was accompanied by what I called 'a nice note!'

372

Next day, after my abortive attempt to influence Beveridge I went to spend a few days with the Giles'. To be at the Master's Lodge again brought back a host of memories of Elspeth and my first initiation into Cambridge as apart from Girton in that magical summer of 1919 my presence must have brought back the same memories of that exuberant blooming when, so full of life, hope, the world seemed at her daughter's feet, Elspeth died in the February of 1923[1], her vitality drained away, little by little by some incurable disease. In the old days I had not been totally at my ease with Mrs Giles but now I found her more expansive than I remembered her to have been in the past. In other ways too the past was recreating itself but with a difference. The Master had some freshmen in, and I, who had been so shy, did my best to entertain them. Writing that night I realized how good it was to be back in Cambridge, declaring:

'I love it as much now as I did ten years ago.
Cambridge is a good place to be in.'

Next day I went out to Girton and discovered that if Cambridge had not changed Miss Jones had.

'I thought she looked very old and tired, but she was
very good and nice to me. I think she is really fond
of me. She is a dear but so altered. She was not too
hopeful about jobs but I think something will happen
and I pray it may.'

I had some grounds for hope. I had kept myself as much in evidence as I could by attending various society meetings held at LSE My research was doing well; the material I had collected was falling into place and the outlines at least of an article were forming in my mind. If it fulfilled my hopes Laski said he would get it published in Economica but that would be too late to help me find anything immediately. Mrs Wootton too, when I went to see her, could only suggest that perhaps I might give a few W.E.A. lectures on an unpaid basis.

[1] See plate section

'But she told me that nothing could happen this year. Personally I thought her softer than my Girton memories when I definitely found her inapproachable, though indeed my only contact with her had been through the debating society where I definitely had been outclassed. EEP too I knew would do what she could to help me find something immediately but the only practical fruits of her benevolence was to get me some coaching which an Indian student wanted in modern history. At least it brought in a few guineas which in the state of my finances was not to be despised.'

But though my day-to-day life was very pleasant I was at times so worried about the future that I almost considered returning to teaching. This was in consequence of a couple of visits to Reigate where my ego had been comforted by my welcome. At my return after my first visit I wrote

'Went to Reigate this afternoon. It was looking rather perfect. They all seemed really pleased to see me, even Miss Aitkin, the Headmistress and wherever I went there were hordes of welcoming girls. Little Mildred Offer followed me round and my own erstwhile form gave me a special greeting. I have promised to go to a house party on Thursday and a picnic on Saturday. Anyway I was a success there!'

After my next visit I pronounced it

'really quite fun. They gave me flowers and mobbed me for dances and at the end twelve of them at least escorted me to the bus. I wonder why I was so popular because there was not any doubt of it. It made me wonder if I ought to go back to teaching. Yet the staff looked tired and jaded.'

On more than one occasion in the future I was to annoy my colleagues when they moaned about their heavy work load by telling them that university teaching was money for jam compared with teaching school children. I am glad I taught for two years before licking the jam. It taught me not to be lordly in my attitude towards those of a lesser status in the academic hierarchy. Dedicated teachers and Headmistresses contribute more to the youth of a country than any don however eminent. For many years a recurring nightmare was that I had resigned my lectureship and returned to teaching. How great was my relief when waking to find that it had all been but a dream. Even when my prospects looked most unpromising, I felt that teaching was not my destiny. If I did not get a lectureship this year than I would next. My luck was bound to change if I soldiered on.

Soldiering on however was only possible if we gave up our London flat and my mother returned to a more frugal life at Old Hutton. For the first time I was on my own and my London background and my pattern of life suffered a sea change, salutary but less comfortable. Yet in fact my luck had turned. This however was not yet apparent. My account of these last decisive months must be brief and sketchy, more or less a matter of milestones than a description of the journey which was to end in the fulfilment of my dreams. This is because I either gave up keeping my diary or over the years it has been lost. So I have only my memory on which to depend and ruefully I must admit though the milestones are clear enough the details of that journey may be open to question. My first problem was to find somewhere to live and, how or why I know not, I landed up in a girl's residential hostel in Bolsover Street I think it was a benevolent institution subsidised by Bourne and Hollingsworth, or one of the other big department stores in Oxford Street for their young assistants. It provided me with adequate accommodation and an interesting sidelight into how the other half lived. My memory of the weeks I spent there are dim. I had a tiny spartan bedroom and joint facilities on the landing. In the dining room in the basement we ate our breakfast and our evening meal. I recollect very little about

375

the inmates but have a vague impression that I got quite friendly with one or two of them but remained something of a fish out of water. My pleasantest memory was of Marylebone High Street that boasted of a wonderful continental cafe where, when I felt extravagant on Saturday mornings I had the best hot chocolate with lashings of whipped cream that I have ever drunk.

How or why I left Bolsover Street I can no longer remember. Probably it was someone at LSE who suggested that I went to the Crumps as a paying guest. Mr Crump had just retired from the Public Record Office and he and his wife, like so many retired and gentle folk in the twenties, planned to spend the winter months in France or Italy where sunshine was plentiful and for the English where the cost of living was low. The Crumps had a daughter who, like myself was a budding historian and her parents wanted somebody to keep her company and to make an addition to the modest expenses of their modest house in the Hampstead Garden Suburb. Even had it been only a change or environment I should have welcomed it. The Suburb was a pleasant place in which to live and, as a bonus, I was in easy walking distance of the Golden Green theatre where all the London hits either began or ended their run. But the key to my future lay in the fact that Helen was a research assistant at the London Institute of Historical Research of which many of the leading London historians were frequenters. As a fellow research student through Helen I gained the entry to that charmed circle. Before the building of the new and magnificent Senate House the Institute was housed in a ramshackle building where I came to meet many interesting people. Several of the other research assistants later became eminent professors themselves, men like Bindoff of Tudor fame. It was there that Pollard, that grand doyen of English sixteenth century constitutional history held court. He was a commanding and irascible figure who when he presided over his seminar had his attendant satellites scurrying like frightened rabbits to find the books he wanted and then listen to the words of wisdom that fell from his lips. J. Neals, who later was to become himself a professor of History and the author of a standard life of

Elizabeth the First was always in respectful attendance as heir apparent to Pollard's throne. I was lucky to sit, a silent listener to such seminars. They were stimulating, exciting evenings and my introduction to some of the most important historians of London University, either made or in the making. At LSE I had never really belonged. I had been a hanger-on to the group of Smellie and his friends. At the Institute I had my own admittedly small niche. This wasn't the only way in which my prospects were beginning to be seem brighter. Whatever the distractions that London had to offer I had worked steadily on my domestic servants and reaped my reward when in the form of an article *Domestic Servants in the Eighteenth Century* Economica was published in the April of 1929. I had intended it to be the nucleus of a longer book but fresh ideas turned my interests elsewhere. However I can fairly consider it as a small pioneering contribution to social history as it was re-issued as one of the pamphlets by the Historical Association in 1940 and re-printed in 1968. Though I had failed to secure an appointment the two years since I had returned from South Africa had not been wasted.

Nor was I completely jobless. Though my beloved Miss Jones had been far from hopeful when I had seen her on my visit to Cambridge, I had the feeling that, like a conjurer, she would somehow produce a rabbit out of a hat. This in 1929 she did. How the trick was worked I do not know. It may have been a sudden influx of First Year students who wanted to read History, but to my delight she asked me to do some coaching in Economic History. As I have no diary to which I can refer and my memory is lamentably bad I do not remember how often I came down to Girton to see students but to be back in Cambridge and spend the night at Girton was a joy. It was an even greater accolade to be treated by Miss Jones as a colleague and to discuss the students whom I was tutoring. Selecting students for admission was already becoming difficult as demands for places were increasing, steadily. Already the criteria for success was depending more and more on school reports and examination results. But occasionally Miss Jones would put her money on an untrained colt from an unknown stable and in one instance proved brilliantly justified. The dark horse among the students I tutored romped home with an outstanding First and I count her as the first of the select students that I taught who afterwards were high achievers. At Vassar, and even more at the Witwatersrand I had learnt my craft, mainly by trial and error and to work with Miss Jones had been valuable training.

How far this renewal of my connection with Girton helped me to get my first full time lectureship I do not know. Certainly Miss Jones backed my application for the junior lectureship that became vacant at Bedford College with a testimonial that it would make me blush to include. But I suspect that it was once more a case of 'not what you know, but who you know' and that my personal contacts at the Institute of Historical Research was the deciding factor. I remember Professor Mackey as a kindly avuncular figure who I used to see there from time to time. His academic career was almost at its end as he was retiring from the chair of Modern History that he held at Bedford College where in 1930 he was succeeded by Lillian Penson. Her appointment and his retirement coincided with a vacancy for a junior lecturer. One never knows what goes on behind the scenes but I think he must have recommended me and, as they wanted someone to be in residence at least I was not faced by any male competitor. For the next four years I was secure. The lectureship was for four years only and not renewable but four years meant four years of security and in fact the luck was with me. Until I retired from University College, Cardiff in 1971 never again was there a hiatus in my academic career. The apprenticeship was over, my wanderings finished the door at last was opened, I entered the castle of my dreams and life was good.

CHAPTER FOURTEEN: AN EPILOGUE

This chapter in reality is an epilogue, and is not written by Dr Dorothy Marshall, but by her nephew David Edge Marshall. Indeed it is being written some six years after she died on the 13th February 1994. However ironically it completes the century, as the real author, my Aunt Dorothy Marshall was born on the 26th March 1900 and the year now is 2000.

Eleven months before she died, in March 1993, Joan Perkins for the Historical Association, London, interviewed her on video. In this recording she said that she had made friends with all her students, some of whom had remained friends for life. This chapter very much summarises what she said in this interview. Now it is these friends, former students, who are so keen for her memoirs to be published.

It will have been noted that during her life she met, influenced, and was influenced herself by many well known and politically famous people, Beveridge and Professor Laski to name but two. In turn she influenced some of our better known politicians, such as James Callaghan and Lord Jenkins. Indeed Lord Roy Jenkins, in his autobiography, paid her the most glowing praise. On page 24 of his A Life at the Centre *he says in his memoirs about his short time at University College, Cardiff,*

> *'My most vivid memories from that interlude are of the hour's bus journeys to and from Pontypool (for I lived at home) and of a great deal of coffee drinking in the Kardomah Café in the*

middle of Cardiff. I was privately tutored by a young assistant
lecturer called Dorothy Marshall, who subsequently taught
at Vassar and Wellesley and was the author of several good
early-nineteenth-century biographies. I never encountered her
again, although I read her books, but I think her teaching may
have been crucial. I desperately needed coaching in the writing
of Oxford-style history essays. Even she could not get me a
scholarship, but with her help I secured in March 1938 my
entry to Balliol, which was then the only Oxford men's college
with competitive entry for commoners.'

In fact she did meet him again at his home in Oxfordshire, but only after his
autobiography had been published.

Roy Jenkins mentions that she taught at Wellesley College in the United
States. This she did in 1960. It had always been her hope to return and teach at
Vassar, which she had intended to do upon her retirement. Unfortunately after all
the arrangements had nearly been completed, she had to cancel the trip in order to
enter hospital for a hip replacement here in England.

However this did not stop her literary career. In total she had ten books
published. These included The English Poor in the Eighteenth Century
which of course she mentions in her autobiography, but in addition she wrote
The Rise of George Canning, The English People in the Eighteenth
Century, Eighteenth-Century England, John Wesley, Dr Johnson's
London, Industrial England 1776-1850, Life and Times of Queen
Victoria, Life of Lord Melbourne, *and* Fanny Kemble. *Most of the*
copies of The Rise of George Canning *were destroyed in the London blitz,*
and I would imagine hard to find these days.

She even had ideas about trying to write a novel based on the life of Fanny
Burney, the author of Evelina, *and had made notes on this subject which are now*
in the archives at Girton along with all her other documents. The idea to do this
came while she was researching into material for Fanny Kemble.

At the time of her retirement, she had been Reader in History at the University of Wales at Cardiff, and her previous posts included the universities of London and Durham. By rights she should have been awarded a professorship. It is the opinion of at least some, that the reason she was not awarded such a title was because she was a woman. However she was made an Honorary Fellow of the University of Wales, College Cardiff.

Neil Kinnock, who is also a Fellow, had a very narrow escape on one occasion. He had made some historical reference, which she thought inaccurate, and she had intended to challenge him on this matter. However he was spared by a snap General Election, and he could not as a result attend the Fellows Dinner.

Once she had retired, she gave up her flat in the Castle Court Flats, Cardiff. which at that time overlooked the Glamorgan Cricket Ground (at the far end of these buildings it was possible to look into Cardiff Arms Park), and made her permanent home in Old Hutton on the banks of the River Bela. Between Old Hutton and my mother's home near Folkestone, Kent, she did most of her writing. Folkestone was for her more convenient for research at the British Museum as it was much easier for her to travel up to London from there than it would have been from Cumbria. She also had many friends in London.

On the 4th December 1984, she was awarded an Honorary Doctorate in Literature at Lancaster University. The other recipients of honorary degrees at Lancaster on that day were Dr Norman Nicholson, Mr Robert Fisk and Nelson Mandela. HRH Princess Alexandra, who is Chancellor of the university presented the awards to all except Nelson Mandela who, of course, was still in prison in South Africa at that time.

Dorothy was very proud of the reception she received at these awards, as she made an acceptance speech on behalf of all the recipients, but especially on behalf of Nelson Mandela. I have tried hard to find out what she actually said, without success Lancaster University only keeps a video record for four years after the event, and nobody there now appears to remember. I have scanned back copies of both the Westmoreland Gazette and Lancaster Guardian without finding comment on what was said. The Lancaster Guardian reported the speech given by the Public Orator, Mr Colin Lyas who said of Nelson Mandela.

> 'Those who live in countries where the basic rights that Dr
> Mandela seeks for his people have been won: owe at the very
> least a duty of sympathy for those who have no such rights.'

Of my aunt he said,

> 'Dr Marshall, who has written many books on 18th Century
> British social history, has never forgotten her origins –
> apparently delighting undergraduates during lectures by including
> sudden bursts of famous seaside songs from her childhood in
> Morecambe.' He also said, 'In telling her story Dr. Marshall
> has been committed to the belief that history is on the whole
> rather too precious to be left entirely to professional historians.
> Recognising the interest that many non-professionals had
> increasingly begun to show in learning about and understanding
> their predecessors, she sought to attract the attention of the
> general reader and to stress the claims of history to a place
> among the mental recreations of intelligent people.'

In an effort to try and find out what she actually said, I contacted Professor Harold Perkin, who originally nominated her for this award. He told me that she may have met Nelson Mandela when he was a young man. It was an honour and why she felt so strongly about the injustice of his imprisonment. He also said that she had greatly impressed Princess Alexandra and had sung one of the old Morecambe pier songs, which was greatly acclaimed by the audience. It was his wife who interviewed her in March 1993, and she was therefore the last person to do so.

Her other great joy was to travel. Nobody in the family was really allowed to travel abroad without her, and Folkestone was very convenient for that also. Very often abroad we would meet former students, either by design or by accident. I remember on one occasion meeting a professor from the Hebrew University in Jerusalem. He told me how he had totally confused the lodging authorities when he arrived in Cardiff as an Empire student after the war. They had expected all

382

empire students to be black. He came from what was then British Palestine, which is now mostly Israel and was not what they had expected.

At other times we would stay with two former students Bill and Joy Farr in their home near Geneva. Bill had been a student of Dorothy's after the war, when he was reading for an economics degree at Cardiff. He later became an International Civil Servant working with the ILO (International Labour Organisation) Geneva, ending his career as Director of Personnel at the ILO.

They had a house in the Swiss village of Coppet, which was on the shores of Lake Geneva. Coppet has a chateau made famous by Madame de Stael, who was forced to flee from France for being a constant thorn in Napoleon's flesh. Her salons were frequented by great writers, like Benjamin Constant, and our own Gibbon who completed his The Decline and Fall of the Roman Empire at the chateau. In a well-known passage he described his sadness in parting from an old friend, as he paced the gardens of the chateau looking at the reflection of the moon in the lake.

Madame de Stael was a great conversationalist and had many heated love affairs despite the fact that she was no beauty. This place and the character of Madame de Stael being no mean conversationalist herself intrigued Dorothy, as a historian. Madame de Stael is now buried in a garden near the chateau.

Bill also took us over the Palais de Nations in Geneva twice. Whenever my wife, Joan, and I see conferences taking place in that building, we say, 'do you remember that room?' Somewhere we also have a photograph of Joan sitting on the bonnet of the car belonging to the Secretary General of the United Nations.

After Bill had retired, he and his wife Joy, made their main home in East Sussex, buying a converted oasthouse. They also bought a flat in Divonne-les-Bains, which is still close to Geneva, but is actually just in France. When we visited them there, we would stay in a hotel. However from the balcony of their flat, which was probably less than a mile from the border hedge which separates France from Switzerland, you could see across Switzerland, Lake Geneva, back into France and on to Mont Blanc in the distance. We could see the snowy whiteness of that mountain.

On one occasion, as the sun was setting, this snow turned first to crimson, and then it deepened to a flame red. Imagine that reflected off the still waters of the lake. Alas, I had left my camera in the hotel bedroom.

After Mother died, and my brother and his family gave up their Kentish home to move to Cumbria, Dorothy of course spent more time at Old Hutton.

It was therefore perhaps fitting that the final great gathering of all her family, former students, colleagues and friends, should have been at Claridges where she celebrated her 90th birthday on the 26th March 1990. This was the last time I saw my mother outside of a hospital ward. She died in June of that year. Since my Father, Dorothy's only brother, was killed in action on the 10th May 1944; they had given each other considerable support. Neither ever got over his death and it also shortened her mother's life.

Dorothy's last journey abroad was with Joan and me. We took her to Normandy in the autumn of 1993, where at Pegasus Bridge Madame Gondree insisted that she sign her visitor's book. You may recall that the cafe by Pegasus Bridge was the first building in France to be liberated in 1944. Madame Gondree told us to bring her back the 50th anniversary of that liberation. Alas she did not make it.

Joan and I last saw her getting on the train at Milton Keynes Central. She somewhat prophetically said, 'This is my last visit south.' It was. As usual upon boarding a train, she was like an ill-sitting hen, not satisfied with her pre-booked seat. We saw her wandering up the coaches before the train had even left the station.

Dorothy had been to see a fortune-teller early in her life, and was told that she would come to a sticky end. She never forgot this prophecy. We therefore supposed it might be that she would fall down the very steep dangerous stairs in her cottage, The Fold, Old Hutton.

I think we all agreed, including possibly Dorothy herself, that during the winter months of 1993-4 she should reside in some residential establishment. Nicholas and his family then lived at Braithwaite near Keswick in Cumbria.
384

Nick's wife Leila, persuaded her to move, just for the winter months, to Millfield a residential establishment in Keswick, bearing in mind this fortune-teller's prophecy. She took some items of furniture with her plus her favourite picture painted by a well-known Lakeland artist Grieg Hall.

On the 12th February 1994, I received a telephone call from her saying that she had just decided to go on a cruise up the Norwegian fjords during the summer months. This was just prior to Joan and I visiting our daughter Valerie for her birthday on St Valentines Day. On our arrival in Norfolk, Valerie had received a telephone call from Nick to say that our aunt had fallen while crossing a road and had been taken to Keswick Cottage Hospital. She had very badly banged her head, and she was worried that she might have damaged her eyesight. Blindness or even poor sightedness was one of her great fears. During that night her condition worsened, and she was transferred to the Cumberland Infirmary, Carlisle where she died.

Even this is not quite the end of her story. Because of the circumstances of her death there had to be a post-mortem. It appears she was returning from buying a bottle of vodka from what she called the chemists, which in fact was Threshers, the well-known purveyors of wines, spirits and beers. Threshers to us now are known as that well-known chain of chemist shops. She tripped while crossing the road and tried to save her precious bottle. In that she succeeded.

She would have been flattered to know that she had an obituary in The Times, and also The Westmoreland Gazette.

Her funeral was early in March. The residents in Old Hutton wanted a full funeral service in the village church of St Johns. First however she had to be cremated. This was done at Carlisle Crematorium. For this to happen in one day meant that she had to be first to be cremated. We all had to set off early from Braithwaite, before most people had left their beds. It was cold, and the shores of Bassenthaite were frozen.

The vicar of St Johns Keswick took the first service of the day, which was the church she attended during her stay in the town. The congregation at the crematorium was for just a few close friends and family. However we were touched

385

when an ex vicar of Old Hutton made the effort to attend, especially as he and she had had a theological disagreement. Apparently he had made a reference in a sermon that it had never rained before Noah and the Great Flood. She had told him that was ridiculous and that just because rain was not mentioned in the Bible before Noah did not mean that it did not rain. Perhaps this shows a historian's attention to practical detail, as opposed to a clergyman's attention to faith?

After the service at the Crematorium we set off, through a snowstorm, to cross Shap to Kendal. Dorothy was taken for one last visit to a pub, the Station Inn at Oxenholme, where later we were to have the reception.

For the service we had chosen two hymns. The first was Onward Christian Soldiers, because before the war, Dorothy owned the one and only car she ever possessed. It was an old Bullnose Morris. The only way she could change gears via an old-fashioned crash gearbox was to sing Onward Christian Soldiers. Think about it. Go through the motions, and you will see how it works.

The second hymn was Cwm Rhondda, because of her long association with Wales, and especially Cardiff. It is for this reason that I have also given it its Welsh title. The opening lines are Guide me Oh Thou Great Redeemer.

The lesson was read by a former student, Brian Watkins, and was taken from I Corinthians chapter 13. It is the chapter that deals with love, and ends with the verse

> *'And now these three remain: faith, hope and love. But the greatest of these is love.'*

Brian said that he was tempted to read it in Welsh because he was sure that everybody would know that passage in whatever language it was read. It would be nice to think that he was right.

The vicaress in her sermon told us that Dorothy kept a special savings account for her old age. At 93 she was apparently still too young to touch it. Now there is encouragement if not hope!

386

Once the indoor part of the service was over, we ventured out into a howling blizzard to the graveyard. By now the snow was horizontal. A path had been dug to the place where her ashes were to be interned. This was in her mother's grave. It seemed appropriate to us. You will recall that during her academic experiences of the twenties, Vassar and Witwatersrand, her mother always accompanied her. On that gravestone, therefore are both their names plus our mother's. That too seemed appropriate. Since my father was killed in action in 1944, the two of them had supported each other as well as Nick and myself. Mum had rented half a farmhouse near the town of Tenbury Wells in Worcestershire, and whenever we were ill, such as the time we caught chicken pox, it was to Cardiff that we went to be nursed.

Mum's ashes are in a graveyard in Kent, but I think she would have liked being together at Old Hutton. Inside the church there is a wooden cross upon which are brass plaques containing the names of all from the parish who died in the wars. At the east end of the church there is a stained glass window, put there as a memorial to those who fell. It seems to me therefore, that in the parish of Old Hutton and Holmscales there will be for ever a piece of ground that will be Marshall, our roots and history are attached to this parish. In addition my brother Nicholas was born in Bela House, Bridge End, Old Hutton on the 24th September 1944.

Bridge End, we were told in the 1940s, was where the Peasey Beck ended and the River Bela started. Indeed the deeds of Dorothy's cottage stated that it stood on the banks of the River Bela. According to modern Ordnance Survey maps, this does not appear to be the case.

In 1944 my father was killed and her mother, my grandmother, died in the December, thus the end of so much. The birth of my brother Nicholas was the start of something new. History teaches us about endings and new beginnings, true not always for the better. If you have lost a war or battle, things could be very much worse, and Dorothy never really recovered from the loss of her brother (my father). However she was always full of history, life and laughter and she would have been thrilled to know that her great-niece Sarah Marshall obtained a BA (Hons) this year, 2002, at Lancaster University. This degree was for Sociology, *not History, but that would not have mattered to her, for she was truly a 20th century woman and knew that history could be fun.*

Her memoirs started a hundred years ago in 1900, and I have now ended them 102 years later in the year of 2002.

David Edge Marshall , March 2002.

Post Script:

Since completing this chapter Lord Roy Jenkins has died on 5th January 2003. In the Daily Telegraph *obituary of 6th January it says:*

"Roy, meanwhile, was purusing a competent but by no means exceptional career at Abersychan Grammar School. His father, though, was determined that he should go to Oxford and a short spell under the tutelage of Dorothy Marshall at University College, Roy secured a place at Balliol."

APPENDICES

Appendix 1: Extracts of an interview with Dr. Marshall by Dr. Maxine Berg and Lois Reynolds on 20th December 1991.

26th March 1900: Born in Morecambe, only daughter of a schoolmaster, John Willis Marshall and his wife.

Education:

1907-12:

Moved to Leighton Hall in 1907, a stately home of the Gillow (furniture) family, rented out as a boys' school. From age 7 to 12 educated with boys. Grandfather died in 1912, leaving a house to her mother, in Thornton, just outside Blackpool, then in the country.

1912-18:

Various schools for ladies. Considered St. Andrews, but the war intervened. Decided on Park School at Preston. Headmistress, Miss Stoneman, an old Girtonead, persuaded DM's father than DM should go on to Girton, not to Manchester, which was his own university. DM wanted to go on the stage and was persuaded to wait until after her degree.

1918-22:

History Tripos, Girton College, Cambridge plus an additional postgraduate year. First two years' tutor, Eileen Power, and Gwladys Jones during the last two years. Eileen Power directed DM's research in 1921-22.

1922-24:

Two years at LSE, seconded from Girton, working on the Poor Law, supervised by Professor Lillian Knowles.

1924:

Cambridge PhD (titular), one of the first awarded to a woman in History. Published in 1926 as *The English Poor in the 18th Century*.

1985:

Honorary D.Litt., University of Lancaster. Others honoured by Lancaster that year were Robert Fisk and Nelson Mandela.

Employment:

1924-25:

Lecturer at Vassar College, (Poughkeepsie, NY) accompanied by her mother. Spent Thanksgiving in Boston, Christmas at the estate of General Johnson in Virginia and travelled in Canada on the way home. Visited Niagara (shot the rapids on the old river boats).

1925-27:

Taught at the Redhill and Reigate County School for Girls.

1927-28:

One year lecturing at the University of Witwatersrand, Johannesburg, returning in October 1928.

1928-30:

Various money-earning jobs, including visiting tutor in Economic History at Girton, every fortnight from 1929, arranged by MG Jones, Eileen Power's successor as Director of Studies.

1930-34:

Lecturer at Bedford College, 4 year, non-renewable appointment if no vacancy in department.

1934-36:

Durham. "Two part time salaries; two full-time jobs." Moral censor (part of the title of Senior Tutor at St. Mary's College, for women) and lecturer at the University. DM liked her students, the College and Durham itself. She was not happy because she didn't like her Head, "an awful snob". Most of her students were of working class origin from the mining community.

1936- 67:

Lecturer and Reader in History at Cardiff, one of the constituent colleges of the University of Wales.

1962-63:

Visiting Professor, Wellsley College, Massachusetts. Travelled extensively in the US and returned to England via Canada, visiting Vancouver Island, Lake Louise and the Canadian Rockies.

Extracts from an interview with Dr. Dorothy Marshall, 20th December 1991.

Educated with boys: "I was the only girl in the school, you know. Of course, I was naturally spoilt. But I was brought up with boys… It means that later when I had to go to a girl's school I didn't know how to get on with the creatures."

DM had read a lot of historical novels in her school days, e.g. "Cloister and the Hearth" and those by Marjorie Bowen based on the House of Orange from the time of William the Silent.

Arriving at Girton at 18:

"a nasty little intellectual snob"

"quite above clothes"

Girton's History Tripos:

Part one was Political Science A and the second part was the history of political thought through the Middles Ages. Decided to be an academic during Part II. Attended ordinary university lectures and some tutorials at men's colleges.

Girton and chaperons, 1918-22

In 1918, two or more students could have two or more young men in their rooms to tea on Saturdays and Sundays, with permission of the Mistress in the presence of a chaperon. Rules eased over the period to include a picnic in the grounds with no chaperon and in a punt with parties of four, but not alone with a man in a canoe. By 1921-22, one could meet a young man alone for tea in a café without permission and without a chaperon. DM credits this change to servicemen returning after the Armistice, particularly American GIs, recently out of the trenches, not standing any nonsense.

A popular chaperone was Miss Dean. When asked "why not Miss Power" DM replied "Oh no! She is far too attractive."

Miss Power was a popular chaperone for dances as she left her charges at the door and collected them afterwards.

Eileen Power:

Great debt owed. "She has been absolutely the one person in my life who has had more influence on my whole academic life than anybody else." "She touched my life at every angle. I was a very emotional young woman in those days."

Everyone thought EP got her clothes from Paris, but she died in a department store (Bourne and Hollingsworth). (Maxine Berg noted that EP's sister Rhoda died in the same place in 1957.)

"Beautifully dressed, beautifully turned out" "Well, if it was good enough for Eileen Power, it is alright for me. She probably saved me from ever becoming an intellectual frump."

EP set her students at ease during a tutorial, seated at the edge of a chair, offering chocolates.

"She would give a lecture that was so simple, that you have no difficulty in remembering it and also so straightforward, so simple, so just right. … She had go the essence out of every one of those books she had told us to read and presented it there in a simple form."

Dr. Lillian Knowles:

Took over supervision of DM on arrival at LSE. Lillian Knowles was praised for spotting "nasty gaps" in evidence and for her attitude towards career women:

"Any woman can have a career if she has, A, a good husband, and B, a good housekeeper."

Mrs. Knowles was also sympathetic towards DM's inability to spell, as her son, William Cunningham Knowles, had the same difficulty.

Michael Postan:

Rode with Postan on the top of a bus one Sunday on the way to Harold Laski's tea parties. He told her a story about getting digs in London, ringing round a list of landladies. One asked him what colour he was. He hadn't a clue what this meant and replied "Red" on account of his red hair.

K.B. Smellie:

Met in October 1923 at LSE, outside Dr. Knowles' lecture room.

KBS   "I believe we used to go to the same lectures at
             Cambridge."

DM   "Yes, I believe we did."

Smellie provided DM with her social contacts, introduced her to the Junior Common Room, to his friends.

Harold Laski:

A personal friendship.

"I think he thought I would make a nice wife for Smellie."

DM went as often as possible to Laski's Sunday afternoon open house because it was interesting. She got to know his best stories, which were introduced into the conversation by his wife.

"A thin man, if you can imagine a thin flame with two flashing eyes."

Laski took the trouble to find her odd jobs which would pay money. Suggested Economica for the publication of "the Domestic Servants".

Accommodation:

DM's last year at LSE, 1923-24, was spent as a paying guest at the Crumps. Father was important at the Record Office and the parents wintered abroad. They wanted a companion for their daughter, Helen, who was a research assistant at the Institute of Historical Research when "it was still in those old tin houses". DM attended meetings there ("Pollard with Neale as heir apparent"); met Denis Brogan there. Attributes her appointment at Bedford College in 1930 to her link with the Institute. When Lillian Penson got the chair at Bedford College (Professor of Modern History from 1930 and first and only woman Vice-Chancellor of the University of London, 1948-51), a retiring Professor from Bedford who had known DM from the Institute recommended her to Lillian Penson. After all that effort made by Laski and Beveridge.

John Hicks:

DM met John Hicks in Johannesburg while teaching at Witwatersrand in 1927-28. Hicks had been sent by LSE as a temporary replacement for Professor R.A. Lehfeldt (1868-1927), physicist and the first professor of economics in South Africa, who had committed suicide. DM was on friendly terms with Hicks, not an easy man to know. The friendship was renewed in England and she occasionally went to dinner and the theatre in London with Hicks.

Cardiff:

Eileen Power saw the post advertised and told DM to apply for it.

"I went there. I did not expect to get the interview. And they did not mean to appoint me either. Apparently I interview very well and the man they were going to appoint didn't. And so, somehow, they found that they had appointed me instead."

Eileen Power's advice on research

How to organise research:

"Always keep your notes on (the size of paper, writing only on one side)... always put your dates and references on, which I don't always do and I give myself endless trouble. And then she said when you begin to get a whole pile on one subject, then separate it out in piles so that the different aspects- if it is work houses- then shuffle them round. That will give you the structure of your book. Then, you see, you don't have to worry about that because it will do itself if you put things in the right piles. She never, alas, told me really how to write footnotes."

"Now get yourself a typewriter, and learn to think on your typewriter, which was invaluable." and scissors and paste. How to manage if they had the desire to do research.

"I'm not really a scholar, in the sense that I'm interested in the minutiae of scholarship. What I like, and... I suppose I'm a teacher more than anything else. I like synthesis, so that I can then present it and it will go over."

LSE and equality of the sexes:

"What I did notice at LSE ... was, after Cambridge, the equality of the sexes at LSE, which is so utterly different than at Cambridge, both among the staff and among the students."

"It was Mrs. Mair who was the driving force behind Beveridge."

Economic History Society:

DM not at the inaugural meeting because she did not return from South Africa until October 1928. DM was an original subscriber to the journal. Perhaps she will leave her copies of the journal to the University of Lancaster who had bestowed upon her an honorary D.Lit. in 1985.

Extract from Dorothy Marshall's Diary, pages 13-15, undated.

"From 11-12 we had Miss Power, familiarly known as EEP, for Economic History. Women were not really supposed to lecture to the men as they were not part of the University. But at that time there were very few men to lecture to and no man, since Professor Watkins died, to lecture to them *(on Economic History)*. So since Miss Power was brilliant she was allowed the privilege. She was the best lecturer we had and her A was A, and her B, B. Not that she was dull for all her method, instead she would flash one charming smile round the room, take you all into her confidence and then start lecturing in her low thrilling voice. She seldom joked or played to the gallery more than most lecturers but when she did, however feeble that tale might be in aftertelling, it swayed you to mirth or indignation just as she wanted, not only us but also the men. I think it was her voice and that smile that commanded and entreated us at the same time. I can see her sitting there now with her long pale face unrelieved by any touch of colour and made brilliant only by her eyes. In her eyes dwelt the whole life of her face, they were deep blue grey with dark lashes which she had a trick of lifting suddenly and sweeping you with her gaze. Then she would smile so that her whole face lit up and at that moment she had put her head a little on one side and said "Miss Marshall I should like the moon", well, you would be a hard-hearted cynic not to charter an aeroplane and go off after it. Her hair was dark with the tiniest wave in it. She wore it parted down the centre and it naturally gathered itself into a coil just above the nape of her neck. She was always beautifully dressed, like a Princess out of a medieval story book. One dress she had was deep blue with gold brocade and sometimes out dancing she would sit in Kitt's carved chair[1], her hand resting on one pale long-fingered hand, her eyes searching into space. Of course she posed, but she did it so obviously, so perfectly and somehow with such a trick of childish glee that you could only love her for it. Laugh at her, love her, stand in awe of her, and yet work desperately hard for one flashing smile and a few words. "This is a very good piece of work Miss Marshall" in her beautiful voice. Such was EEP, at least in my eyes. Some called her "pacifist"; "agnostic" and "poseure". She was all those things, dangerous and seductive in charm. But for me, who was not "a superior person", it was enough that she should smile. At any rate, her economic notes were enough to inspire a dunce or pull a stone wall through Tripos. So, whatever her moral attributes, I am in no position to quarrel with her. It is certain that she has a kind heart and a humorous outlook on life. One would not dare to go to every Don and ask if one could do a Time Paper[2] on another day "because one had a tea party". Even EEP had been known to turn and when at the end of a long term's frivolity Gwen Wright sent her Med. paper in later she received the following writ. "Dear Miss Wright, If you have time to go to dances you have time to do your work. The sooner you learn this the better. Yours sincerely, E. E. Power". In fact when she's good she's very very good and when she's bad she's horrid, but she's always EEP".

Notes:

[1] "Dancing was a college phrase for an occasional informal dance in Hall in the evening after dinner which was an occasion for fostering the social integration of the First Year during their first term. It was an all female affair with the Second Year as main hostesses, though some Third Years might come, and which dons sometimes graced with their presence. The allusion to Kitt's Chair was to the Mistress's chair at High Table." Letter, May 1992.

[2] "A time paper was an essay which you wrote without supervision, but which must be written within a time limit, i.e. probably 2 hours, and always within the stated time from start to end." Letter, May 1992

"This was the end of my wanderings. My first head of
department was Professor William Rees, my second Professor
S.B. Chrimes. For my first two years I had a young man, twelve
years my junior, who came to specialise in Constitutional
History while I concentrated on Economic and Social, who
was to have a distinguished career first as a writer and historian
and then as Master of Balliol, Christopher Hill. We were a
happy department and when, at the beginning of the Second
World War, Professor Brogan asked me to come into the
Ministry of Information I was not tempted. As a consequence
I, whose dancing partners at Cambridge had been men from the
trenches, was coping with ex-servicemen in the second war.

During my thirty years at Cardiff no woman was appointed to
a Chair but I did become a Reader in the University of Wales
and after my retirement, an honorary Fellow of the College,
a distinction that I shared with Geraint Evans and Lord
Tonypandy. When I retired in 1967 Wales was very dear to me.
My flat had a balcony which looked over the Glamorgan Cricket
Field and Cardiff Arms Park was next to our block of flats,
and except when the match was against England, my loyalty
was to Wales. I was proud too that men and women who in
life had made their mark as historians, as administrators, in the
Church and in Industry, had once been students of mine. The
most eminent of these was Roy Jenkins, who was putting in six
months at the College while hoping to go up to Oxford and
whom a colleague of mine asked me to give a little attention.
Therefore I was surprised and very touched that after so many
years he should write in his autobiography:

"I was privately tutored by an assistant lecturer called Dorothy
Marshall, who subsequently taught at Vassar and Wellesley
and was the author of several good early nineteenth century

biographies. I have never encountered her again, but I read her books, and I think her teaching may have been crucial. I desperately needed coaching in the writing of essays, Oxford-style history essays. Even she could not get me a scholarship, but with her help I secured in March 1938 my entry into Balliol, which was the only Oxford college with competitive entrance for commoners." *A Life at the Centre,* Macmillan, 1991, p.24.

If without my help he might not have gone to Balliol then I feel that I too have a minute place in History."

Appendix 3: Transcript of the orations given for Dorothy Marshall and Nelson Mandela on 4th December 1984, at the ceremony to bestow upon them honorary degrees from Lancaster University. Reproduced with the kind permission of Lancaster University.

Your Royal Highness and Chancellor:

The eminent social historian, Dorothy Marshall, was born in 1900 in Morecambe, into the then very different local world of horse drawn trams and penny bazaars. I have to add however, that different though that local world may have been in other respects, the weather was then apparently no better; one of Dr. Marshall's first recollections being the destruction of the Morecambe North Shore Pier in a violent storm. As a child Dr. Marshall would take a daily walk with her governess to see the various entertainments on Morecambe Pier. Upon those visits was based her ability to delight generations of undergraduates by embellishing her lectures on the social history of holidays with impromptu bursts from famous seaside songs.

Dr. Marshall had a distinguished career as an undergraduate and post-graduate at Cambridge and after various teaching appointments of a temporary nature both here and abroad, she was appointed to a post at University College Cardiff where she was to remain for the rest of her teaching career. In recognition of her very many contributions to her College she was made, on retirement, an honorary Fellow of University College Cardiff, a distinction shared with such luminaries as Lord Tonypandy, James Callaghan and Geraint Evans.

Dorothy Marshall achieved distinction as a social historian at a time when social history did not have its present popularity. When she began her work, Eighteenth Century history, under the magisterial influence of Sir Lee Namier largely meant Eighteenth Century political history. It was, however, Dr. Marshall's pioneering conviction that political history is only a part, though an important part, of a larger story, a story shaped by the everyday social lives of countless men and women.

In her many books, Dr. Marshall has told us much about the ways of life and the satisfactions which were open in the Eighteenth Century to members of various classes of society. And since the Eighteenth Century stands at the threshold of the Industrial Revolution, her work has helped us to understand the forces shaping the great revolution that was to so influence our own present culture.

In telling her story Dr. Marshall has been committed to the belief that history is on the whole rather too precious to be left entirely to professional historians. Recognising the interest that many non-professionals had increasingly begun to show in learning about and understanding their predecessors, she sought to attract the attention of the general reader and to stress the claims of history to a place among the mental recreations of intelligent people.

Generations of readers have read Dr. Marshall's books with profit and pleasure. Generations of students, too, have been in the debt of a remarkably popular teacher and friend. I am told, for example, that despite teaching the superficially unpromising subject of Victorian sewers and drains her classes invariably attracted a large following. To these followers she was able to offer the fringe benefit of exquisite hospitality in a flat with the most precious commodity in Cardiff- a view over the Cardiff Arms Park.

Your Royal Highness and Chancellor,

It is my privilege to present to you, on behalf of the Senate, the name of Dr. Nelson Mandela, the imprisoned leader of the African

National Congress, as one eminently worthy of the degree of Doctor of Laws.

Dr. Mandela's life has been devoted to the effort to secure for all the citizens of South Africa regardless of their colour, certain simple yet basic rights, the most fundamental of which is the right of each of those who must obey the law to an equal voice within the political system under which the law is created.

Those who live in countries where the basic rights that Dr. Mandela seeks for his people have been won owe, at the very least, a duty of sympathy for those who have no such rights. And they owe, too, the duty of respect to those who, like Dr. Mandela, have unceasingly striven in the face of hardship and danger to claim those rights. But in addition to what is owed to Dr. Mandela by the citizens of any free nation, any university in a free society owes him a special tribute. For Dr. Mandela has unswervingly asserted the centrality of an open education to the cultural life of any nation. He has insisted, as the Charter of the African National Congress puts it, "that the doors of learning and culture shall be open". He has emphasised that in a healthy society, young scholars are to be thought of as a credit to their nation and not merely as a threat to its rulers. He has insisted upon the profoundly liberalising effects of the meeting of the world's peoples in open institutions of learning. And to use his own words, he has resoundingly affirmed that, "for centuries universities have served as centres for the dissemination of learning and knowledge to all students, irrespective of colour and creed". "In multi-racial societies," he continues, "they serve as the centres for the development of the cultural and spiritual aspects of the life of the people".

The Charter of this University commands that no test related to sex, race, colour or creed shall be imposed upon any person in order to entitle him to be admitted as a member, teacher or student. For us, this charter enshrines a victorious principle, and the fruits of that victory can immediately be seen in the international community of scholars that has graduated here today. Their presence has enriched this university and this country, and they will return, hopefully, to enhance their own nations. But those who can live by the principles of such charters owe a special duty of testimony to those for whom the fight to achieve a recognition of those principles has not been won: whose allegiance to the principle of an open educational system in an open society is a confession and a proclamation to be paid for in the coin of imprisonment, separation and even death. And Nelson Mandela has, of course, been willing to pay that price.

Your Royal Highness and Chancellor:

At all times there have been women and men whose lives and words have taken on a special meaning to innumerably many of their fellow human beings. Their lives embody and their words articulate the legitimate aspirations of the deprived, the suffering and the slighted. Nelson Mandela has become one such. And I can think of no better way to commend him to you than to use his own words, spoken in court at the end of his final trial, when he was indeed facing the possibility of a sentence of death. He said to them:

"During my life I have dedicated myself to this struggle of the African people. I have fought against white domination and I have fought against black domination. I have cherished the ideal of a democratic and free society in which all persons live together in harmony and with equal opportunities. It is an ideal which I hope to live for and achieve. But if needs be it is an ideal for which I am prepared to die."

I therefore present to you the name of Nelson Mandela, in absentia, as one eminently worthy of the award of the degree of Doctor of Laws, *honoris causa*.

Further Reading

1988   Angela Holdsworth *Out of the Doll's House - The Story of Women in the Twentieth Century* BBC Press

2000   John Parker *The Parish of Old Hutton and Holmescales- a Millennium survey* Stramongate Press

2001   Maryann Bruno and Elizabeth A. Daniels *Vassar College* Arcadia Publishing

Index

A

Abbot, Minnie 13
Africa 332, 364
Afrikaners 349
apartheid 8

B

Balliol 402
Bantu Social Settlement 362
Barrie, James 20
Bedale, Joan 105
Bedford College 378
Belloc, Hilaire 112
Beveridge, William 236, 370
Bonham Carter, Lady 107
Boston 272
Breakell, Ethel 27
Butcher, Polly 318

C

Caernarvan Castle, The 330, 331
Cairns 183
Caius Ball 228
Callaghan, James 379
Cardiff 396
Carews 309
Coulton, Dr 59
Crawshaw, Kenneth 19
Crumps 376

D

Dalton, Hugh 116, 368
doggerel 326
Dr. Johnson's London 7

E

Economica 377
Edge, William 22
Eighteenth Century England 7
Ellery, Miss 280, 311
English Poor in the 18th Century 7

F

Fanny Kemble 7
Farr, Bill and Joy 383
first class 182
First World War 17
Footlights 82, 153
Freaken, Wanda 267

G

George, Lloyd 109
Gibbs, Philip 305, 308
Gilbert and Sullivan 28
Giles, Dr 88
Giles, Elspeth 66
Gillies, Miss 302

410

Girton 20, 30, 32, 41, 66, 70, 98, 118, 128, 140, 210, 229, 324, 352
Graces 209
Gypsy Moth 8, 350

H

Haaroff, Professor 355
Haldane, Lord 110
Harvard 245, 277
Hebrew University in Jerusalem 382
Hot Springs 281
Humphries 228

I

Industrial England 7

J

Jenkins, Lord 379, 401
Johannesburg 24, 333, 346, 351
Jones, Gwladys 352
Jones, Miss 378

K

King's College Chapel 105
King, Martin Luther 290
Kitts 211
Knowles, Lillian 63, 231

L

Labour party 115
Lamlash Bay 17
Lancaster University 11, 381
Laski, Harold 237, 395
Leifeldt, Professor 359
Leighton Hall 17, 23, 28
Liberal party 109
Llewellan Davies, Theodora 51
London School of Economics 215, 231, 360

M

Mandela, Nelson 382, 403, 404
Marshall, Sarah 387
Martin, Mr 73, 83
May Week 155, 181
McMahons 252
Melbourne, Lord 7
Morecambe 11, 13
Morecambe Pier 13

N

New York 250
New Zealanders 35

O

obituary 385
Old Hutton 8, 34, 323, 366

P

Park School 25
parties 124
Penson, Lillian 378
Perkin, Harold 382
Peterhouse History Society 124
PhD 230
Philadelphia 282
Philips, Anna Jane 313, 318
Poor Law 209
Poughkeepsie 256
Power, Eileen 56, 183, 187, 189, 215, 231, 236, 311, 323, 352
Pretoria 355
Princess Alexandra 382
Pryor-Wandesforth 138
Publications 7

Q

Queenstown 243

R

Radclyffe 277
412

rapids 319
Raymond Lodge 345, 356
Reigate County School 322, 365, 366
Research 189
Reyburn, Francis 314, 318
Round Room 367
Rugger 224

S

S.S. Caragyer 319
S.S. Olympia 280
S.S. Sagneny 321
scholarship 215
Smellie, Kingsley 233, 367, 371
South Africa 8, 353
de Stael, Madame 383
Stoneman, Miss 31
Swindley, Ian 240

T

Tawney, H.R. 236
tennis 346
The Cam 140
The English Domestic Servant in History 7
The Life and Times of Victoria 7
The Long 159
The Rise of George Canning 7
Thornlea 29
Toronto 320
Tripos 152, 179

U

University College, Cardiff 378
University of Manchester 30
University Rag 176

V

Vassar 241, 247, 263, 292, 312, 318, 352, 380
Vignoles 165

Vingt et Un 137, 144, 219

W

Warm Springs 283
Washington 306
Waterman, Faith 267
Webb, Sidney and Beatrice 236, 371
Wellesley 263, 275
Wellesley College 14, 380
Wesley, John 7
Whitmore, Mary 27
Witwatersrand 330, 334, 352, 353
Woolworth Tower 253
Wycombe Abbey 240